Current Perspectives in Clinical Treatment & Management in Workers' Compensation Cases

Edited By

Chris E. Stout, Matt Kruger and Jeff Rogers

EDITOR AFFILIATIONS

Chris E. Stout, PsyD

ATI Physical Therapy
and
College of Medicine, University of Illinois-Chicago
E-mail: chris.stout@atipt.com

Matt Kruger, MS, CSCS

ATI Physical Therapy
E-mail: matt.kruger@atipt.com

Jeff Rogers, BA

ATI Physical Therapy
E-mail: jeff.rogers@atipt.com

DEDICATION

To all those who committed to find justice and help for the injured worker. – CES

To my partners, Greg Steil and Dylan Bates, thank you for a long, productive partnership and staying true to the core values of our company – providing a level of care that exceeds people's expectations. We have always treated the injured worker like a person, with dignity and respect. Without this, protocols and techniques mean nothing. Thanks for helping in sharing this "secret" with countless patients, employees, and referral sources. It has changed many lives.

To TEAM ATI, thank you for your hard work, long hours, and dedication in providing an excellent service to the injured worker. It is because of this team effort that ATI has achieved outstanding outcomes, growth and reputation. I hope that you are proud of your accomplishments, as I know the days get long and the tasks can sometimes be mundane. Your efforts make a difference in people's lives on a daily basis.

To my co-editors, thank you for translating my words into something both A.) readable and B.) fit for public consumption. This project is both a great accomplishment and a true contribution to the field. Thanks for making it happen.

To my family, thank you for your love and support.

Finally, to all the injured workers that we have been fortunate enough to treat at ATI – please know that we have tried our best. You deserve it. – MK

To all of those who have lost their loved ones and friends in a work related injury. In memory of all who died in the 1909 Cherry Mine fire in Illinois, one of the country's worst mining disasters. The fire killed 259 men and boys and left 465 children without fathers. This disaster prompted the first workers' compensation laws in Illinois.

To my family, Ryan, Katelyn, Erin and my loving wife, Kathleen.

To Greg Steil, Dylan Bates and Matt Kruger. Thank you for giving me the opportunity to work for such a great company. ATI continues to live by its mission statement every day by exceeding customer expectations by providing the highest quality of care in a friendly and encouraging environment. This mission statement has enabled thousands of injured workers to return to gainful employment. – JR

eBooks End User License Agreement

CONTENTS

CHAPTERS

PART 1: A Look Back, A Look Around and A Look to the Future

PART 2: Invited Specialty Chapters

APPENDICES

FOREWORD

It is a great feeling to see this book project come to fruition. In a way it is a natural and evolutionary progression from my perspective. That is, back in 1996, I founded the Athletic and Therapeutic Institute, or ATI, literally in my basement. Not unlike a proverbial "garage start-up"—my focus was not that of technology hardware or software development, but rather developing a unique approach to help injured workers regain their strength, their confidence and thus their jobs and their lives.

This book provides an amalgam of perspectives—not all necessarily in accord with one another either. The editors, Chris Stout, Matt Kruger and Jeff Rogers, come to work with the injured employee population from differing perspectives themselves, in fact they wanted to be "professionally ecumenical" in the opinions and point of views they present, and as a reader, I am sure you will see that they accomplished this.

As ATI has grown from my basement into a national company in five states as a provider of outpatient physical therapy and related services to injured patients and workers, we currently have over 100 clinics in Illinois, Wisconsin, Delaware, Maryland and Pennsylvania. Early on, ATI worked to distinguish itself by incorporating a comprehensive treatment philosophy in all types of care and clinical services that incorporate best practices from traditional physical therapy, exercise physiology and strength/athletic training, synthetic with relevant evidence-based findings from the scientific literature. In fact, while much of the unifying thread of this book is based on evidence-based practices, it was just that concept that our flagship and pioneering F.I.R.S.T.™, or Functional Integration of Rehabilitation and Strength Training program was born. (F.I.R.S.T.™ is a work conditioning/hardening treatment based program.) When I started F.I.R.S.T. ™ and ATI, I was driven by the necessity to develop a far more effective rehabilitative treatment option than standard rehabilitative programs. So, in developing the F.I.R.S.T. ™ model, I first sought "ecumenical" input from orthopedic surgeons, physical therapists, athletic trainers, exercise physiologists, attorneys, occupational medicine specialists, and bio-mechanists in architecting an optimal and unique return to work program. Over the past 10 years, the F.I.R.S.T. ™ program has successfully returned over 5,000 post-therapy patients back to work.

A similar perspective of identifying problems, finding solutions, and considering differing perspectives is the formula that Chris, Matt, and Jeff have used while writing their book, and I applaud them for it—for I know another similarity is that it was not an easy nor a fast project to complete. And to their credit, I believe it is a success.

Gregory F. Steil
ATI Physical Therapy
Bolingbrook, IL
USA

PREFACE

This book is the result of a thoughtful request by the publishers at Bentham eBooks. Had it not been for their suggestion, this project would not have been started. While the editors of this book are quite active and always interested in publishing, a book was not something that had been considered before this suggestion from Bentham.

As with all book projects, and especially with edited works, there are many important people involved. First and foremost, the editors would like to thank the publishers at Bentham for their generous invitation. In formulating the structure of this book, the editors additionally developed a new questionnaire and posted it online for interested workers' compensation professionals to frankly and anonymously weigh-in on the various aspects involved in working with the injured employees. Had it not been for those respondents, there would be no Part Two of this book or the fascinating insights provided by their answers.

Next, the editors are thrilled to have some of the sharpest thinkers involved in the workers' compensation arena who have generously contributed their time and talent in authoring their chapters. This powerhouse includes Robert Aurbach, JD, Martha Gely-Kruto, JD, Gregory Krohm, PhD, Richard W. Lenkov, JD, Gregory Moore, MPH, Joseph Paduda, Kim Presbrey, JD, Brian A. Pryor, PhD, Peter Rousmaniere, Dongchun Wang, Kathryn Mueller, MD, Dean Hashimoto, MD, Sharon Belton, PhD, Richard A. Victor, JD. PhD, and Maureen Kohl Bennington, MS.

In the production process there are many of the proverbial moving parts—ensuring that the proper style is used, formatting, proofing, version control, and a myriad of other details that are all equally important in making this project a success. In recognition of that support, the editors would like to thank Hema Burra, Jillian Richardson, MA, and Marissa Webb, without their help, this work would still not be finished.

Finally, the editors would like to recognize the injured worker. While there are many and often opposing perspectives involved in the workers' compensation "industry", it is important to keep in mind and recognize that the person in need is the one who is ultimately the focus of our concern, our trust and our responsibility.

Chris E. Stout
Matt Kruger
Jeffrey Rogers
ATI Physical Therapy and College of Medicine
University of Illinois-Chicago

LIST OF CONTRIBUTORS

Robert M. Aurbach

Uncommon Approach, Inc
819 Suzanne Lane SE
Albuquerque, NM 87123
Tel: (505) 681-4607
E-mail: Bob@uncommonapproach.com

Sharon Belton

Workers Compensation Research Institute
955 Massachusetts Ave.
Cambridge, MA 02139
Tel: 617-661-WCRI (9274)
Fax: 617-661-9284
E-mail: sbelton@wcrinet.org

Maureen Kohl Bennington

8138 E. Sprucewood Avenue
Orange, CA 92869.
Tel: 714-350-7952
Fax: 1-360-933-6616
E-mail: mbennington@buildingpeopleinc.com

Hema Burra

ATI Physical Therapy
790 Remington Blvd.
Bolingbrook, IL 60440
Tel: 630.296.2222
E-mail: Hema.burra@atipt.com

Martha Gely-Kruto

MGK Law
7343 W. Howard St.
Chicago, IL 60631
Tel: 773.807.0644
E-mail: migely16@yahoo.com

Dean Hashimmoto

Partners Occupational Health Services
101 Merrimac St., 4th floor
Boston, MA 02114
Tel: (617)726-4792
E-mail: dhashimoto@partners.org

Gregory Krohm

International Association of Industrial Accident Boards & Commissions
5610 Medical Circle, Suite 24
Madison, WI 53719
Tel: +1-608-663-6355

Fax: +1-608-663-1546
E-mail: gkrohm@iaiabc.org

Matt Kruger

ATI Physical Therapy
790 Remington Blvd.
Bolingbrook, IL 60440
Tel: 630.296.2222
E-mail: Matt.kruger@atipt.com

Richard Lenkov

Bryce Downey & Lenkov LLC
200 North LaSalle Street
Suite 2700
Chicago, Illinois 60601
Off: (312) 377-1501
Fax: (312) 377-1502
E-mail: rlenkov@brycedowney.com (email)
http: www.brycedowney.com (Web Site)

Gregory Moore

Harbor Health Systems, LLC
One Venture, Ste 130
Irvine, CA 92618
Tel: (949) 273-7020
E-mail: gmoore@harborsys.com

Kathryn L. Mueller

Professor, Department of Emergency Medicine, School of Public Health, University of Colorado at Denver
7742 S. Glencoe Ct.
Centennial, CO 80122
Tel: 303 318 8759.
E-mail: Kathryn.Mueller@ucdenver.edu

Joseph Paduda

Health Strategy Associates, LLC
292 Neck Road
Madison, CT 06443
Tel: (203)-314-2632
E-mail: jpaduda@healthstrategyassoc.com

Kim Edward Presbrey

Presbrey & Assoc PC
821 W. Galena Blvd.
Aurora, IL 60506
Tel: 630.240.0051
E-mail: kim@Presbrey.com

Brian A. Pryor

LiteCure, LLC
250 Corporate Blvd. Suite B
Newark, Delaware 19702

Tel: 302-709-0408
E-mail: brianp@LiteCure.com
http: www.litecure.com

Jillian Richardson

Adler School of Professional Psychology
17 North Dearborn
Chicago, IL 60602
Tel: 309.826.0735
E-mail: jilliannicolerichardson@hotmail.com

Jeff Rogers

ATI Physical Therapy
790 Remington Blvd.
Bolingbrook, IL 60440
Tel: 630.296.2222
E-mail: Jeff.rogers@atipt.com

Peter Rousmaniere

Consultant, entrepreneur and journalist
29 Church Hill Rd.
Woodstock VT 05091
Tel: 802-457-9149
E-mail: pfr@rousmaniere.com
http://www.peterrousmaniere.com

Greg Steil

ATI Physical Therapy
790 Remington Blvd.
Bolingbrook, IL 60440
Tel: 630.296.2222
E-mail: Gregory.steil@atipt.com

Chris E. Stout

ATI Physical Therapy and
College of Medicine, University of Illinois-Chicago
790 Remington Blvd.
Bolingbrook, IL 60440
Tel: 630.296.2222
E-mail: Chris.stout@atipt.com

Richard Victor

Workers Compensation Research Institute
955 Massachusetts Ave.
Cambridge, MA 02139
Tel: 617-661-WCRI (9274)
Fax: 617-661-9284
E-mail: rvictor@wcrinet.org

Dongchun Wang

Workers Compensation Research Institute
955 Massachusetts Ave.

Cambridge, MA 02139
Tel: 617-661-WCRI (9274)
Fax: 617-661-9284
E-mail: dwang@wcrinet.org

Marissa Webb

Adler School of Professional Psychology
17 North Dearborn
Chicago, IL 60602
Tel: 708.205.0552
E-mail: marissa.webb81@gmail.com

ABOUT THE AUTHORS

Robert Aurbach

Robert Aurbach is a 1979 graduate of Cornell Law School and served as a General Counsel for the N.M. Workers' Compensation Administration from 1990 to 2005. He is currently the CEO of Uncommon Approach, Inc., which provides consulting services on a wide range of workers' compensation and related issues in the United States and Australia. He has prior experience in private practice, as a state prosecutor and state Prosecutor Coordinator.

He is a 1991 honors graduate of the International Association of Industrial Accident Boards and Commissions (IAIABC) Workers' Compensation College and has participated as a lecturer for the College on a variety of issues. He has published articles on workers' compensation issues in the IAIABC *Journal*, Burton's *Workers' Compensation Policy Review*, Larson's *Workers' Compensation News* and the Inside OSHA website. He has served as chairman of the IAIABC Standing Committee on Regulation and Enforcement, chairman of the Task Force on Tribal Sovereignty and Co-chairman of the Coverage and Compliance Committee and International Committee. Bob has been the Editor of the IAIABC *Journal*, the only peer reviewed workers' compensation professional journal published in the United States, since 2003. Bob is an Associate of the American College of Occupational and Environmental Medicine (ACOEM), and has presented at ACOEM's American Occupational Health Conference in 2008, 2009 and 2010.

Bob has served as one of three U.S. delegates for the Working Group on Cross-Border Workers' Compensation Issues formed by the Commission on Labor Cooperation, North American Agreement on Labor Cooperation. He wrote the administrative rules for the State of New Mexico workers' compensation system. He has assisted the Navajo Nation with two rewrites of the Tribal workers' compensation act, written the administrative rules for the U.S. Virgin Islands and authored a complete scheme redesign for the State of Delaware. He served as a consultant to the evaluation of the Federal Longshore and Harbor Workers Compensation program. He has presented at the Personal Injury Education Foundation (PIEF) graduate program on "Scheme Design" in Sydney, and PIEF seminars in Sydney, Melbourne and Perth. Bob spent five weeks in residence as a Visiting Fellow at Curtin University of Technology in Perth, Australia in 2009.

Bob's research and writing includes chapters on American workers' compensation system in the *International Labor and Employment Laws,* published by the American Bar Association, and the interaction of the legal system upon behavioral health concerns in *The Handbook of Behavioral Health.* Other recent research topics include the avoidance of unnecessary disability, effects of attorney involvement on workers' compensation programs, reformation of the treatment of workers' compensation claims in Federal Bankruptcy Court, and tribal sovereignty law issues. Bob has also worked with Australian workers' compensation professionals on three pending publications dealing with international comparative workers' compensation issues. Bob is a member of the National Academy of Social Insurance, the Workers' Compensation Research Group, and the Advisory Panel of the Workers' Compensation Policy Review, and is a technical reviewer for the Workers' Compensation Research Institute.

Sharon E. Belton, PhD

Dr. Sharon E. Belton is a Senior Public Policy Analyst at the Workers Compensation Research Institute (WCRI). She is currently completing a study which examines changes in Wisconsin's workers' outcomes. Sharon returned to WCRI in 2004 and was previously employed during 1995 to 2000 as a policy analyst on WCRI's CompScope™ team. From 2001 to 2004 she was the Executive Director of the Wausau Health Foundation located in Wausau, Wisconsin, and a consulting research scientist on "Targeted Change Strategies for Improving Workers' Compensation Medical Care," an initiative funding in 2002 by the Robert Wood Johnson Foundation and housed at the University of Massachusetts Center for Health Policy and Research. She also served as a Co-Deputy Director of the Robert Wood Johnson Foundation's "Workers' Compensation Health Initiative" during 2000 and 2001. Sharon is a Ph.D. in Public Policy Analysis/Political Science from the University of Illinois at Chicago and a B.A. in International Relations and French from Duquesne University in Pittsburgh, PA.

Maureen Kohl Bennington, M.S., CCM, CDMS, CPUR, CRC

Maureen Kohl Bennington is a Southern California based managed care consultant. She is also a published writer, experienced speaker and educator in workers' compensation and disability management.

Bennington began her career with a well known large workers' compensation managed care company. She began as a medical case manager and vocational consultant before moving into sales and operations management. As operations manager, responsibilities included opening multi-state medical case management and vocational service field operations with responsibility for both sales and management. She opened one of the first cost containment units for the company which included medical bill review, provider networks and utilization review. This cost containment unit became a center of excellence dedicated to servicing national accounts and remains so today. These accomplishments were recognized and Bennington transitioned to senior management where she continued to thrive and contribute to the growth of the corporation.

Bennington's desire to make a difference in the industry was the catalyst for her transition to consulting, educating and publishing. Bennington has over twenty years experience in workers' compensation and disability management. She also has extensive knowledge related to all managed care products. Bennington's goal has been to help payers and employers understand cost containment services and utilize them effectively to improve claims outcomes and decrease workplace injury.

As a consultant, Bennington has created customized case management, medical bill review and utilization review programs for payers. She has also created return-to-work programs and completed job descriptions, including essential functions, to address ADA compliance issues for employers. Bennington is experienced in ergonomic assessment and work design with the focus of her work placed on minimizing workplace injury by creating a healthy work environment. As a consultant, Bennington has conducted audits of large public entity managed care programs. Public entities have contracted her to create, disseminate and manage their RFP process for managed care services. Bennington provides similar services to payers in auto, general liability, long term and short term disability.

Bennington consistently writes industry related articles for a number of workers' compensation on-line news sites. Most recently, she wrote a chapter on Return-to-Work Programs for the Larson Series, Occupational Injuries and Illnesses, published by LexisNexis.

Bennington earned her M.S. degree in Rehabilitation Administration from DePaul University in Chicago, Illinois. She is a Certified Case Manager (CCM), Certified Disability Management Specialist (CDMS), Certified Professional in Utilization Review (CPUR) and a Certified Rehabilitation Counselor (CRC).

Martha Gely-Kruto

Martha Gely-Kruto is a legal consultant for ATI Physical Therapy in the area of Workers' Compensation. She has assisted and helped coordinate several attorney CLE seminars hosted by ATI as well as a Work Comp Case Manager Seminar.

Prior to joining ATI, Martha worked as a respondent's attorney for the Liberty Mutual Insurance Group for several years. She handled complex litigation cases in the area of Workers' Compensation for corporate clients like Nation Pizza and UPS. Martha was an instrumental member of the UPS Settlement Team.

Martha also represented Liberty Mutual as a mentor for the INROADS Internship Program and was an active member of the company's diversity program.

Martha earned her law degree from the Indiana University Law School in Bloomington and is licensed to practice in Illinois. She is active within the Workers Compensation Lawyers Association and other organizations.

Dean Hashimoto

Dean Hashimoto is a physician and lawyer. His scholarship focuses on the interfaces between law, medicine and science. He is the Chief of Occupational and Environmental Medicine for Partners HealthCare System, which is the parent corporation of the Massachusetts General Hospital and the Brigham and Women's Hospital. He serves as the primary medical adviser to the Massachusetts Department of Industrial Accidents and is the chairman of the Health Care Services Board which oversees the quality of healthcare within the state workers' compensation system. He is the principal investigator for the Partners research project associated with the NIOSH Center for Work, Wellness and Wellbeing at the Harvard School of Public Health.

Dr. Hashimoto is an associate professor at the Boston College Law School. He has academic appointments at the Harvard Medical School and the Harvard School of Public Health. He is a graduate of the Yale Law School and the University of California, San Francisco, School of Medicine. He is a former law clerk for Justice William Brennan of the U.S. Supreme Court and worked for the law firm of Ropes & Gray before joining the law school faculty. He is board-certified in occupational medicine and received his post-graduate medical training at the Brigham & Women's Hospital and the Harvard School of Public Health.

Matt Kruger

Mr. Kruger holds a Masters Degree in Kinesiology, Biomechanics, and Exercise Physiology from the University of Wisconsin LaCrosse. He has a double Bachelor's Degree in Biology and Political Science/Criminal Justice from Buena Vista University in Storm Lake, IA. While obtaining his Master's Degree, he served as the Assistant Strength and Conditioning Coach for the University of Wisconsin LaCrosse, training all 19 intercollegiate athletic teams. At ATI, he helped Greg Steil formalize the FIRST Program, initiated the Research

Department, and trained FIRST Program & FCA providers. He holds a vast amount of practical experience with the treatment of Workers Compensation clients – with WC/WH clinical experience and 1100+ Functional Capacity Assessments (FCAs) performed for WC case closure. He has published/presented 40+ research abstracts on ATI's Workers Compensation outcomes at venues such as the North American Spine Society, National Strength and Conditioning Association, American College of Sports Medicine, American College of Occupational and Environmental Medicine, etc. He has performed 40+ presentations for Workers Compensation groups in over 10 different states regarding the efficacy of ATI's WC/WH Program and FCAs. Currently, Mr. Kruger oversees the following ATI departments – Workers Compensation Clinical Programs, Workers Compensation Services, Research & Development, and Preventative Medicine, and he is ATI's Senior VP of Workers Compensation.

Richard W. Lenkov

Richard W. Lenkov is a partner at the law firm of Bryce Downey & Lenkov LLC. He represents companies ranging from Fortune 100 corporations to small businesses across the civil litigation spectrum, concentrating in workers' compensation (heading up the firm's Workers' Compensation department), premises liability, products liability and personal injury. Since joining the Illinois bar in 1996, Richard has developed a specialty in representing retailers in these practice areas. Richard has become an expert in such issues as slip and fall accidents, spoliation of evidence, false arrest/imprisonment and food contamination.

Richard is a frequent lecturer on these and other civil litigation topics including: Obtaining a Winning Medical Opinion; Managing and Closing Workers' Compensation Claims in a Cost-Effective Manner; Closing the Nightmare Case; Top 10 Ways to Lose Your Workers' Compensation Claim; Litigation 101; Turning the Tables: How To Use An Employee's Own Actions As A Defense To Their Workers' Compensation Claim; Protect Your Business, Your Employees and Stay Afloat; Evaluating Permanency; Illinois & Indiana Workers' Compensation Issues; and Top 10 Misconceptions About Illinois Premises Liability.

Richard is an active participant in organizations such as the Illinois Retail Merchants Association, Illinois Manufacturers Association, Illinois Association of Defense Trial Counsel, Illinois Chamber of Commerce, Illinois State Bar Association, Illinois Workers' Compensation Lawyers Association, National Retail & Restaurant Defense Association, Counsel on Litigation Management, Workers' Compensation Claims Association and Risk Insurance Management Society (RIMS). Richard is also active with Northern Illinois University College of Law, serving on its Board of Visitors. In addition to participating in these organizations, Richard is currently in the process of starting up the National Workers' Compensation Coalition, a not-for-profit national organization dedicated to representing the interests of employers in workers' compensation.

Rich is a graduate of Northern Illinois University law school and is licensed to practice in Illinois. When not practicing law, Richard enjoys spending time with his family and playing basketball.

Gregory Moore

Gregory Moore is the founder of Harbor Health Systems, and currently serves as its President and CEO. Since 2001, Greg has led Harbor Health's effort to develop the systems and operations for building and managing outcomes based networks. Greg's efforts in outcomes based networks began while a graduate student at UCLA in 2000. His research led to an early model for predicting provider outcomes based on claims and billing data. Upon graduation, Greg founded Harbor with the vision of using outcomes based measures as a foundation for making intelligent quality based decisions for managing networks and directing care.

Over the past 9 years, Greg and his team have racked up many industry firsts including the first outcomes based network, the first network management system with integrated benchmarking, and the first provider contracting model with tiered performance based reimbursement.

Greg's background includes serving as the Executive Vice President of Tera Health, a medical software company with a core focus on large medical practice optimization and data integration. Mr. Moore was also a Healthcare IT consultant for Darwin Partners in Boston, MA, where among other projects he led a team on one of the Largest HIPAA initiatives in the late 90's for Columbia HCA. Mr. Moore holds a Masters degree in Public Health (MPH) from UCLA, and a B.S in Optics from the University of Rochester.

Kathryn Mueller, M.D., M.P.H., F.A.C.O.E.M

Kathryn Mueller, M.D., M.P.H., F.A.C.O.E.M., has served as the Medical Director for the Colorado Division of Workers' Compensation since the inception of this position in 1991.

Dr. Mueller is board certified in Occupational Medicine and was previously certified in emergency medicine. She is a Professor in the Department of Preventive Medicine and Surgery at the University of Colorado Health Science Center, the former developer and Director of the Student/Occupational Health Service Clinic and currently the Residency Director for the Occupational and Environmental Residency. In her position with Colorado Workers' Compensation she has been incharge of the development of ten medical treatment guidelines which are evidence based, to the extent possible.

Her educational efforts include directing the Level I and II accreditation courses, which focus on training and certification of doctors in impairment rating. She also directed the development of the Colorado supplemental guidelines, which provide a rating system for psychiatric impairment, apportionment of spinal range of motion and cumulative trauma. At the University she serves as course director for a year round masters level course in occupational and environmental topics and chairs a thesis committee. Her activities with ACOEM are numerous. She has recently completed her two year term as Secretary/Treasurer after having been elected for two terms on the Board of Directors. She contributed significantly to the current ACOEM Occupational Practice Guidelines being used in California Workers' Compensation.

Dr. Mueller helped develop the original ACOEM course on impairment and served as faculty. Her recent research funded by Robert Wood Johnson Foundation, focused on clinical practice patterns after training on low back, hand hand and wrist American College of Occupational And Environmental Medicine occupational practice guidelines. She also served as a reviewer for the 5th edition of the AMA Guides to the Evaluation of Permanent Impairment and continues as a reviewer and contributor to the Guides Newsletter, published by the AMA and section editor for the 6th edition of the AMA Guides to the Evaluation of Permanent Impairment.

Kim Presbrey

Kim Presbrey is a graduate of Northwestern University and Vanderbilt Law School. He has spent the last 32 years practicing almost exclusively in the field of workers compensation in the state of Illinois. He has been the senior, managing partner, in his law firm since 1981. During that period of time he has had over 80 cases argued in the Appellate Court Industrial Commission Division. He is a frequent lecturer and author on the subject of workers compensation.

Kim Presbrey has served on the board of managers for the Illinois Trial Lawyers Association since 1992. He served as president of this Association in 2001-2002. He has also served as a governor for the Illinois State Bar Association from 2003-2009. He has been a sustaining member for WILG since its inception in 1993.

Kim Presbrey has been chosen as a Super Lawyer and a Leading Lawyer in the state of Illinois every year since the inception of these two organizations. In 2008, Kim Presbrey was chosen as one of the top 100 trial lawyers in the state of Illinois.

Brian Pryor, PhD

Dr. Pryor is a founder and the Chief Executive Officer of LiteCure, LLC in Newark, DE. He completed his undergraduate studies in Mathematics and Chemistry at Salve Regina

University in Newport, RI. He then continued his studies at the University of Pennsylvania where he received a PhD in Physical Chemistry. His thesis work was developing laser spectroscopic techniques to study the structure of molecular complexes. He is well published (> 25 papers) in the areas of chemistry, physics, laser development and application as well as laser applications in medicine. In addition to medical laser development, he has aided in the development of various laser sources for application in semiconductor manufacturing, telecommunications and military operations. Over the past 10 years, he has studied how light and lasers interact with tissue, leading to the development of medical devices in the areas of aesthetics, diagnostics, and therapy. Dr. Pryor has been the principle investigator in many research studies and developments sponsored by National Institutes of Health, US Department of Defense, and the National Institute of Standards and Technology. He has recently published "Clinical Overview and Applications of Class IV Therapy Lasers". Dr. Pryor frequently lectures about light and laser sources and their uses in medical applications.

Jeff Rogers

Jeff Rogers is the Director of Workers' Compensation for ATI Holdings. Jeff oversees the workers' compensation department for ATI which manages and tracks all of its workers' compensation patients across 5 states in 82 different clinic locations. He has been instrumental in building ATI's first EMR software for the their work conditioning/hardening program, building an online real time access to patient information and patient outcomes, and enhancing their billing and scheduling purchased software package. Also during his 4 years with ATI Jeff has become an integral part of ATI's revenue cycle by increasing cash collections and reducing ATI's accounts receivables. Prior to joining ATI Jeff worked for one of the largest property and casualty insurance companies and has 9 years of experience handling workers' compensation claims. Six of those years handling workers' compensation claims in 9 different states and 3 of those 9 years in management. Jeff has a Bachelors degree of Science from Western Illinois University.

Peter Rousmaniere

Peter Rousmaniere is consultant, entrepreneur and journalist in the field of risk. His special focus is workers compensation. He has consulted with over 100 insurance, employers, service providers and information technology firms in the United States and Australia. Rousmaniere has written and spoken on many risk and insurance topics. He is a columnist for Risk & Insurance Magazine and writes frequently for that magazine on workers compensation. Rousmaniere has a BA and MBA from Harvard University. He lives in Woodstock, VT. He can be reached at 802-457-9149 pfr@rousmaniere.com. His webpage is at http://www.peterrousmaniere.com

Greg Steil

Greg is the founder and Chief Executive Officer of ATI Physical Therapy. He established the practice in 1996, focusing on functional capacity evaluations and work conditioning/hardening for workers' compensation patients. By 1998, Greg became the number one provider in the nation for providing KEY functional assessments. Greg has

14 years of experience within the industry, beginning with the founding of the Company and has worked in all facets of the business during that time.

Greg grew ATI from one clinic in 1996 to 82 clinics in 2009, and currently employs over 1300 employees today. He enjoys continuing to build a Company that allows people to grow and develop. Additionally, he continues to focus on developing a team that leads to ATI's continued success and growth through acquisitions and new clinic openings.

Chris E. Stout, PsyD

Dr. Stout is a licensed clinical psychologist and serves as ATI/PRO's Director of Research and Development, where he brings a diverse background perfectly tailored to moving the research agenda forward. He has both impressive track record of publications and presentations along with entrepreneurial experience in various healthcare enterprises.

He also is a Clinical Professor in the College of Medicine at the University of Illinois, Chicago, and a Fellow in their School of Public Health, he holds an academic appointment in the Northwestern University Feinberg Medical School, and was a Visiting Professor at Rush University. He was appointed by the Secretary of the US Department of Commerce to the Board of Examiners for the Baldrige National Quality Award. He holds the distinction of being one of only 100 world-wide leaders appointed to the World Economic Forum's Global Leaders of Tomorrow – joining the ranks of Tony Blair, Jody Foster, Bill Gates, R. J.

Rowling, and Lance Armstrong and he was an Invited Faculty at the Annual Meeting in Davos. He has been invited to work with the Club de Madrid and Safe-Democracy.

Dr. Stout has published or presented over 300 papers and 30 books, including the popular Evidence-Based Practice (Wiley & Sons, 2005, with R. Hayes). His works have been translated into 8 languages. He is currently co-editing Current Perspectives in Clinical Treatment and Management in Workers' Compensation Cases with Matt Kruger and Jeff Rogers for Bentham Books. He has served as the Director of Research and Senior VP of an integrated healthcare system during a 15 year tenure. He was then recruited into the public sector and worked for five years in the Department of Human Services in a Cabinet-level directorship. He also founded a 501(c)(3) to work on international humanitarian projects, and subsequently he has won four international humanitarian awards.

He has lectured across the nation and internationally in 19 countries, and visited 6 continents and over 75 countries. He is frequently interviewed (e.g., CNBC, CNN, NBC, PBS, NPR, Oprah, Eye On Harvard, Time, Chicago Tribune, The Wall Street Journal, New York Times, USA Today, Associated Press, Windy City Sports, Chicago Sun-Times...). He is a fellow in the International Sports Professionals Association and is a columnist for Competitor Magazine formerly (Windy City Sports).

Chris was educated at Purdue, The University of Chicago's Graduate School of Business, and Forest Institute. He obtained post-doctoral experience at Harvard Medical School as a Fellow in neuro-developmental behavioral pediatrics. He was awarded "Distinguished Alumni of the Year from Purdue University" in 1991. Dr. Stout is a Fellow in three Divisions of the American Psychological Association, past-President of the Illinois Psychological Association, and is a Distinguished Practitioner in the National Academies of Practice. He was noted as being "one of the most frequently cited psychologists in the scientific literature" in a study by Hartwick College. He is listed in Fast Co.'s Global Fast 50 nominees and in Richard Saul Wurman's "Who's Really Who, 1000: The Most Creative Individuals in America." He currently serves in an Illinois at the Medical Reserve Corp and is a member of the Disaster Response Network. He hold unique and distinct honor on his being named one of ten Volunteer's of the Year by Pioneer Press, for his global efforts, and both the Illinois Senate and House similarly recognized his work by proclamation of "Dr. Chris E. Stout Week."

Richard Victor

Dr. Victor has been the Executive Director of the Workers Compensation Research Institute (WCRI) since its inception in 1983. The Institute, located in Cambridge, Massachusetts, is an independent, not-for-profit research organization providing high-quality objective information about public policy issues involving workers' compensation systems. Dr. Victor is the author of numerous books and articles on worker's compensation issues.

Prior to working at the Institute, Dr. Victor spent seven years conducting research at The Rand Corporation in both Washington, D.C., and Santa Monica, California. At Rand, he was a principal researcher at the Institute for Civil Justice.

Dr. Victor received his J.D. and Ph.D. (economics) degrees at the University of Michigan, where he was the George Humphrey Fellow in Law and Economic Policy.

Dongchun Wang

Dongchun Wang is an economist at WCRI whose research has increasingly focused on the patterns of medical care delivered to injured workers. She currently is examining area variations in medical practice patterns, especially the use of pharmaceutical and the use of surgery. During her tenure with WCRI, she has been involved in earlier editions of the CompScope™ benchmarks. She did her graduate work in economics and applied econometrics at the University of North Carolina at Chapel Hill.

Marissa G. Webb

Marissa G. Webb is a full time student at Adler School of Professional Psychology. She is working on her Master's degree in Counseling Psychology. She is a member of the American Counseling Association and Illinois Psychological Association for Graduate Students. Marissa has worked as a graduate intern for Dr. Chris E. Stout for the past six months. She has worked on the development of content of the Evidence Based Medicine Institute, has assisted in the development of the National Workers' Compensation certification exam, and has most recently worked with Dr. Stout on the Current Perspectives in Clinical Treatment and Management in Workers' Compensation Cases as the stylistic editor.

Marissa will begin her clinical practicum experience as an intern at Orland Township Youth and Family Services in Orland Park, IL. Upon graduating, Marissa hopes to work in a community mental health facility to further develop her clinical skills. She has a strong interest in working with children and adolescents, but hopes to gain experience in working with multiple populations. She eventually hopes to work in private practice.

Marissa graduated from Illinois State University in 2005 with a degree in Middle Level Education with endorsements in Math and Science. At Illinois State University, she was involved with Delta Delta Delta Sorority and participated in her sorority's philanthropic events to raise money for St. Jude Children's Research Hospital. Most recently, she has participated in both the Avon Walk for Breast Cancer and The Breast Cancer 3-Day Walk, both in Chicago, IL, to raise money for research and treatment of breast cancer.

Marissa taught eighth grade Science and Math for two years at Jerling Junior High School in Orland Park, IL. She was then employed at JP Morgan Chase Bank as a licensed personal banker in Lockport, IL. Marissa was then recruited to work as a Corporate Account Manager for Club Colors Incorporated in Schaumburg, IL.

In her free time, Marissa enjoys spending time with her family and friends and working out. She hopes to continue her support of Breast Cancer research and hopes to find more causes to serve.

KEY WORDS

Comorbidities

Comparative effectiveness

Delaware Rating Bureau

Diagnostic Related Groups (DRGs)

Effectiveness research

Electronic claims management

Electronic Health Record (EHR)

Ethics

Evidence based treatment

Evidence-based medicine (EBM)

Evidence-based practice (EBP)

F. I. R. S. T

Fee Schedules

Functional Capacity Evaluation (FCE)

Health Insurance Portability and Accountability Act (HIPAA)

Iatrogenic disability

Independent Medical Examination (IME)

Malingering

Managed Care

Maximum Medical Improvement (MMI)

Medical errors

National Council of Insurances Legislators

Navajo Nation

Official Disability Guidelines (ODG)

Permanent Partial Disability (PPD)

Rehabilitation

Return to work

Temporary Total Disability (TTD)

Utilization Review

Work Conditioning/Work Hardening

CHAPTER 1

Introduction

Chris E. Stout, PsyD

ATI Physical Therapy and College of Medicine, University of Illinois-Chicago

"Of all the forms of inequity, injustice in health is the most shocking and the most inhumane." **The Reverend Dr. Martin Luther King, Jr.**

Abstract: This book is a novel approach to examine workers' compensation's various and diverse facets. The contributing authors provide a diversity of perspective and opinion that bring richness to this complex debate.

INTRODUCTION

This project was a labor of love. The editors are grateful for the generous invitation from the publishers at Bentham for this venture; without them this book would not exist. Too often injured workers' situations are unknown or ignored or responded to with prejudice and suspicion. It is our hope that this book provides a balanced, ecumenical if you will, offering of differing viewpoints. Our general, uniting thread is that of evidence-based as well as experience-based perspectives. But we have worked hard to be fair-minded in the material presented herein.

I (CES) have had the pleasure of working on writing projects in which I am the sole author, and I have worked on others as the sole editor, writing chapters as well as recruiting contributing authors and editing their submissions. I generally enjoy being an editor more so, and I am reminded of Walter Cronkite's quote that "editorial work allows one to be both pontifical and wrong." In the case of this book, I had the additional pleasure of working with some really sharp co-editors, Matt Kruger and Jeff Rogers. They both bring different yet complementary perspectives and experiences that have made their chapters, as well as the survey we created, along with the selection of the other contributing authors, result in a manuscript we are proud of and hope readers will enjoy.

The book is comprised of two sections. Part One is a look back, a look forward, and a look around at current aspects of workers' compensation issues that includes an inside view of very honest and gloves-off opinions of various professionals working in the area of workers' compensation cases. And Part Two is comprised of chapters from many of the leading thinkers and analysts in the field of workers' compensation today. The book is rounded out with appendices that include a comprehensive list of workers' compensation contact information for all fifty-states, a complete copy of the survey tool that was used for data collection, Fee Schedules for all states in the US that have them, and a listing of workers' compensation studies.

Part One begins with my (CES) chapter entitled "The Role of Outcomes Management and Evidence-Based Practice in Workers Compensation: The Clinical Meets the Practical." This chapter examines the benefits and concerns associated with clinical outcomes-management as it relates to and informs the evidence-based practice of rehabilitation of injured workers. Jeff Roger's chapter, "Workers' Compensation Care is Not the Norm: Why It Is Different," focuses on the common question "Why is workers' comp not reimbursed at the same rate as group insurance?" Herein Jeff explains the difference from the perspectives of treatment, management, and clinical views.

There have been many failed attempts at building better workers' compensation models. So Jeff, Matt Kruger, Jillian Richardson, and I wrote "What's NOT Worked for 50 – 60 Years." It seems that no one is really proud of their state's approach to managing workers' compensation. In fact, it seems that no one is particularly even satisfied with state's approach to managing workers' compensation. The irony is that both "sides" seem to feel this way, that is, those on the "side" of the injured worker as well as those on the "side" of the employer. This examines the history of workers' compensation (in the United States) in the context of problems and attempted solutions, and it offers one perspective as a means toward a solution.

Chris E. Stout, Matt Kruger and Jeffrey Rogers, (Eds)

"Ethical Challenges in Working with Workers' Compensation Patients" authored by the editors, provides an intensive examination of the myriad of ethical challenges and situations that face (and may tempt) most every person involved in a workers' compensation case—from the injured employee to his/her employer to healthcare professionals to legal representatives for employers and employees to case managers. This chapter concludes with various real-life case examples wherein questionable ethical lapses have occurred. This section is rounded-out with "Comorbidities and Workers' Compensation: Responsive Approaches to Work Hardening and Conditioning" by the editors and Maureen Kohl Bennington. They delve into various comorbidities or pre-existing health/medical conditions that may negatively impact injured workers' abilities to gain appropriate rehabilitative milestones. It is surprising to see that such conditions so often go ignored in spite of the dramatic impact they have on treatment and subsequent outcome.

The end of part one concludes with close-to-verbatim responses of an international group of workers' compensation professionals. It turned out to yield a Manichaean-like set of views. Perhaps the anonymity afforded to subjects provided a certain cordon of comfort to really let loose with their opinions and experiences—indeed some folks seemed to have been frothed-up like a cappuccino laced with arsenic. Actually, some respondents' answers reminded me of Garrison Keillor's comment "Militants on either side are outraged, but they enjoy outrage, that is their outrage that is their art form." So, readers will be treated to some magnificent works of art in this chapter, or perhaps at least a good dose of sophistry. The survey, in its entirety, appears in Appendix B herein.

Part Two is comprised of a wonderful set of some of the leading thinkers and doers in the workers' compensation arena. C. Walker Percy would have described them as "Vassar smart and southern shrewd." Robert M. Aurbach kicks things off with "Getting Justice: Unintended Consequences of the Dispute Resolution System" wherein he discusses the adversarial process of dispute resolution in workers' compensation claims that occurs in most American jurisdictions and how it creates significant costs and delays for all parties. These proceedings also have significant unintentional consequences with respect to the long-term outcomes of many injured people. The actions of attorneys in the dispute resolution system are particularly pernicious contributors to problematic phenomena. Thankfully, he offers some mechanisms for adjusting dispute resolution that can improve outcomes.

Next up, Martha Gely-Kruto delves into the "Respondent's Perspective of the Workers' Compensation System" and she describes the many factors that go into determining the outcome of a workers' compensation case. Richard W. Lenkov then discusses "Closing the Nightmare Claim: Practical Approaches for Ending the Most Difficult Workers' Compensation Cases" wherein he notes that every workers' compensation professional has the proverbial "nightmare claim." And, like nightmares, they can literally keep you up at night. But he provides practical techniques on how to turn these cases around, and how to close them quickly and cost-effectively.

The California MPN provides an excellent legislative model for managing an outcomes based medical network in workers' compensation as described by Gregory Moore in his chapter "Practical Application of Outcomes Based Networks." He discusses his managed care model which provides payers with the control to create and certify a medical network from which all injured employees must select physicians and medical services. This containment of patient traffic ensures higher compliance with using trusted providers than typical health care and workers compensation models. Joe Paduda weighs-in with his chapter, "The Ethics of Clinical Guidelines and Other Tales of Evidence-Based Practice: Points and Counter-Points" and he delves into the relatively new (to workers' comp) area of comparative effectiveness and the somewhat less sophisticated but much more common process of clinical guideline development. Kim Presbrey then takes us back to unsettling issues in his chapter, "The Anatomy of a Nightmare Workers' Compensation Case" wherein he examines the complexity of workers' compensation cases. Brian A. Pryor, then educates us as to the clinical applications and "Advances in Laser Therapy for the Treatment of Work Related Injuries" and notes that laser therapy has been used as a therapeutic modality for many years and but has yet to become a standard of care in workers' compensation cases, however he believes that this modality has great potential to be used in the clinic for the reduction of pain, inflammation and to aid in the healing process.

"Persistent problems in clinical practice" is the focus of Peter Rousmaniere's chapter that examines the fact that medical care accounts for 60% of the total cost of workers compensation claims while claims payers under-invest in medical intelligence, thereby allowing medical errors and sub-optimal treatment to happen more than needs be. Similarly, Dongchun Wang, Kathryn Mueller, Dean Hashimoto, Sharon Belton, and Richard A. Victor, consider in their chapter that back pain is a common source of disability, both from work-related injuries and from injuries that occur outside of the workplace, the annual result in the United States is $15 billion and accounts for approximately 15 percent of the costs in workers' compensation medical care. They examine the patterns of medical care for workers with common low back conditions and how the patterns of medical practice compare with evidence-based treatment guideline recommendations.

The Appendices conclude the book with the American Physical Therapy Associations' Workers' Compensation State Resource Guide that was reprinted by permission and actually edited herein by Marissa Webb to ensure accurate links. Following this is the complete, unabridged version of the Survey Questionnaire that was used for data collection in chapter seven. Appendix C provides readers with the Fee Schedules for Workers' Compensation for all states in the US that have them. And a listing of workers' compensation studies rounds out the book in Appendix D.

In closing, the editors would like to note that all royalties for this book will go to a 501(c)(3) charitable foundation devoted to funding healthcare for needy children. We thank you for reading our work, and we hope it will be a help to you in yours.

CHAPTER 2

A Method and Model to Judge Evidence-Bases for Workers' Compensation

Chris E. Stout, PsyD

ATI Physical Therapy and College of Medicine, University of Illinois-Chicago; E-mail: Chris.stout@atipt.com

Abstract: Application of evidence-based medicine and evidence-based practice has not yet completely migrated or been uniformly applied to clinical aspects of workers' compensation. This chapter provides a methodology and model for readers to consider when designing and developing such an approach for their clinical practice with workers' compensation patients.

INTRODUCTION

Evidenced-based treatment guidelines are imperative for assuring that rehabilitative services provided are of value to injured workers. This chapter will discuss a framework developed for identifying evidence-based outpatient rehabilitation services that can be applied idiosyncratically with workers' compensation patients. Such a framework or construct is the initial step for collecting rehabilitation outcomes and driving improved quality of care.

Within the workers' compensation arena, few consensus-benchmarks exist for defining quality care and for measuring outcomes. This author co-authored a book on evidence-based practice within behavioral health (Stout and Hayes, 2005), and now the American Physical Therapy Association has published utilization guidelines for physical therapy services specific to body systems. These guidelines are considered in the functional outcome measurements of many providers, along with reviews of the relevant literature, however, they are not workers' compensation specific.

Folding the criteria for evidence-based treatment guidelines with treatment protocols, and then evaluating efficacy via functional clinical assessment tools (at pretreatment, during treatment, and at discharge) is the foundation of a robust and integrative model. The instruments used to measure outcomes of the provision of rehabilitation healthcare services should be standardized and empirically validated instruments.

Many professionals have varying opinions as to what constitutes an appropriate evidence-base. Thus, this chapter will not dictate a dogmatic "my-evidence-base-is-better-than-yours" but rather herein readers are provided with a tool or annotated guideline for reviewing guidelines. This can be applied to any type of healthcare service provision—workers' compensation cases, general physical rehabilitation, orthopedics, etcetera.

Maja Jurisic, MD, the Regional Medical Director for Concentra, in a 2009 presentation on "Treatment Guidelines, Changing Physician Behavior, and Cost Effective Treatment" noted that while the best approach to getting an injured worker back to work as soon as possible makes a huge difference in outcomes and costs, the application of medical treatment guidelines to do so in workers' compensation patients is generally lacking in sustained success.

ONE PRACTICE'S APPROACH

The organization for which this author works organization incorporates various outcome management components. These include:

- Pre- and post-treatment assessments using standardized clinical tools to measure treatment response/outcome based on body part/injury (e.g., Oswestry, DASH, Knee Outcome Survey, etc.).
    - These are scored in real-time and immediately become part of the patient's Electronic Health Record (EHR).
- Post-treatment patient satisfaction and quality improvement surveys with both quantitative and qualitative questions.

Chris E. Stout, Matt Kruger and Jeffrey Rogers, (Eds)

  - The data are electronically scanned and entered into a database. These data are then compiled and aggregated on a quarterly based with comparisons provided for prior quarter.
  - The forms are bar-coded and the organization has the ability to investigate any untoward comments or ranking to a granular level of clinic and provider, if need be.
  - This instrument and process then is not only a useful quality management/improvement tool, but serves as a keen risk management tool as well.
- In workers' compensation cases, there is a concern vis-à-vis the impact of co-morbidities on outcomes and length of care.
  - Thus, a comprehensive Medical History Form was developed and automated that allows the clinician immediate knowledge of any such factors in real-time via the EHR.
  - These data are also available if the clinician has to deal with a utilization reviewer in order to argue the need for approval for additional services or a longer time in treatment.
  - Over time, the plan is to evaluate the relative impact of various co-morbidities (e.g., smoking, diabetes, obesity, alcoholism, etc.) on care and to subsequently develop "customized" treatment plan modifications that best address these factors in order to maximize current and future outcomes.
- An off-the-shelf tool, SharePoint (published by Microsoft), is used in the organization's intranet. Therein, it is a repository of evidence based article reprints, live web-links to various evidence-based practice websites (including tutorial sites), various research tools, statistics, and clinical instruments. This provides clinical staff with a fast, efficient, and comprehensive tool-box in order to access most any clinical resource they would need.
- Follow-up studies. A new instrument was developed in order to evaluate longer term treatment outcomes (e.g., 2 years post-treatment). It is planned to be introduced in the near future, following a beta-test.
- Internal, specific studies. Many of the clinical leadership have interests in specific aspects of care and/or outcomes. An example of this would be a double blind examination of workers compensation patients' quality of life, fear avoidance/confidence, and depression that is currently underway.
- Fulltime Research Department. This organization believed having such a department was critical in managing all of these various components and aspects. Literature reviews are available to be done "on-demand" for requesting clinical staff (and then also published on a SharePoint site for everyone's access and use). Collaborations with referring physicians, universities, and students are also then norm–with the goals of presentation, publication, and/or education.

EVIDENTIARY ISSUES IN EVALUATING GUIDELINES

The National Guideline Clearinghouse of the United States notes that although randomized clinical trials can make an important contribution to the evidentiary base for treatment guidelines, a single experiment from one setting does not provide sufficient evidence of efficacy. Replication across multiple studies, multiple settings, and by independent investigators is desirable. In addition, clinical leaders should consider the complexity of the research question when evaluating the import of a given literature. Some questions are easier than others to address in controlled clinical trials. For example, short-term, diagnosis-focused treatments lend themselves more readily to controlled studies than do longer-term interventions aimed at more multifaceted concerns and complex patients with co-morbidities. Consequently, the extent of the available scientific literature may vary depending upon the ease with which the intervention can be tested using controlled clinical trials. Easily researched questions may have more literature supporting them than hard-to research questions. Paucity of literature does not necessarily imply that an intervention is ineffective.

The following is a discussion from in Schreiber and Stern (2005), which further a dresses these concerns:

> "Some authors have suggested that physical therapists only read and utilize Randomized Clinical Trials (RCTs) when seeking out evidence for practice and to disregard lower levels of evidence (Maher, Sherrington, Elkins, Herbert, & Moseley, 2004). However, there are inherent difficulties in

applying evidence generated by RCTs to a clinical population (Bithell, 2000). For example, the array of unique clinical circumstances a therapist treating a child with cerebral palsy must take into consideration is daunting. These include, but are not limited to, the child's age, type of cerebral palsy, motor ability, cognitive ability, behavior and motivation, family involvement and support, home environment, and educational placement. The results from highly controlled RCTs often are not directly applicable to an individual patient. Thus the practitioner is required to make an interpretative 'leap' in determining whether the results from any research, including RCTs, yields the best evidence to support a clinical decision (Baxter, 2003; Difabio, 1999) As noted by Bithell (2000), '...There is no intrinsic reason why a clinical experiment developed to prove pharmacological efficacy should be the best way to demonstrate effectiveness of therapies which depend so much on human interaction.' The concept of a hierarchy of evidence, as derived from medicine and pharmacologic investigations may not always be applicable to the array of factors that influence physical therapy outcomes because of the variability inherent in these types of patients, in patient- therapist interactions, and even in statistically significant results (Difabio, 1999; cited in Schreiber and Stern, 2005)."

"Several other limitations related to the perceived 'gold standard' of RCTs have been identified (Bithell, 2000; Difabio, 1999; Ottenbacher and Hinderer, 2001; Ritchie, 2001; Rothstein, 2001; Wakefield, 2000). In physical therapy, RCTs are typically efficacy studies involving distinctly selected patient subgroups in university medical facilities. This information is not always relevant to real-world clinical practice (Ottenbacher and Hinderer, 2001; Wakefield, 2000). In addition, the research procedures of randomly assigning patients to an experimental or control group, using standardized outcome measures that may not have real-world relevance, and the difficulty of blinding investigators and clients to the research procedures all make RCTs difficult for physical therapists to implement, interpret, and utilize (Ottenbacher, and Hinderer, 2001; Ritchie, 2001; cited in Schreiber and Stern, 2005)."

"Along with the methodological limitations, there is often a difference between an optimal and objective research outcome, and an optimal individual clinical outcome. Physical therapy intervention is typically complex, long term, and specifically related to the patient. Translating research results, even those results from high quality RCTs, into specific clinical decisions for an individual patient or client is challenging (Difabio, 1999; Harrison, 1996; Ritchie, 2001). Teasing out one aspect of a clinical intervention for study in isolation may lead to what has been termed a Type III error, whereby the interactive effects of an intervention are not considered (Wade, 2001). The scientific method focuses on one variable at a time across a given number of identical research subjects to determine a single generalizable outcome. Clinical practice deals with countless variables at a time with one person in order to generate a range of outcomes intended to satisfy that person's goals, needs and desires (Ritchie, 1999). Oftentimes, efficacious research regimens that work under ideal research conditions are not implemented if they do not address relevant clinical issues and cannot be applied to individual patients. (Harrison, 1996; Hurley, 2000; Pomeroy, 2003). A recent review of research and review articles in four national physical therapy journals during a 12-month time period produced a relatively small yield of articles containing scientific evidence that was both clinically useful and of high quality (Miller, McKibbon, & Haynes, 2003). An important and ongoing challenge for researchers is to generate clinically relevant findings that subsequently influence practice (Foster, Barlas, Chesterton, & Wong, 2001; Harrison, 1996; cited in Schreiber and Stern, 2005)."

"Given the ambivalence about the relationship of RCTs to physical therapy practice and the inherent bias in inferential statistics, perhaps a re-thinking of what constitutes 'evidence' is in order (Baxter, 2003; Difabio, 1999; Gibson and Martin, 2003; Ottenbacher and Hinderer 2001; Ritchie, 2001; Wakefield, 2000). As Di Fabio noted, 'I think we need to abandon the quest for absolute truth and look, instead, at clinical research as a way to develop a reasoned philosophy about patient care' (Difabio, 1999). A high quality RCT may provide strong scientific evidence, but its relevance to clinical practice may not be clear (Bithell, 2000; Ottenbacher and Hinderer 2001; Wakefield, 2000). Some have argued for an emphasis on "pragmatic" or needs-led RCTs in contrast to "explanatory" RCTs which are more appropriate for traditional laboratory studies and focus on the underlying physiology for a particular intervention (Bury, 1996; Wakefield, 2000). Pragmatic RCTs evaluate a treatment itself, rather than the underlying physiology (Wakefield, 2000). In addition, a less direct but perhaps more useable approach may be to integrate the findings from a variety of studies and a variety of methodologies into a theoretical framework for practice. In this way, the theory guides practice, and results of one specific study or group of studies supports and aids in the development and revision of the theoretical framework (Harrison, 1996; cited in Schreiber and Stern, 2005)."

> "Some have argued that there is little point in practitioners even reading research studies that do not meet basic criteria such as true randomization, blinding where possible, and acceptable follow-up (Herbert, Sherrington, Maher, & Moseley, 2001; Maher, Sherrington, Elkins, Herbert & Moseley, 2004). This implies that clinicians should not read case reports, single case research designs, or qualitative research studies. This is especially problematic since there may be a relatively small number of articles in physical therapy or related journals that are clinically relevant and provide strong research evidence (Miller, McKibbon & Haynes, 2003). In contrast, others have argued that the standards for evidence may be set too high, and that the RCT gold standard established in medicine is not always directly relevant to the complex interactions and clinical decision making inherent in clinical practice for physical therapists (Bithell, 2000; Miller, McKibbon & Haynes, 2003; Ottenbacher and Hinderer 2001). In addition to utilizing RCTs and systematic reviews, qualitative methodologies, single subject research designs, and case series research should continue and must be valued by our profession (Baxter, 2003; Bithell, 2000; Gibson and Martin, 2003; Herbert, Sherrington, Maher & Moseley 2001; Ottenbacher and Hinderer, 2001; Ritchie, 1999). While these methodologies may not appear to ascend to the level of 'high-quality' scientific evidence as currently defined, the information and knowledge generated by these types methodologies is valuable to practicing clinicians and should contribute to the evolution of the practitioners' theoretical framework as noted above (Baxter, 2003; Gibson and Martin, 2003; Ritchie, 1999; cited in Schreiber and Stern, 2005)."

Furthermore, the aggregate data produced by controlled group-comparison trials do not necessarily predict individual patient response. Even the most effective treatments may not work with every patient. In addition, some patients may respond best to a treatment that is not effective with the majority. Therefore, good treatment guidelines allow for some flexibility in treatment selection to accommodate individual responses.

Finally, any study is the product of many subjective judgments concerning whom to treat, how to treat them, and how to measure change. Each of these decisions can affect the study's construct validity (the extent to which the experiment truly addresses the underlying clinical question). As a consequence, even a treatment that is well supported in randomized controlled experiments may turn out to be of little relevance to the clinical population and its needs. The clinical leader has a fundamental responsibility to evaluate all these considerations when evaluating a guideline, program, or practice.

Clinical Utility

The clinical utility dimension addresses (1) the ability of health care professionals to use, and of patients to accept, the program/practice under consideration, and (2) the range of applicability of that treatment/program/practice. This dimension reflects the extent to which the intervention will be effective in the practice setting where it is to be applied, regardless of the efficacy that may have been demonstrated in the clinical research setting.

The evaluation of clinical utility involves the assessment of interventions as they are delivered in real-world clinic settings. Many aspects of clinical utility are themselves increasingly the focus of systematic evaluation and even controlled studies.

Generalizability

The term "generalizability" refers to the extent to which an effect of a treatment is robust and therefore will be replicated even when details of the context are altered. Relevant factors include patients' characteristics, clinicians' characteristics (e.g., experience with a particular injury, training, etc.), variations across injuries, and the interactions among these factors.

Feasibility

Feasibility refers to the extent to which a treatment can be delivered to patients in the clinic actual setting. Feasibility evaluation addresses such factors as the acceptability of the intervention to potential patients, patients' ability and willingness to comply with the requirements of the intervention, the ease of dissemination of the intervention, and the ease of administration of the intervention.

RATING OR WEIGHTING SCHEMES

It is recommended that a rating or weighting scheme be used in order to consider the differences in the level of empirical evidence offered for any particular method of program/practice. The following is a suggested model to be considered:

Criteria for Identification of Empirically Supported Therapies

A. Well-Established Treatment (Chambless *et al*, 1998)

I. At least two good between-group design experiments must demonstrate efficacy in one or more of the following ways:

A. Superiority to placebo, or to other treatment

B. Equivalence to already established treatment with adequate sample sizes (Replicated RCT with placebo/nonspecific/attention control or empirically-supported tau comparison)

OR

II. A large series of single-case design experiments must demonstrate efficacy with:

A. Use of good experimental design and

B. Comparison of intervention to another treatment (Large clinical replication series with good internal validity and current-program/practice-comparison)

PLUS

III. Experiments must be conducted with treatment manuals or equivalent clear description of treatment (Demonstrated Treatment Validity/Fidelity)

IV. Characteristics of samples must be specified (Identified population)

V. Effects must be demonstrated by at least two different investigators or teams

B. Probably Efficacious Treatment

I. Two experiments must show that the treatment is superior to waiting-list control group (Replicated RCT with wait list/no treatment control)

OR

II. One or more experiments must meet well-established criteria (controlled study),

III. Experiments must be conducted with treatment manuals or equivalent clear description of treatment (Demonstrated Treatment Validity/Fidelity) and

IV. Characteristics of samples must be specified (Identified population)

BUT

V. Effects must be demonstrated by at least two different investigators or teams (Transportability and absence of allegiance effects) is not met

OR

VI. A small series of single-case design experiments must meet well-established treatment criteria (Large clinical replication series with good internal validity and sufficient-program/practice-comparison)

C. Experimental Treatment

Treatment not yet tested in trials meeting criteria for methodology (e.g., Single group, Waitlist comparisons with no fidelity check, nonrandomized).

D. Promising Interventions (Spirito, 1999)

I. There must be positive support from one well-controlled study and at least one other less-well-controlled study

OR

II. There must be positive support from a small number of single-case design experiments

OR

III. There must be positive support from two or more well controlled studies by the same Investigator.

CONCLUSION

Evidence-Based Practice has demonstrated promise as well as challenge in workers' compensation as well as medicine. However, there is growing indication that clinicians and clinical organizations are not only becoming more open to considering integrating such approaches to care, but also integrating when possible. There is no currently accepted universal clinical guideline for most injuries that employees suffer in workers' compensation situations, per se. But, as more tools and a growing scientific literature become available, the ease of application in workers compensation cases will become more prevalent–this will benefit payors, employers and, most importantly patients and their families.

Furthermore, as for the future, Dr. Jurisic suggests that while most current evidence-based practices in workers compensation have focused on clinical aspects of care and procedures, further impact can be made if we also focus our attention on process management in order to maximize case outcomes. In such a model, the frequency and timing of appointments, communication between involved professionals, timing of referrals and ancillary tests are the critical components to process management as applied to workers compensation cases.

Looking forward in the workers' compensation field, we hope to see an integration of various approaches–clinical, technological, processional, and so forth, trialed and evaluated for efficacy and effectiveness in differing payor situations, practices, and patient/employees. It is through such a quasi-experimental approach that quality and value can be born, altered, and replicated to various situations. One size does not fit all in medicine, nor should it in workers' compensation.

REFERENCES

Baxter, D. The end of evidence-based practice? Physical Therapy Review. 2003;8:3-4

Bithell, C 2000, 'Evidence-based physiotherapy: Some thoughts on "best evidence"', *Physiotherapy,* vol. 86, no. 2, pp. 58-60.

Bury, T. Evidence-based practice: Survival of the fittest. Physiotherapy. 1996;82:75-76.

Chambless DL, Baker M, Baucom DH, Butler LE, Calhoun KS, *et al.* 1998. Update on empirically validated therapies, II. Clinical Psychology. 51(l):3-16.

Difabio, R. Myth of evidence based practice. Journal of Orthopedic and Sports Physical Therapy. 1999;29(11):632-634.

Foster, N., Barlas, P., Chesterton, L., Wong, J. Critically appraised topics (CATs): One method of facilitating evidence-based practice in physiotherapy. Physiotherapy. 2001;87(4):179-190.

Gibson, B., Martin, D. Qualitative research and evidence based physiotherapy practice. Physiotherapy. 2003;89(6):350-358.

Harrison, M. Evidence based practice: Practice based evidence. Physiotherapy Theory and Practice. 1996;12:129-130.

Herbert, R., Sherrington C, Maher C, Moseley A. Evidence-based practice: Imperfect but necessary. Physiotherapy Theory and Practice. 2001;17:201-211.

Hurley, M. Linking research with practice: The missing link-collaboration. Physiotherapy. 2000;86(7):339-341.

Maher, C., Sherrington, C., Elkins, M., Herbert, R., Moseley, A. Challenges for evidence-based physical therapy: Accessing and interpreting high-quality evidence on therapy. Physical Therapy. 2004;84(7):644-654.

Miller, P., McKibbon, K., Haynes, R. A quantitative analysis of research publication in physical therapy journals. Physical Therapy. 2003;83(2):123-131.

Ottenbacher, K, Hinderer S. Evidence-based practice: Methods to evaluate individual patient improvement. American Journal of Physical Medicine & Rehabilitation. 2001;80(10):786-796.

Pomeroy, V., Talls, R. Avoiding the menace of evidence-tinged neuro-rehabilitation. Physiotherapy. 2003;89(10):595-601.

Ritchie, J. Using qualitative research to enhance the evidence-based practice of health care providers. Australian Journal of Physiotherapy. 1999;45:251-256.

Ritchie, J. Case series research: a case for qualitative method in assembling evidence. Physiotherapy Theory and Practice. 2001;17:127-135.

Rothstein, J. Evidence based guidelines: Application to clinical practice. Physical Therapy. 2001;81(10):1620-1621.

Schreiber, J & Stern, P October 2005, 'A review of the literature on evidence-based practice in physical therapy', *The Internet Journal of Allied Health Sciences and Practice,* Vol. 3, no. 4, viewed 7 June 2010, http://ijahsp.nova.edu/articles/vol3num4/Schrciber-Stern.htm.

Spirito A, ed. 1999. Empirically supported treatments in pediatric psychology. Journal of Pediatric Psychology. 24:87-174 (special issue)[ISI]

Stout, CE & Hayes, R 2005. *The evidenced based practice: Methods, models, and tools for mental health professionals.* John Wiley and Sons, Hoboken, NJ.

Wade, D. Research into the black box of rehabilitation: The risks of a type III error (editorial). Clinical Rehabilitation. 2001;15:1-4.

Wakefield, A. Evidence-based physiotherapy: The case for pragmatic randomized controlled trials. Physiotherapy. 2000;86(8):394-396.

CHAPTER 3

Workers' Compensation Care is Not the Norm: Why It Is Different

Jeff Rogers

ATI Physical Therapy; E-mail: Jeff.rogers@atipt.com

Abstract: This chapter focuses on the common theme that is brought up by some stakeholders within workers' compensation – "Why is workers' compensation not reimbursed at the same rate as group insurance?" Herein this author explains the difference from the perspectives of treatment provision, management, and clinicians as they relate to this topic. The perspective provided stems from the author's experience at the "ground level" rather than from a top-down management point of view. Additionally, the differences will be explored in the form of responding to a question so that the complexity of such a topic can be more clearly understood.

For the past year, this author has been heavily involved in the revenue cycle and reimburse of all payers for a national physical rehabilitation company. The payers included group, Medicare, Medicaid, auto, personal injury and, of course, workers' compensation. This responsibility covered a five state area and over 100 different group contracts. The result is a very non-theoretical but rather realistic perspective.

INTRODUCTION

It has been estimated that workers' compensation medical care represents 2 to 3% (Coppelman, 2009) of the total medical costs in the United States. While workers' compensation medical care is not frequently discussed at the federal level it is nevertheless a highly debated topic among all the stakeholders in every state—regardless of statute within each state and its administration. This author has had the unique experience to work for a very large property and casualty insurance carrier within the claims department and leave to then join a growing outpatient physical therapy company. While this author is not an attorney and (fortunately) has never been an injured employee, this author has had vast experience in dealing with both of these groups and thus has a good understanding of how they view the system and how it is administered.

PART 1, QUESTIONS CONSIDERED:

At what rate do we get reimbursed if we do not have a fee schedule? Is it Medicare based? Is it based off a HMO or PPO plan?

Currently 33 states' fee schedules use some form of Medicare reimbursement to calculate their fee schedule rates. With the recent changes and the new health care plan it will be very interesting to see how reimbursement will change for Medicare. Throughout late 2009 and 2010 there was the possibility of a 21% decrease in Medicare reimbursement. Such a decrease would have been devastating to those who provide a substantial amount of their practice in caring for those receiving Medicare. Such carryover to the workers' compensation population would drive providers away from seeing injured workers' and would have created an access-to-care issue for those who are hurt on the job.

When considering workers' compensation fee schedule based on group health, it has been this author's experience in dealing with over 100 contracts, that the reimbursement per visit or Clinical Procedure Terminology (CPT) code is dramatically variable (payment contract language prohibits disclosing the agreed upon rates for the company that he works for has). Suffice it to say that this author's company accepts such varying rates based on expected increases in patient volume, capacity, and geographical area and being able to serve patients from local referral sources.

Irrespective of the payer contracts/rates and regardless of the patient's ability to pay, the practice organization this author works for will provide care for any patient that comes to one of its clinics. The author's practice organization does not market specifically to each contract that it has. It is important for referral sources to know that that the practice organization's clinics are willing to treat any patient. This is important to the referring physician as he/she is concerned about the continuity of post-operative care vis-à-vis the outcome of his/her patient. If a physician has to start thinking about where to send the patient for post-operative clinical/rehabilitative services, there is the risk that he/she will stop managing the whole course of care. And if the physician does not manage the case, there is an increased risk of poorer outcomes.

Perhaps the key issue of how to effectively manage workers' compensation cases is communication. The communication between the patient, the physician, the nurse case manager, the adjuster and the employer is a critical piece to effectively managing a workers' compensation claim. Most large medical providers understand the importance of this and in doing so they develop an infrastructure to manage these cases. They thus employ workers' compensation coordinators and internal nurse case managers. They develop scheduling preferences to cut down on Temporary Total Disability (TTD). They enlist research activities track and investigate outcomes. All of this is done with a goal of rapid turnaround times. In some states there are requirements placed on medical professionals to provided requested information within certain, specified time frames.

All this extra work and effort is definitely warranted for the practice organization. However, it comes with a concomitant additional cost to the provider. All of these aforementioned activities (and costs) are not present in managing group insurance payer cases. Furthermore, in group insurance payer situations, typically medical records do not have to be included with the medical bills. There are no incoming calls from adjusters or nurse case managers requesting information. (Too frequently, once called back, they inform the provider that they did not receive a fax containing needed information that was, yes, already sent…twice.) Once the information is received, the provider may receive a call requesting further clarification and he/she must then defend the course of care in order to justify services provided or needed in order to mitigate the payer's challenge to reduce the cost of the workers' compensation claim. There is a requirement by some individual or group payers to prepare the bills. For most carriers all bills must include all medical documentation in order to be paid—even after such documentation has already been sent, following the appointment.

Of course, this opens up yet another Pandora's Box as medical paper billing has all the drawbacks that one would expect. The requested supporting documentation attached to the bill is separated by the workers' compensation carrier's mail room staff and paper bills are sent for scanning (usually to another company) where data are (hopefully) transposed correctly and linked to the correct claim. Next, the bills either go through an automated process or are reviewed manually. Of course, the more processes that a bill goes through, the greater the opportunity (and likelihood) for errors to occur (and for the bills to be lost). This author knows from his experience that the most frequent response that a billing collector is told when calling as a follow-up to a late/unpaid claim is that the payer "… has no record of having received the claim…." In this author's experience, this situation occurs in approximately half of all accounts receivable.

Based on this author's recent attendance at the International Association of Industrial Accident Boards and Commissions (IAIABC) conference on the topic of electronic billing in workers' compensation it is clear that workers' compensation payers are not ready for such a move from traditional, paper billing. Given the fact that there are usually hundreds of insurance companies licensed to do workers' compensation business in each state (and actually over 400 in the state of Illinois), it is unlikely that participation and consistent administration is possible. Actually, there have been several states that have mandated electronic claims management with the hope of reducing administration costs and thereby lowering the cost of medical care, but thus far the results have not met expectations.

This author is not, per se, advocating electronic claims management at this point in consideration of the poor results thus far. In fact, there are additional connectivity issues that exist between medical providers and insurance companies that may involve two or more clearinghouses in the middle. There are problems in the ability to send and keep medical records attached to bills, and there are yet to be uniform billing practices adopted. Unless there is a clear information technology structure for use by both provider and payer expectations that providers will be reimbursed at the group rate is unlikely.

As an outpatient physical therapy company, this author's company sends its bills electronically to Aetna, BC/BS, and others. Such access saves the company a considerable amount of resources. In addition to the initial billing, this company is also able to:

1) Confirm within less than 24 hours that the bills that were sent were approved and accepted by the payer,

2) receive a rejection notice for a claim that allows the organization to address any issue and resend the bill back to the payer within 24-hours. If this were to happen with a workers' compensation claim, it would result in a bill that would be "in processing" for 30 to 60 days only to find out that it would not be paid because of missing information. The provider would receive an explanation of benefits (EOB) that is difficult to comprehend. An appeal would then take place and the result of such an appeal is not always positive. Most bills are "duped-out" because they have already been received. Furthermore, the appeal process is just as long as the billing process because there is no statutory requirement for appeals to be processed within a certain time frame.

3) The provider is paid by electronic fund transfer (EFT) within 2 to 3 weeks. For workers' compensation, it is all paper-based and the company receives an actual "live check: at the bank.

When the company's collectors call a group health customer service line in order to enquire about an unpaid date of service, the call is usually picked up within three-rings. From time to time there is a two-to-five-minute waiting period. Once the caller contacts a proverbial "live body," the caller usually can discuss up to five different patients and as many dates of service that apply to each patient. The resolution for these cases is usually 90% or more. But for workers' compensation cases in general there is usually a wait time on all calls placed. Once one gets a "live body" on the phone, the caller is limited to discuss a small number of outstanding claims and limited to only be allowed to talk about only one patient's account balance per call. The resolution rate is thus low and the only recourse is to file a written appeal or to discuss the problem with the adjuster. This author is not sure if this is set-up purposely, but it definitely puts a burden upon providers, and where balance-billing is allowed, puts unnecessary frustration on the patient.

It is this author's opinion that one of the major reasons why injured employees seek out attorneys is to gain help resolving with their unpaid medical claims. The unpaid medical bill issue could be easily resolved if workers' compensation payers had similar customer service departments available with a goal in resolving unpaid bills versus the seemingly Byzantine labyrinth that providers must deal with.

There are also a number of workers' compensation carriers who have no dedicated customer service line for billing issues. These calls are then placed directly to the adjuster handling the file. Given the amount of email, other phone calls, best practice guidelines to be met, and postal mail, this author knows that returning a provider's call on unpaid medical bills is a low, low priority. It is also very often that a billing customer service representative refers a provider back to the adjuster. It is also a fact that most adjusters do not have a good understanding of medical billing, CPT codes or reimbursement.

Most states prohibit the practice of balance billing or they require notice and a certain period of time to resolve any unpaid balance to first pass. In the group health arena, providers submit bills to the payers on behalf of the patient. Lack of payment because of a payer's error can affect the patient by putting the responsibility on the patient to resolve the bill directly with the carrier.

This author believes that workers' compensation carriers have just entered into an age of having robust data. The advancements have been made in order for insurers to attract new business and make claims data available for their customers (employers/business owners). However, there still appears to be a real void in the ability to access medical data and clinical outcomes. Because of the lack of focus on medical data this author is sure that there has been no genuine improvement in the process or investment into the management of medical billing and reimbursement. If workers' compensation carriers view customer service on billing issues to be costly, they could easily provide the ability to look at claims status online and to access EOBs. Some insurance carriers have tried, but from the provider's perspective, such advancement has taken place in the group insurance side industry and, perhaps ironically, Medicare has one of the best online tools for such.

It is often very difficult to find a contact name with a workers' compensation carrier to address large reimbursement issues. Of course, it is much easier for both payer and payee to handle this in bulk rather than piecemeal. An example of this is the annual increase in reimbursement. In Illinois the fee schedule is adjusted to Consumer Price

Index-Urban (CPI-U) as of January 1 each year. For 2009, CPI-U was 215.303 (ending 2008) and the medical fee schedule increased by 3.8%. For the first three months of the year a number of payers did not adjust their fee schedule in their payment systems. For this author's company, the result was in 1227 dates of services being shorted the 3.8 % increase. Adding insult to injury is the fact that these payers had full knowledge that these shorted payments occurred and nevertheless did not go back to correct the errors once the problem was made public. From a staffing standpoint this took this author's company's collections department over 480 man-hours to correct the reimbursement shortfall.

For group insurers, such problems can be addressed with a few calls and a case inquiry is opened by the group health payer. Providers are given a contact name and phone number of a liaison or payer relations representative to handle such requests. If workers' compensation payers want to build a closer relationship with healthcare providers, such a position should be created.

PART 2

In Part 1, much of what was discussed concerned reimbursement and the difficulties providers faced in getting reimbursed for services. In Part 2, this author will discuss some of the fundamental issues that are seen in the medical and disability management of workers' compensation cases and how such improvements and philosophical changes could positively impact the outcome of the workers' compensation case. To begin, Paduda (2010b) addresses the reasons behind the quandary "Why don't workers' compensation payers change?" with the following thoughts:

> "... by no means is this situation unique to that one payer. If anything, resistance to change is a consistent thread throughout the workers' comp payer/buyer/service industry. There is a cultural issue in comp, and perhaps in the larger property and casualty industry that has significant negative influence on the ability of companies to evolve and improve.
>
> "That gravy train is fueled by managed care fees, fees that in many cases are larger than the earnings from claims administration, and can represent a big chunk of an insurer's profit margin. Fees, whether from case management, utilization review, bill review, networks, or other services, contribute to the overall organization's financial results, making it tough to consider programs that might actually reduce the amount 'earned' by managed care programs. Never mind that these new programs will also reduce medical costs. In fact, I can, and often have, made the argument that the current large generalist PPO reimbursed on a percentage-of-savings basis is actually driving up workers' comp medical expenses, and the data I've seen bears that out. Yet the vast majority of payers are still wedded to this old model."

While Paduda touches on a lot of managed care points in his blog, if this author puts on his "insurance adjuster's hat" there are many reminiscences from having worked for an insurance company. Insurance companies, by nature are conservative, and thus do not easily adapt to change, and perhaps certainly do not spur it. Nevertheless, insurance companies must adapt to changes in the law, but it is usually those changes that modify how an adjuster would handle a file. Most companies set a standard of "best practice" and if files are handled in compliance to those best practices, the adjuster is then considered to be doing a great job. However, this kind of best practice does not take into consideration the issues of managing a case for an early return to work, effective medical cost containment measures, or even the overall ability to turn around a case that is going down the wrong path.

This author's experiences that it a rare event for an adjuster to "step outside of the box" or the commonly accepted practices/standards of the insurance industry in conducting his/her work. In today's world of workers' compensation there is much greater involvement by the employers of injured workers'. Data are on now available for employers to actually view adjusters' notes and action plans in their workers' compensation cases. It is not this author's intention to advocate that there should not be a strong relationship between the employer and adjuster, but this relationship has forced times to change, and now an adjuster's greatest concern in a workers' compensation case is the employer.

Joe Paduda wrote another great blog on the differences between work compensation and group medical insurance. Given more space he probably could have turned his explanation an entire chapter, but his summary is excellent (Paduda 2010a).

"The biggest difference is in the type of coverage; WC involves both medical and wage replacement while individual/group is only concerned with medical coverage.

"Work Comp:

- Regulated by states and mandatory in every state except TX
- Only covers injuries/illnesses occurring during or arising out of the course of employment
- Return to Work is critical...
- Mix of injuries and illnesses is different, mostly Musculoskeletal/orthopedic, trauma and some cardiovascular (public safety in a handful of states
- Coverage is "first dollar, every dollar"; No copays, coinsurance, or deductibles, and no caps
- Drug "Formularies" tend to be fairly open...
- Comp docs only treat the occupational injury, NOT the 'whole person'

"Individual/Group Health:

- Not mandatory or required by law...
- Covers all types of injuries and illnesses
- Wide range of provider types
- Physicians treat the 'whole person' for all conditions and co-morbidities
- Unconcerned about Return to Work
- Covers treatment delivered during the policy year only
- Employs cost sharing and seeks to affect patient behavior via deductibles, copays, coinsurance
- Drug formularies are dictated by payer and PBM, can be highly restrictive."

As a provider who handles injured employees, this author's company has made a move to focus on what the patient can "do" as opposed to focusing solely on the disability. As a result, clinical progress notes clearly outline the patient's baseline (or "first week"), as compared to the previous week or progress as opposed to the current week or progress note. This is a move that should continue and it is supported by the recent law changes in Delaware supports this concept (State of Delaware Department of Workers' Compensation 2009):

2.3 ACTIVE INTERVENTIONS Emphasizing patient responsibility, such as therapeutic exercise and/or functional treatment, are generally emphasized over passive modalities, especially as treatment progresses. Generally, passive interventions are viewed as a means to facilitate progress in an active rehabilitation program with concomitant attainment of objective functional gains. All rehabilitation programs must incorporate "Active Interventions" no later than three weeks after the onset of treatment. Reimbursement for passive modalities only after the first three weeks of treatment without clear evidence of Active Interventions will require supportive documentation.

2.4 ACTIVE THERAPEUTIC EXERCISE PROGRAM Exercise program goals should incorporate patient strength, endurance, flexibility, coordination, and education. This includes functional application in vocational or community settings.

It must be understood that the treatment process of therapeutic exercise and functional strength gains does have an associated cost. Such steps require the skilled services of a physical therapist and therapeutic exercise is best done via one-to-one treatment conditions. Of course, the one-on-one time spent with the patient will cost more; however the resultant functional gain will only be accomplished in such a condition. The alternative, lower cost approach is the use of passive care and modalities.

The focus for all who treat workers' compensation cases should be return-to-work. This is perhaps the primary fundamental difference between workers' compensation and indemnity insurance cases. In indemnity care, the patient may only need enough treatment or therapy to return to their activity of daily living (ADL), but in such cases there is no concern with getting the patient back to a pre-injury level of function and back to gainful employment. If it was a "dual benefit" system (like workers' compensation) wherein the carrier was paying medical and short term disability/long term disability, one could expect that there would be additional care authorized.

When comparing the patient population in workers' compensation versus indemnity, there are two distinct differences that manifest: 1) the workers' compensation patient has a job that is usually medium duty (i.e., required to lift 50 lbs) or higher and are post-surgical, as compared to the proverbial "weekend warrior" who has a job that is not as physically demanding as the workers' compensation patient and most are not post-surgical. (In a study of 2.5 years of data conducted at this author's company, only 17% of non-workers' compensation patients had a history of surgery, verses 33% of workers' compensation cases.

This then raises the question as to why workers' compensation patients are more likely to have surgery. Of course, there is a potential contaminating variable of reimbursement. However, there could be several other reasons as well. The first being the pressure put on the physician by those who handle workers' compensation claims, to quickly make a decision and to go forward with whatever treatment that will bring the patient back to work and be discharged from care as soon as possible. Considering surgery while someone is off work is often a sore-spot for many employers, nurse case managers and adjusters due to cost concerns. Second, if a doctor can return the patient back to work and the best possible means to do so is with surgery that is then more likely to be the option versus prolonged, "conservative" care. Lastly, today's advancements in medicine and surgical procedures have shown a decrease in recovery time and there are better outcomes than that were ten to fifteen years ago post-operatively.

Additional aspects to consider if workers' compensation was handled just like indemnity insurance are:

1) The term "Maximum Medical Improvement" (MMI) is a legal term that is not used nor is relevant in group/indemnity medical insurance,
2) Health Insurance Portability and Accountability Act (HIPAA), does not apply to workers' compensation in most circumstances,
3) That group/indemnity insurance care covers all accidents and diseases. (There is no expectation that workers' compensation should also cover but if workers' compensation carriers are also paid for underlying co-morbid conditions that are negatively impacting the work related injury, imagine the beneficial impact that would have in getting injured workers' better and back to work),
4) The choice of medical/care provider from a larger list other than a panel of one to three physicians, versus this authors' experience with small workers' compensation paneled providers that are picked based on the insurance companies' or employers' ability to influence the doctor or put pressure on the providers into reduced rates. (This additionally contradicts the patient-doctor relationship and payment based on performance.)

Over the years there have been numerous reports showing the inflation of workers' compensation medical costs and how medical costs have exceeded indemnity costs. While this may be based on fee schedules and utilization, there is also a concern that workers' compensation carriers and those who handle workers' compensation claims have not kept up with actual medical costs. Indeed, it is not unusual for a nurse case manager or adjuster to tell a physical therapy provider that they want the patient in three times per week rather than two times per week, or to continue physical therapy until the patient is able to return to work, or to get an MRI immediately instead of waiting. Such factors all conspire to increase actual costs, which tend to exceed CPI-U rates.

CONCLUSION

This author is often reminded while at workers' compensation seminars and during the talks given by administrative law judges and arbitrators, that the workers' compensation system was advantageous for both the employer and injured employee. The injured employee receives the medical care that is necessary to return back to work and paid TTD to pay the bills and support one's family. In return the employer gets "exclusive remedy" which then prevents the injured employee from filing a civil suit and providing the opportunity for the possibility of a potentially high jury award.

The cost of workers' compensation medical reimbursement varies from state to state. The factor that is most often overlooked is that access to quality care is critical in the rehabilitation of an injured worker. With the problems discussed earlier in this chapter concerning reimbursement, the continued need to focus on return-to-work and the concomitant difficulties in appropriately handling injured workers', a reduced fee schedule acts as short term gain but is not effective as a longer term solution.

REFERENCES

Coppelman, J 2009, 'Health care reform and the cost of comp', *Workers' Comp Insider*, 23 March, viewed 19 July 19, 2010, http://www.workers'compinsider.com/archives/001023.html.

Paduda, J 2010a, 'How workers' comp and group differ', *Managed Care Matters,* 19 January, viewed 19 July 2010, http://www.joepaduda.com/archives/001726.html.

Paduda, J 2010b, 'Why don't comp payers change?', *Managed Care Matters,* 14 June, viewed 19 July 2010, http://www.joepaduda.com/archives/001843.html.

State of Delaware Department of Workers' Compensation 2009, Delaware administrative code, viewed 19 July 2010 http://dowc.ingenix.com/info.asp?page=pracguid.

CHAPTER 4

What's Not Worked for 50 – 60 Years

Matt Kruger, MS, CSCS, Jeff Rogers, Chris E. Stout*, PsyD and Jillian Richardson, MA

ATI Physical Therapy; E-mail: Chris.stout@atipt.com

Abstract: It seems that no one is really proud of their state's approach of managing workers' compensation. In fact, it furthermore seems that no one is particularly even satisfied with state's approach of managing workers' compensation. The irony is that "both sides" seem to feel this way, that is, those on the "side" of the injured worker as well as those on the "side" of the employer. This chapter will consider the history of workers' compensation (in the United States) in the context of problems and attempted solutions, and it will offer one perspective as a means towards a solution.

INTRODUCTION: COST CONTAINMENT PROBLEMS

It seems that there is no area in just about any type of healthcare today that does (or did) not suffer from being considered too expensive. To go into the history of third party payors for medical claims, or the use of insurance companies to offer healthcare benefits to employees at the employer's primary expense, or that of workers' compensation insurance is too far afield for this chapter, and perhaps this book.

THE CONCERNS WITH USING TPAS AND THIRD PARTY PAYORS IN WORKERS' COMP

While it may seem a compelling argument that the transfer and application of traditional "group insurance" models to workers' compensation would offer a direct and robust solution to cost containment due to the superficial similarities (e.g., healthcare), such an argument is fraught with problems. Rogers (2011), in his chapter herein notes many of the differences. In this chapter we will address those vis-à-vis payment.

Third party administrators (TPAs) are in business. They remain in business by making a profit. They do not provide clinical care, nor do they ensure outcomes, quality, or value. They are nevertheless intimately involved in care decisions. TPAs make money by charging their clients. The only reason a client would pay a TPA is less than what they would pay a healthcare provider. The basic business formula then is that the TPA negotiates a lower rate for the healthcare provider's services and reduces the frequency of visits (i.e., limits access to care) or types of services (e.g., diagnostic tests, a limitation of service).

However, in a workers' compensation situation, clinicians' fees are already governed (reduced/limited) by a state fee schedule. Thus, the only other way to decrease costs is via limiting access; which is what they then do. The problem for the TPA is how to do so. Their solution is generally to create a massive infrastructure that can be made-up of:

- Adjusters
- Training departments
- Management support
- IT infrastructure
- Defense Attorneys
- UR/UM Departments
- IME Physicians
- Peer reviewers
- Second opinion specialists
- Medical directors

- Subrogation teams
- Telephonic nurses
- Field nurses
- Catastrophic teams & examiners
- PPO specialists
- Private investigators
- Surveillance operations
- Occupational medicines experts
- Loss prevention experts
- Injury prevention programs
- Bill review departments
- Return to work programs…

This infrastructure can cost and enormous amount to run, so the unintended consequence of managing care this way is that healthcare costs go up, NOT because of the healthcare provider, but ironically because of the charges resultant from those (supposedly) managing the costs! For example, in the Canadian healthcare system, costs associated with services such as those noted above, account for 1% of their healthcare costs. In the United States, they account for 11%. Paduda (2010b) gives an example of this, in that there are "misaligned incentives for work comp managed care programs, and payers' increased reliance on managed care program revenue and profits. This leads to a focus on processing bills (which generate fees) and doing utilization review (which generate fees) and using huge provider networks (which generate fees) and sending lots of claims to case management (which generates fees), instead of actually managing the medical components of the claim."

The offered offset to the decrease in usual and customary fee structure for healthcare providers is the promise of increased patient referral volume. Sometimes this is the case, and sometimes it is not. In reality, many high quality providers try out being contracted providers in a network. They find that the utilization review is too cumbersome or frustrating (see the chapter on Ethics by Kruger, Rogers & Stout, herein, 2011, for examples of this), and as a result, they drop out. This then leaves the TPA to resort to recruiting lesser and lesser quality healthcare providers as they are then the only ones willing to participate as they are desperate for any type of referral at any fee. Indeed, it is common for quality healthcare providers to purposely incorporate fewer and fewer patients whose case management is problematic or time consuming, and/or have poorer fee schedule reimbursement levels. Indeed, Paduda (2010a) has verbalized the concern that "low fee schedules disincent provider participation in workers' comp thereby reducing access to care, or the inability of the regulatory process to keep pace with medical innovation, or bill review vendors charging some payers merely to reduce provider bills to an inordinately-low fee schedule" more on this below.

INSURANCE COMPANIES INCENTIVIZED TO BE SLOPPY

Payors may actually have incentive to reduce the amounts they pay providers below what is agreed upon in regulated state fee schedules. Delinquent, improper, or late payments in spite of laws to the contrary, have little to no consequence for the erring payor. Late fees are more often than not left unpaid in spite of being owed. Rebilling costs the provider in real dollars, time, and morale-breaking frustration. The longer payors do not pay what is proper; the greater the economic gain they reap in interest and potential for bills that will never be paid as a result of outlasting the provider. An additional problem is that an EOB may say that the fee paid is based on the Fee Schedule, but in actuality it is not, either by shorting or denying payment.

Information from the first annual Survey of Workers' Compensation Bill Review (Paduda 2009) discovered that "the range of pricing for payers using external bill review vendors is over four dollars per bill…A majority of respondents voiced concern about their vendor's inability to keep up with fee schedule and regulatory changes, and the negative impact this has had on the payer….Most respondents view bill review as unnecessarily complex, difficult, time-consuming and expensive. The perception is much more of the bill intake, triage, review, repricing, and transmittal processes should be automated, with far fewer bills requiring human intervention." So, adding layers of costs help the payor, rather than the employer or provider. These (utilization review, nurse case managers, etc.) are *de facto* revenue streams for workers' comp cases that may be helpful in managing cases, however, each time such services are used, they increase the subsequent fees and thus add to the profit of the insurance company. Ironically, these are bandied as cost control methods. While not per se a conflict of interest, the addition of such services, at the insurance company's discretion, nevertheless increases the profit of the insurance company.

Another reason costs are increasing for us is that the system for dealing with many of the problems herein is that workers' compensation payor's systems are not automated, and thus no systems are active to catch this problems in a timely fashion. The "insurance side" is automated and has the capability to catch such errors. It is thus puzzling as to why providers have to then go thru a Byzantine maze of payment hurdles in order to get correctly paid in a timely fashion. It seems that it would be more cost and time effective for all parties involved if the workers' compensation payors would revise as a whole, not on a one-by-one at a time. This is evidentially a widespread concern as noted in a recent industry posting that noted:

> "workers' comp payers spend hundreds of millions of dollars each year on medical management - pre-cert, utilization review, peer review, case management, clinical guidelines, and the variations and permutations thereof. Dozens of companies from mom-and-pops to regional players to industry giants like Coventry and Genex employ highly trained professional medical personnel to watch over the care delivered to injured workers', carefully reviewing and approving or not approving thousands of medical procedures. Then, the medical bills come in to the payer. The frightening/amazing/ unconscionable truth is that many determinations are not automatically fed into the bill review system's database, and/or the bill review system can't link the determination to the bill/provider/claimant. How much of this actually occurs on a national basis is impossible to say, and there's no doubt some payers have the links in place to ensure most if not all medical management determinations are linked to the right claimant/provider/event. But many payers do not have this link in place and/or it doesn't work very well and/or it requires a human to make the link, dramatically increasing the opportunity for error. I've seen anecdotal evidence of this non-connect in audits performed for payer clients, but this is the first evidence I've seen of an industry-wide issue" (Paduda 2009).

DO FEE SCHEDULES DRIVE COSTS UP?

Many workers' comp wonks like Joe Paduda and Greg Krohm (both contributing authors herein) have wondered aloud as to the impact, merit and value of regulated fee schedules in workers' comp. Krohm (2010) believes "...that payment rules like fee schedules are devoid of financial incentives for good medicine and good treatment outcomes, including early return to work....I can think of no reason for a clinician – other than professional and moral values – to put in the extra time it takes to counsel and manage patients on tricky issues like return to work, pain management, therapeutic programs, and the prevention of re-injury. The payment is a flat rate per billing code without regard to quality or care given."

Furthermore, Krohm's (2010, reprinted with permission) concerns note that:

> "The levels of compensation are set by political considerations, which seldom have any relationship to the market rate for medical services in general, or for services provided to injured workers'. In many markets, the fee schedule amount is quite generous relative to the amount paid by group health insurance, and higher still than Medicare payment levels. Sure, there is justification for paying a bit more than group health, but the increased reimbursement should be based on time and cost of treating workers' compensation cases.
>
> "In many states, surgeons and other specialty providers have successfully lobbied regulators and lawmakers for payment advantages over "evaluation and management" CPT codes, i.e., office visits and primary care. It is troubling that fee schedules offer markedly higher payments than all other payers for invasive and sometimes risky medical treatments.
>
> "Compounding the problem, some states do not allow payment above the fee schedule. Many reason that payment above the fee schedule provides a financial incentive to offer treatment that favors the

payer versus the injured worker. This seems like a misplaced fear. The bigger problem is restricting the ability of the payer to offer incentives for quality care and compliance with recognized treatment guidelines.

"By making the maximum fee a public number, some providers (or their office managers) can set it as the target for charges. Thus, the ceiling becomes the floor. Medicare based fee schedules are the best of the lot, but too often these become politicized as well. Income conversion factors for specialists are typically set at 200-500% of Medicare. Also, administrative rules often fall grossly out of sync with Medicare codes and payment rules, e.g., Minnesota and Pennsylvania still use payment rules from the early 1990's when their Medicare fee schedule rules were written. Notwithstanding smart computers that look for code shifting and unbundling of services, the opportunities for manipulating treatments to maximize revenue are ever present in a fee for service environment.

"Fee schedules might be rehabilitated, or their faults mitigated, if they paid a uniform percentage amount over Medicare (say in the range of a 25-40% premium). The target should be set to mimic the prevailing payment level for group health. A small extra margin could be justified by the increased paperwork and reporting that often goes with workers' compensation cases.

"In addition, special codes and appropriate payment levels should be offered for special/idiosyncratic reports (return to work forms, etc.) required or expected by the workers' compensation system. For example, a special code could be created for submitting a functional rating for return to work purposes.

"Given the drawbacks of traditional fee schedules, is there a better way to control the cost of medical treatment for occupational injuries? The answer may not be in government price controls but in establishing a framework for allowing market mechanisms to work. However, there are inherent problems for a payer of medical services to intelligently buy medical services. Among the problems leading to market failure are:

"The fact that in states giving workers' free choice of providers, the payer cannot materially control the choice of vendor that will provide the service; even in states where the payer can direct care to a selected panel of providers, the so-called managed care networks are a shame. They are at most contractual discounts from stated charges on a per procedure basis. There is little public or private information that can meaningfully guide purchasers of medical service to the most effective providers.

"Most insurance claims departments have a common knowledge of notoriously idiosyncratic and high cost providers operating in a given state. This seldom rises to the level of a formal system of scoring or rating doctors on performance.

"A few large payers have amassed good data on providers involved in their own claims. For example, the California Fund has an extremely sophisticated system to identify providers with good and bad claims experience. The metrics have appropriate to adjustments for the mix of claims being presented to each provider. Unfortunately, in most cases even if all the adjusters in department named a doctor as a serious bad actor, there is no way for the claims department to control access to that provider. Purchasers fear law suites from providers that they sanction or delist as providers.

"With rigorously developed metrics of provider performance in hand, the payer has a better basis for negotiating purchase contracts with individual providers or large clinical groups. To make such a contract worthwhile for both the payer and provider, the law must allow a clear requirement for injured workers' to use the payer's negotiated network. Of course, such a system must protect the workers' freedom of choice within the network.

"The other ingredient to efficient markets is to allow payers to freely negotiate with providers on terms of compensation without regard to fee schedules or other cost containment mechanisms. Also important is the freedom for a payer to not contract with a particular provider based on poor outcome data. The ability of payers to individually refuse (not collectively boycott) to trade with anyone they regard as a poor provider can be a powerful discipline to the supply side of the market.

"There are a few bright lights on the horizon. There have been some individual payers who have invested long hours to track provider outcomes and treatment practices. Unfortunately, it remains to be seen how successful these payers will be in maintaining these lists and if they have the authority to limit participation in the system by unsatisfactory providers."

WHY FEES SCHEDULES DON'T WORK

There is a compelling, albeit false, logic in thinking that fee schedules control costs. Furthermore, fee schedules do not eliminate cost differential between workers' compensation and group health insurances. Workers' compensation patients typically have labor intensive jobs, thus the "activities of daily living" must be adjusted to account for the physically demanding nature of their daily activities as well. At best fee schedules provide short-term relief as costs eventually rise due to network abuses.

In response to this, the next evolution was to apply managed care-styled approaches to contain costs. Generally, these have resulted in delaying access to care and degrading the subsequent quality of care. Ironically (and iatrogenicly), such an approach ultimately *increases* costs at the backend due to increased indemnity awards. Bernacki et al (1998) note that "containing medical costs is not an end in itself. If the cost of containment adversely affects the quality of medical care, workers' will be negatively affected, and the cost to the employers and insurers will increase as indemnity benefits rise to compensate for the consequences of diminished care."

Peele and Tollerud (2001) note that managed care techniques were developed within group health plans with the objective of health at the lowest cost. However, in workers' compensation cases, managed care must address a different objective-restoring a worker to health and productivity at the lowest cost. It is this fundamental difference that makes the application of managed care techniques to workers' compensation plans contentious and at times inappropriate. The real promise of managed care for workers' compensation plans is to discover through utilization review and outcome evaluation how to alter provider practice patterns to better deliver care and obtain the objective of a healthy, productive worker at the lowest cost. However, achieving that goal requires more than just decreasing medical expenditures; it requires evaluation of the quality and appropriateness of care, and a timely return to work by injured employees (Boden, 1995).

Although perhaps seen as a more radical philosophy, an elegant approach would be for managed care insurers to put quality of care first, no matter what, with the expectation that doing pays off—both in terms of patient outcome and payor coats. To the extent that an injured worker can be rehabilitated, there would in fact be a concomitant reduction in the ultimate payment that would have to be made (Atcheson, et al, 2001; Bernacki et al 1998; Bradford et al. 2001; Bois et al, 1999, Gatchel et al 2008, Smith, 1995).

FEE SCHEDULES NOT IMPACTING COSTS

California and Texas utilized fee schedules in managing workers' compensation costs and when evaluating its effectiveness, found that costs did not decrease. One of the main reasons costs did not decrease was due to the fact that each hospital's costs and services offered vary from once facility to the next. To help reduce some of the discrepancies between facilities

> Diagnostic Related Groups (DRG) were established. The DRGs created (Wilson et al. 2001) detailed fees for certain procedures and each was designated by a specific number. Despite their best efforts, the Division of Workers' Compensation was still unable to address several issues.

First, certain DRGs were found to have negative fiscal impacts on the providers and threatened patient access to state of the art inpatient surgical care (Wilson et al. 2001). A specific example would be spine surgeries coded 496-500 (Wilson et al. 2001). The fees associated with these codes were not high enough to cover the actual cost of the facility, personnel, instrumentation, and the surgical procedure. Second, DGRs are unable to predict new medical technologies. As a result, the fees associated with their implementation are often much higher and exceed the reimbursement schedule (Wilson et al. 2001). Finally, outpatient surgical facility fees were not addressed in current fee schedules. This is due in large part to the fact that outpatient surgery facility fees are highly variable and there is limited information to determine the appropriate fee level for outpatient surgery facility fees (Wilson et al. 2001).

WHY NOT CONTRACT DIRECTLY?

There is a certain quality of the Emperor-Has-No-Clothes in asking the provocative albeit obvious question of "Do PPOs really save money in workers' compensation?" The answer may be "sorta" or "initially they did," but today as things have evolved, it seems worthwhile to at least puzzle the question.

Initially managed care approaches to cost containment were pretty primitive—reduce fees paid to clinicians and reduce the amount and/or types of services provided. It was a pretty basic formula. But there were some problems with this initial, wholesale set of cuts. Certainly there was an outcry from clinicians, but few were too concerned or sympathetic to their complaining as the public generally harbored the thought that healthcare providers were already overpaid and likely were wasteful in ordering tests and procedures. But in order to be competitive with one another, managed care entities had to perform by showing continuing coats savings to the employers buying their services with the hope at healthcare benefit cost containment. This was then usually borne on the backs of healthcare providers via more cuts to their usual and customary fees (that had already been cut pretty close to the bone over the preceding years).

So, utilization reviews began to come on the scene- as yet another way to insinuate non-healthcare providers into the healthcare system. This then did result in cost savings for the employer, but the restrictive pinch was being felt more so by the insured employee, resulting in complains back to their employer, and the problem became so pronounced and ubiquitous that it raised audience cheers in Hollywood feature movie, *As Good As It Gets*, when a character played by Helen Hunt bemoans the limitations of her very ill son's utilization review denial of needed care.

For lack of a better model, workers' compensation insurers adopted managed care techniques as a means of cost containment for employers and increased profitability for themselves tapping a new market with old tools. At face value, it may seem that workers' compensation clinical situations are similar to those of injured employees. There is an employee-patient with a health problem, there are doctors and healthcare providers providing services. So what's different? Plenty! Forty-six states have already established fee schedules, which then lock-in healthcare service fee rates for workers' compensation cases, making it totally unnecessary to have a managed care product to cut provider fees.

In general healthcare it is to feel better, cure an illness, etc., but in workers' compensation, the goal is to not only be returned to well being, but also to return to work. There is generally not an adversarial process in general healthcare that can exist in workers' compensation. Ditto that for attorneys on employee and employer's sides that may occur only in workers' compensation situations.

Additionally, there is the question as to whether utilization in workers' compensation actually reduces overall utilization. True, it may postpone services (which is another whole ethical/outcomes mess), but more often than not, the needed services are eventually provided. This being the case begs the question as to whether workers' compensation utilization review really decreases costs.

It would seem that directly contracting with qualified providers who must continually demonstrate their ability to deliver high-quality outcomes would be an elegant solution to cost-containment, especially in states where there are workers' compensation fee schedules. As noted earlier, most workers' compensation managed care organizations have grown internally to have massive amounts of costly staff, but in spite of this, profits remain high.

Furthermore, it seems curious that insurance companies have multiple Preferred Provider Organizations (PPOs). At one point in time there was only one major player in the workers' compensation PPO field, First Health/Coventry. Over the last 10 years the market has exploded with additional PPO/Networks, but most being specific to a given area of medicine. Some manage only diagnostics, others only physical therapy and others still for durable medical equipment and prescription drugs. While competition is great for the market place this can cause confusion for medical providers. What makes it even more confusing is many of the large workers' compensation carriers contract with all PPOs to try and capture as much savings and generate as many dollars as possible. This leaves providers with many questions–Which one do I sign up for? Which network with the adjuster, employer, or case manager used to send me referrals? There are 50 providers within a 10 mile radius; will I be the 1 of 50 to be chosen?

A LOOK AT THE WORKERS' COMPENSATION LEGAL LANDSCAPE

While questioning the value of applying managed care approaches to workers' compensation cases, it is worthwhile to also consider that there are a number of indicators present nationally that should be taken into consideration.

LAWSUITS

FirstHealth PPO was sued by Drs. Lawrence Shipley, Richard Coy, and Kathleen Roche as a result of the claim of "unjust enrichment" with providers. In this case, they sued FirstHealth over what they alleged were improper PPO discounts that deprived them and other health care providers of fees they were owed (Flood 2009). The plaintiffs alleged that FirstHealth "illegally reaped huge savings for themselves and their customers, and pocketed substantial revenues in customer fees, while giving no consideration to preferred providers in exchange for PPO discounts" (Burke 2009). FirstHealth accomplished this by inappropriately applying PPO discounts to workers' compensation and automobile accident bills that did not qualify for PPO discounts. This harmed the plaintiffs economically as it cheated them out of money that was rightfully theirs for services they provided. By engaging in these behaviors, FirstHealth broke contracts with the plaintiffs, and other providing physicians, which is a violation of the Illinois Consumer Fraud and Deceptive Business Practices Act (Burke 2009).

OUTLAWING SILENT PPOS

In what may be foretelling, albeit bold moves, the legislatures of Connecticut, Colorado, Florida, Indiana and Ohio have all passed laws that in some way limit or prohibit unbridled third-party network access to a prior contracted PPO network. In fact, the authors of this chapter were successful in altering the Insurance Code in Illinois by having the following language added in the JCAR Administrative Code, TITLE 50: INSURANCE:

> CHAPTER I: DEPARTMENT OF INSURANCE, 50 Ill. Adm. Code
>
> 2051.290(h)
>
> A provision stating that the rights and responsibilities under the contract cannot be sold, leased, assigned, assumed or otherwise delegated by either party without the prior written consent of the other party. Similarly, the provider's written consent must be obtained for any assignment or assumption of the provider contract whenever an administrator or insurer is bought by another administrator or insurer. A clause within the provider contract allowing assignment will be deemed consent so long as the assignment is in accordance with the terms of the contract. The assignee must comply with all the terms and conditions of the contract being assigned, including all appendices, policies and fee schedules;
>
> And
>
> 50 Ill. Adm. Code 2051.300(d)
>
> No preferred provider program may be sold, leased, assigned, assumed or otherwise delegated to another administrator without the prior written consent of the providers contracting under the program. A clause within the provider contract allowing assignment will be deemed consent so long as the assignment is in accordance with the terms of the contract. The assignee must comply with all the terms and conditions of the contract being assigned, including all appendices, policies and fee schedules.

CONCLUSION

It is obvious that workers' compensation is a troublesome albeit necessary part of the contemporary healthcare landscape—filled with differing perspectives, opinions, and approaches. It is hoped that this chapter has been able to articulate in a balanced, fair, and yet frank way the various machinations and aspects in play. Perhaps readers may feel the need to take up the good-fight and offer their talent in moving forward innovative approaches to solving the problems inherent in workers' compensation.

REFERENCES

Atcheson, SG, Bigos, SJ, Brunner, RL, Cox, JC, Greenwald, EJ, Rivera, VG, Stanley, J 2001, 'Paying doctors more: Use of musculoskeletal specialists and increased physician pay to decrease workers' compensation costs', *Journal of Occupational and Environmental Medicine,* vol. 43, no. 8, pp. 672-679.

Bernacki, E, Green-McKenzie, J, Parkerson, J 1998, 'Comparison for workers' compensation costs for two cohorts of injured workers' before and after the introduction of managed care', *Journal of Occupational and Environmental Medicine,* vol. 40, no. 6, pp. 568-572.

Boden, LI 1995, 'Workers' compensation in the United States: High costs, low benefits', *Annual Review of Public Health*, vol. 16, pp. 189-218.

Bois, MD, Donceel, P, Lahaye, D 1999, 'Return to work after surgery for lumbar disc herniation: A rehabilitation oriented approach in insurance medicine', *Spine,* vol. 24, no. 9, p. 872.

Bradford, CO, Davin, JS, Ford, LF, Linz, DH, Nightingale, MJ, Shannon, PL, Shepherd, CD 2001, 'Care management of work injuries: Results of a 1-year pilot outcome assurance program', *Journal of Occupational and Environmental Medicine,* vol. 43, no. 11, pp. 959-968

Burke, R 2009, 'Fairness Hearing Set In First Health Class Action Settlement, media release', *Plaintiffs V First Health,* 27 May 2009, viewed 12 June 2010, http://www.lawcash.com/class-actions/first-health-lawsuit/5346.

Flood, A 2009, 'PPO plaintiffs again ask judge to approve First Health settlement, media released', *The Madison Record*, 8 October 2009, viewed 12 June 2010, http://www.stclairrecord.com/news/221547-ppo-plaintiffs-again-ask-judge-to-approve-first-health-settlement.

Gatchel, RJ, Mayer, TG, Neblett, R, Theodore, BR, Towns, BL 2008, 'Chronic widespread pain in patients with occupational spinal disorders: Prevalence, psychiatric comorbidity, and association with outcomes', *Spine,* vol. 33, no. 17, pp. 1889-1897.

Krohm, G 2010, 'Are Fee Schedules Effective in Workers' Compensation?', *Thoughts from Greg Krohm*, 12 April 2010, viewed 23 July 2010 http://www.iaiabc.org/i4a/headlines/headlinedetails.cfm?id=158.

Paduda, J 2010a, 'Are workers' comp fee schedules driving up costs?', *Managed Care Matters, 14* April 14, http://www.joepaduda.com/archives/001796.html#comments

Paduda, J 2010b, 'Work comp medical costs - heading up... ', *Managed Care Matters*, 26 January, viewed 23 July 2010, http://www.joepaduda.com/archives/001731.html.

Paduda, J 2009, 'Workers' comp bill review survey - initial highlights', *Managed Care Matters*, 17 April, viewed 23 July 2010, http://www.joepaduda.com/archives/001493.html.

Peele, PB & Tollerud, DJ 2001, 'Managed care in workers' compensation plans', *Annual Review of Public Health,* vol. 22, pp. 1-13.

Smith, JL 1995, 'The best care, not the cheapest, it pays off', *Health Systems Review,* vol. 28, no. 2, pp. 50-52.

Wilson, J C, Davenport, A, Dulich, J A, McLeod, L C, Rankin, T, Schwenkmeyer, K, Steinberg, R B, Thacker, D 2001, *The California Commission on Health and Safety and Workers' Compensation 2000-2001 Annual Report, media release,* The California Commission on Health and Safety and Workers' Compensation, State of California, viewed 10 June 2010, http://www.dir.ca.gov/chswc/AnnualReport00/2001annrpt.html#60.

CHAPTER 5

Ethical Challenges in Working with Workers' Compensation Patents

Matt Kruger, MS, CSCS, Jeff Rogers and Chris E. Stout*, PsyD

ATI Physical Therapy; E-mail: Chris.stout@atipt.com

Abstract: This chapter provides an intensive examination of the myriad of ethical challenges and situations that one faced (and may tempt) almost by every person involved in a workers' compensation case—from injured employee to employer to healthcare professional to legal representatives to case managers. The chapter concludes with various real-life case examples wherein questionable ethical lapses have occurred.

INTRODUCTION

Ethics in workers' compensation, beyond personal professionalism and moral code, seem to be fundamentally based on their needs and incentives. There are different ethical conflicts at all phases of a case. The world of workers' compensation can be a complex maze for the injured worker, filled with ethical pitfalls for the professionals working with them. This illustration depicts this maze.

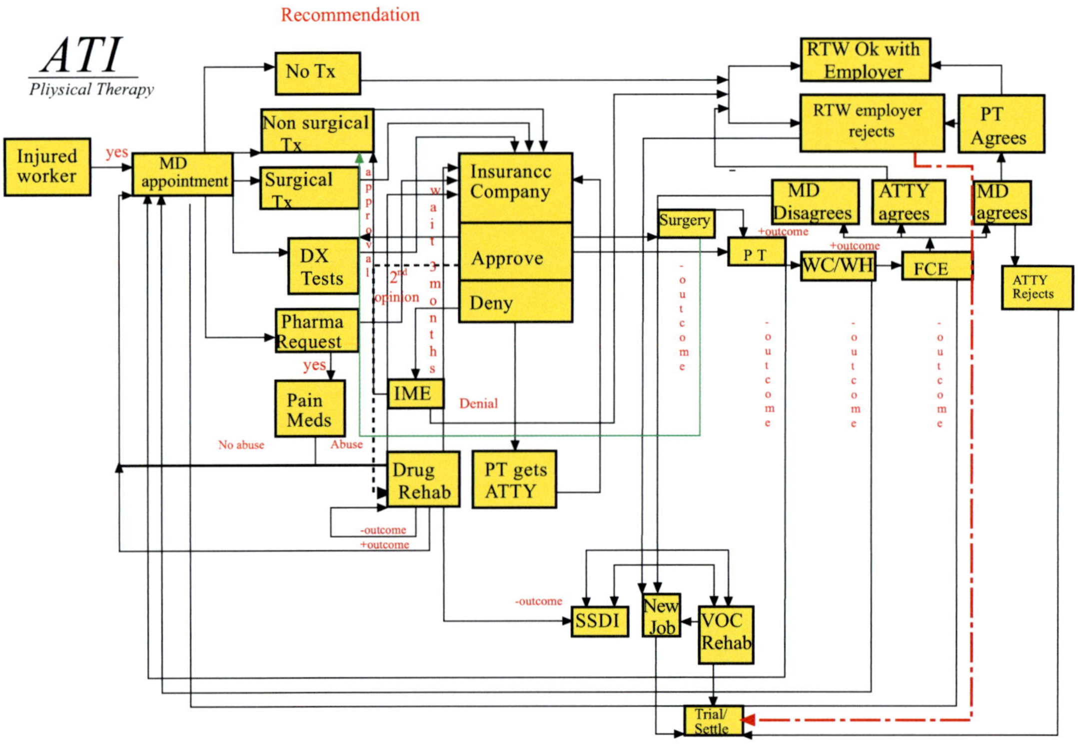

FEELING THE PINCH IN REHAB

Rehabilitation professionals often feel as if they are caught in the middle between the workers' compensation patient, and his/her physician and attorney, as well as the workers' compensation patient's employer, and the employer's attorney and insurer, and the insurer's managed care organization and/or third party administrator, and their adjusters, utilization reviewers, independent medical examiner, consulting physician(s), peer reviewers, subrogation teams, telephonic nurse case managers, field nurses, catastrophic loss examiners, private investigators, occupational medicines experts, loss prevention experts, and so on.... Often there is such a diffusion of responsibility, and not necessarily purposely, that the patient may even be confused as to who the "go-to" person actually is.

So, as a result, if the patient is in rehabilitation, most likely he/she has the closest contact with their rehabilitation specialist. In the program that the author's of this chapter are a part of, the contact level is daily, for approximately 4 – 5 hours, for generally 4-6 weeks. Thus, but default, the rehabilitation therapist becomes the most frequent and intimate clinical and professional contact that the injured worker has. The therapist then becomes a de facto champion or advocate for the case. Indeed, it is not unusual for physicians and attorneys to abdicate their leadership role—unless there is something that comes up that is disagreed with—ergo, the resultant ethical concern.

For example, a rehab professional may be finished with clinical services, conduct a Functional Capacity Evaluation/Assessment (FCE/A) and find that the worker is functional for a medium physical demand level job (50 lbs. occasional lifting). And, this person's job demand level is at a medium physical demand, and therefore he/she can go back to work from a functional standpoint. However, this may also result in the employee's attorney getting a smaller (to no) fee. So, the employee's attorney argues that the patient cannot go back to that job or equivalent position. Sometimes these arguments have merit, and certain semantics of the job or case have been overlooked. Thus, the attorney is providing a true service to their client. More often than not, the resulting argument occurs because of misaligned incentives and desire for payment, justifying that the patient deserves monetary compensation for this injury (and then they get paid too). However, you now have a person that cannot ever return to work at their former occupation, usually without transferable job skills to earn a similar wage. This dynamic can occur with all professionals in the WC system. An example would be the MD that releases their patient with a flat "20 lb. lifting restriction" without thinking of their patient's future employment. Sure, 20 lbs. is a safe recommendation and keeps malpractice lawsuits away, but for most manual workers' it severely limits their future earning opportunities.

From the perspective of the rehabilitation professional, there is a successful completion of rehabilitation. Part of this is not just the physical healing and conditioning, but also the psychological as well. In his book "Super Training," Mel Siff (1998) discusses the factors limiting Strength Production, including physical factors and biomechanical efficiencies that improve with proper exercise and training. However, most interestingly he discusses that pain (or fear-of-pain) and injury (or fear–of-injury) as key factors in optimal functioning. As everyone in the workers' compensation system knows, pain and injury (and fear thereof) occur with every patient going through the system--exacerbated by social and monetary stresses that naturally occur. Siff notes (1998, p.12) "It is often largely unimportant if medical assessment pronounces rehabilitation to be complete, return to top level performance will occur only if the athlete perceives rehabilitation to be complete and fear of pain or re-injury is minimal."

This certainly speaks to the power of the human mind, but also lends some insight into the lingering complaints of injured workers' long after they have been deemed "healed," "released," or "fit for return to work." Outside professionals may be ready for the case to close, but the injured worker may still have remaining concerns. It is their pain, their body, their life at stake. They want to be heard. This is an important lesson to be learned when dealing with workers' compensation patients. The authors have found that in the F.I.R.S.T.™ Program, treating injured workers' with dignity and respect allows them to trust, progress, and heal. The fact that someone has heard them plays a powerful curative role.

ISSUES IN COMMUNICATION

The rehabilitation professional often winds up as the default holder of clinical information and thus the linking conduit thereof. When he/she is in contact with a physician's office to give an update, for example, the physician may never learn of the change due to an internal disconnect between the physician's front office and the physician. Maybe the information went directly into an electronic medical record, and the physician was unaware of it. Maybe it was on a Post-It note that never made its way to a paper file or the doctor's desk, and so on… Of course, the same can occur with the plaintiff's attorney, or any of the other many professionals involved in workers' compensation cases.

Communications can be negatively impacted simply by infrequent contact. Busy medical, surgical, or legal practices may simply not have time to keep everyone up to date on the latest or interstitial changes in a client's situation. The problem then is that the non-communicative professional lets something in the case stew until near the end and then acts in a reactionary (and often angry) way.

The authors herein found that a very simple, if not elegant solution to communication issues on their part was to simply type their clinical notes, as at the time, many if not most all of their peers were not doing so. It was learned that well written clinical notes (both in terms of content and legibility) equaled payment. That was a pretty basic reinforcer. It is critical that clinical notes need to tell the story of the patient's care, progress, etc., and not just consist of data or context-less numbers. (NOTE: There have been many instances in these authors' experience wherein the clinical notes were faithfully sent on a weekly basis to the patient's attorney, and the attorney nevertheless said "what's going on in physical therapy?" Thus suggesting that either the attorney is NOT managing the case or communications are not being properly channeled. Similar instances happen with Nurse Case Managers or Insurance Adjusters. Treatment has been approved, but the next week a phone call is given by the same person who is "surprised" they are being treated in PT. As most know, there is too much paperwork involved in the WC system. Written notes need to be clear, concise, and explanatory.

THE PHYSICIAN'S PERSPECTIVE

From the surgeon's perspective, the procedure may have been flawless—the injury has been successfully repaired, no complications, no issues with sedation, no post-operative infection, and the incision is healing well. Likewise the patient is similarly happy to hear that everything went according to plan, and is greatly relieved. The problem in some cases is that the patient's post-operative condition does not relieve the pain. The clinical-ethical problem then manifests in that the surgeon by philosophy, orientation, and training then thinks another procedure is called for. Additionally, the less ethical physician is also financially incented to do more surgery or surgeries. The first treatment for a problem that a surgeon thinks of is generally not medication or physical therapy as they were not trained as pain specialists/anesthesiologists or physical therapists, there were trained to perform surgery. This is not the "fault" of the surgeon; rather, it is a consequence of a system of training and specialization in medicine and healthcare. In lay terms, when you are a hammer, everything looks like a nail.

Additionally, it is rare that a patient would question a surgeon's recommendation. There may be some progress being made in the education of laypeople vis-à-vis the acceptance of questioning a healthcare provider's opinion, but is far short of universal. Indeed, doesn't a patient go to a physician to gain their professional opinion? Why go if one is going to ignore or argue with what's recommended? Again, not to over-generalize, but surgeon's see surgery as the solution to the clinical issue. Informed consent is gaining ubiquity but it may not be uniform in all medical offices. Indeed, many patients are told what the surgery can fix, and that not having the surgery will thus not fix the problem. It is rarer that a full and complete explanation of all treatment choices is articulated along with the concomitant pros and cons for a fully informed choice and consent. This is amplified by the fact that not all of us may fully understand the options even if they were spelled out for us. As a result, a physician during a consult may spend more time with an x-ray film or MRI image than in conversation with the patient, and at the meeting's end, simply tells the patient and his/her nurse to schedule the surgery as a *fait de complet.*

The physician can be further ethically challenged if the patient needs a follow-up procedure, but the case has been settled, there is no longer an employer, thus there is no longer any medical insurance to pay for the procedure. What is the surgeon to do? Pay for the procedure him/herself? Additionally, some physicians have their own testing laboratories or imaging centers. The Stark Anti-Kickback Bill has addresses this issue for many years, however research indicates that if a physician owns his/her own MRI or lab that he/she tends to order more diagnostic tests. Levin and Rao (2004) estimate that the cost of unnecessary self referred imaging to be conservatively $16 billion per year.

HIRED (MEDICAL) GUNS

It is the payor's right to hire a physician to conduct an Independent Medical Examination (IME) of the injured employee in order to have a different medical opinion. Ethically, this individual should function with impartiality and without bias. However, by the simple nature of the situation, there is an inherent expectation that this physician will make decisions and thus recommendations based on the most conservative and cost-saving treatment alternatives.

These may or may not be in the best interest of the injured employee, and they may or may not be in agreement with the patient's physician of record.

The result can be then continuation of an already adversarial and contentious relationship between the injured worker and his employer and all of their affiliated proxies and agents. The ethical challenge nevertheless resides in the IME physician's commitment to impartiality or seduction of the consultation arrangement as somewhere, perhaps even subconsciously, in the IME physician's mind is that the fewer cost saving findings made, the less likely his/her opinion will be asked for in the future.

THE PATIENT'S CONUNDRUM

Unlike any other medical or healthcare situation, workers' compensation law, and thus cases, supersede or preempt any state's confidentiality acts or the federal Healthcare Information Portability and Accountability Act (HIPAA). What this then means is that an injured worker knows that what is said to any healthcare provider is not confidential and is discoverable by their employer, insurer, whomever. As a result, the patient may be ethically tempted to not be fully honest in his/her self-reporting of pain, ability, or functionality to his/her healthcare provider. Such subterfuge, if present, takes the form of exaggerating the problems, pain, and/or limitations. Ironically, this could subsequently lead to iatrogenic problems of true or worsened physical disability, experience of pain, misuse of narcotic and addictive pain medications, and so forth—all of which are real, and were avoidable, had the patient been honest at the start with all parties.

THE BIND OF THE REHABILITATION/OCCUPATIONAL MEDICINE SPECIALIST

Many employers utilize an on-site service of providing employees with occupational medicine on-site services. The ethical challenge for the professionals working in such venues is to over-treat or provide unnecessary treatment, albeit short term and likely benign. The scenario is that say a worker suffers a minor fall. The ethical occupational medicine specialist examines the worker and sees all is well, needing no more than ice, over the counter pain relief medication, and rest for a day. The less ethical counterpart would likely prescribe the same, but in addition, add 2-3 more (billable) visits under the pretext that doing so would prevent a workers' comp issue in the future. This, in reality, would never have manifest anyway. This manipulation is known as "See them in treatment now before they get better." The well intentioned employer is thus duped by an unethical occupational medicine professional.

THE TALE OF TWO LAWYERS: THE ETHICAL CHALLENGES FOR PLAINTIFF AND DEFENSE ATTORNEYS

Ideally, the judicial process should involve a situation in which two attorneys, representing their respective clients' best interests serve as champions and advocates before a court wherein a fair and reasonable decision is handed down. The ethical challenge for the attorney representing the injured worker (plaintiff's attorney), is that fundamentally, he/she is not economically incentivized to settle the injured employee's case quickly, even if given the opportunity to do so. Basically, there is a financial conflict of interest for the attorney to resolve or thus settle the issue "too" soon. The longer it takes, the presumption is that the higher the settlement, thus maximizing the 20% fee of the attorney.

Ethical plaintiff lawyers are indeed interested in the proverbial "protection of the little guy," and they do nothing to staff or inflate their eventual fee. But from the experience of these authors, there are a minority of plaintiff attorneys who are just working for their percentage under the cloak of false advocacy. A recent example of this was a situation in which an injured worker was complete with his rehabilitation and ready to return to work. When his attorney was told of this the attorney responded to the therapist, "... you are messing up my case and my decreasing my 20% compensation."

Plaintiff attorneys do not work in behalf of the healthcare provider; they are not incentivized to help providers get paid for services they have rendered. Attorneys are the first to be paid from a case settlement. Healthcare providers who have rendered clinical services, often months prior without pay, are left to fend for themselves and pursue the former patient—who, too often, has spent much of the settlement dollars, and is left unable to pay for surgical, medical, and rehabilitative services that he/she thought had already been taken care of by the employer or insurance.

Defense attorneys who work for the injured workers' employer may often feel limited in terms of the scope in what they can do, depending on the state in which they practice. For example in Illinois, which is considered to be an employee-friendly-state (as opposed to an employer-friendly-state), defense attorneys nevertheless sell employers on their services of mitigating the damages ("because we cannot pick the MD, the PT, etc…) that could (would) occur without their intervention. This is the ethical rub, as this may or may not be true, unless attorneys making such claims also have powers of clairvoyance. Their role can legitimately be weighing the value of surveillance if there is a sense the employee is faking or malingering, ordering IME if there is a concern over proper diagnosis and treatment plan, and so forth.

The other ethical consideration is that the defense attorney's latter noted actions may result in a delay or protract the injured employee's access to appropriate care. This then worsens potential outcome, and thus can create a horrid, negative spiraling downward of the patient's life—no trivial matter.

THE ETHICS OF FOR-PROFIT STATUS

Joe Paduda has a popular workers' compensation blog. Therein he brought forth an interesting perspective as to not for profit health plans' responsibilities. It seems fitting herein to just mention it, knowing that not for profit organizations have their own limitations, the commentary below underscores some of the inherent misaligned incentives in the "for profit" world of workers' compensation.

"As a not for profit, Harvard Pilgrim doesn't have to deal with the primacy of stockholder returns inherent in the for profit world; that's not to say it doesn't have to ensure financial stability and long-term viability. The difference is in what's most important - profits or patients. The primacy of stockholder returns influences ethical and business decisions, or rather should. For profit companies must consider shareholder returns first and foremost; to do otherwise would be an ethical problem. There are for-profit health plans and insurers that work diligently to deliver services ethically and responsibly, bending over backwards to do the right thing. Aetna is one that comes first to mind. And there are others that don't bend at all."

THE BIG FISH: QUESTIONABLE PRACTICES OF THIRD PARTY PAYORS

Ethical Concerns with Utilization Review: One State's Experience

In 2010, the Illinois Workers' Compensation Commission requested feedback from interested parties concerning any problems and/or recommendations they may have as to utilization review of workers' comp cases. The following section of this chapter will summarize what one clinical organization provided. It is felt that these issues highlight some of the ethical concerns therein, and may be likely be generalizable beyond solely Illinois or the organization. Recommendations for change are also provided, not just critique.

The first problem is the situation in which an adjuster wishes for a case to undergo utilization review; the adjuster requests the provider re-send all of the records to the utilization review (UR) organization. This practice delays the entire process and adds to the costs by requesting the provider to re-send all of the records to the UR organization. Instead, if the adjuster wishes for a case to undergo utilization review, then the adjuster, who already has all the records, could simply forward the records to the utilization review company. The benefits would be improved fairness and equity, greater transparency, improved ethical practice, and likely yield an economic/cost savings.

The inappropriate use of clinical guidelines is the next issue. Simply put, one size does not fit all. Guidelines are a synthesis of averages and do not take into consideration patient co-morbidities, re-injuries, etc.—all of which are reasonable and legitimate factors that should be taken into account in the UR process (as they are in the clinical process of treatment planning). (See more on this in he Differing Approaches… chapter herein.) So, UR needs to consider and appropriately manage each case as a person and a situation and not blindly and ignorantly follow a guideline that does not fit the person. Additionally, UR should accommodate atypical case presentations that do not penalize nor discriminate against a person because their situation was not within the norm of that of a global/general/generic guideline states. The benefits would be improved fairness and equity, greater transparency, and improved ethical practice.

It is often the case that workers' comp patients who have been denied by a UR organization have a difficult time in finding appropriate legal representation. They may not have sufficient personal funds needed to retain legal representation and an interested attorney has no mechanism to be compensated for his/her time and expertise in representing the patient. This creates an additional unjust and unfair hardship for such individuals. In order to better deal with the event of a non-certification by a UR organization, an attorney representing the patient may file for a hearing of that issue, and in the event that they prevail, that attorney's time is paid for by the losing party. The benefits would be improved fairness and equity, greater transparency, and improved ethical practice.

Often appeals from the clinician go unanswered by the utilization reviewer. While sloppy at best and unprofessional at worst, this situation causes an unnecessary increase in the costs for the clinician vis-à-vis accounting, rebilling, etc. Thus, it seems reasonable to establish a practical timeline for UR organizations to respond to clinician appeals. Doing so would result in improved fairness and equity, greater transparency, improved ethical practice and economic/cost savings.

It is inappropriate to retrospectively conduct a utilization review on a case that has previously been denied. Retrospective review is fine, but it makes no sense and is unjust in situations where a case has already been denied. If an employer and insurer have denied liability for an injury, they do not enjoy the practical protection afforded by the statute which allows for utilization review. Since they have denied liability they have no real interest in information about the course of care the injured employee is receiving and no legitimate expectation of influencing or limiting the injured employees treatment options or plan of care. The employer and insurer cannot deny liability for the employee's work related condition, yet assert protection of or demand compliance with utilization review.

Allowing a retrospective review to only be permissible on cases that have not previously been denied seems more appropriate. In doing so, there would be improved fairness and equity, a decrease all costs in general based on a resultant decrease in litigation costs in particular, and thus economic/cost savings.

It is an obvious conflict of interest when an insurer is doing UR on a case it is responsible for payment. There may be a question as to whether the patient's best medical interest is being supported or if UR is more so focused on cost containment. Imagine if a clinical provider also ran a UR organization and completed review on its own cases. To avoid such conflicts, it seems prudent to have all UR organizations be independent of the insurer, if they are reviewing the case. No more foxes guarding hen houses. This would provide improved fairness and equity along with greater transparency.

Many UR organizations provide patient information to an outside vendor or company in order to re-direct patients they are reviewing to a contracted clinical provider. This seems remarkably unethical and a violation of patients' privacy and confidentiality as well. It seems that a more ethical, transparent, and equitable approach would be to not allow any patient information to be released without the prior, informed and written consent of the patient. The purpose of UR is to comment on care, not redirect care. This change would result in improved ethical practice, via greater transparency, and thus, greater fairness to the patient.

Some insurers deny payment if the case did not go through UR. This practice seems overtly manipulative and is not based on reason—UR is not mandatory for payment. Period. So to manipulate or delay payment via this gambit seems absurd. Additionally, the provider can call back the insurance carrier/adjuster numerous times, leave messages, and not have the calls returned while the patient is concurrently being treated. A provider has no control over the responsiveness of the carrier/adjuster. Furthermore, the carrier/adjuster can conduct a utilization review because they already have all of the patient records in their possession. In order to deal with this situation, there should be a prohibition of the denial of payment if a case did not go through UR, as submission to UR is the responsibility of the carrier. Again, this type of transparency would help make things more fair and equitable, and generally be a more ethical practice.

Some of the individuals conducting utilization review have not achieved a similar level of board specialty as that of the provider being reviewed. While those conducting utilization reviews may have the same license as those they are reviewing, they may not have the same or superior level of training and education as evidenced by Board Certification. It is incongruous to have a lesser trained professional directing or contradicting the professional judgment of a more advanced practitioner. This is especially the case when an actual examination of a patient has not been conducted. It seems more logical if the individuals conducting utilization review must have the same Board Certification or superior to that of the actual provider. Requiring this would go far to improving ethical practice, and most likely improve the quality of the review.

Utilization review denials are often vague and indistinct as to why a case is being denied. As a consequence, the clinician has to request from the UR organization their rational as to why a case is being denied in order to adequately mount an appeal along with the full, detailed report by the peer reviewer. The provider should not have to request any additional documentation or rationale. Instead, as a matter of course, UR organizations should provide the clinician with specific reasons as to the logic of the denial and provide all appropriate evidence to support their decision. This is simply establishes a more fair and equitable relationship between provider and reviewer which supports a more ethical practice, and likely would result in a cost savings.

Physicians are overwhelmed with managing a robust practice and the concomitant demands thereof. Most often the utilization reviewer contacts the referring MD, rather than in instances where the actual question lies more so in the purview of the treating healthcare professional (e.g., physical therapist). Thus, the MD may therefore not know the answer and/or may (mistakenly) think that the reviewer would also logically have contacted the physical therapist to get resolution. In reality, this does not happen. The result is potential jeopardizing of the case's approval resultant from communication issues rather than clinical. In order to prevent this if a patient's case is in UR and if the initially treating physician is unable to respond to a reviewer's initial contact, the treating healthcare professional must be contacted directly. The individual conducting utilization review shall make no less than three phone attempts (leaving messages if direct contact is not made), and a certified letter must be sent to the MD with the questions that UR wishes to have answered. Obviously, this is **a f**air and more logical approach, and much more ethical.

Sometimes, a UR staffer overrides the clinician's judgment as to frequency of, say, physical therapy visits (e.g., "...2 visits/week instead of the prescribed 3visits/week), and/or says that the case "...is only certified for the next 30 days or X number of visits..." and/or dictates treatments, for example, approves one injection but not the prescribed 3 that are in the patient's treatment plan. Such restrictions are (may?) not even (be) within the conservative and strict Official Disability Guidelines (ODG). Micro-restrictions such as these result in:

- Delay in patient care (which can lead to compounding problems, unnecessary anxiety and avoidable aggravation)
- Increased costs of UR due to unnecessarily restrictive management (ironically, the initially requested care is subsequently approved anyway—but now with added, albeit avoidable costs of that UR)

It is absurd (and expensive) to conduct three utilization reviews in order to incrementally get to the Guideline threshold point anyway. A typical scenario is to approve 12 visits, then UR, then approve 6 more, then UR and then approve 6 more rather than following the pre-agreed Guideline of "24 visits." This adds delays and costs to both the UR provider and the clinician, all avoidable. Interruptions in care resultant from awaiting UR approvals do nothing to speed up care or improve clinical outcomes; in fact they increase the iatrogenic risk of exacerbation and diminish the likelihood of an optimal patient outcome.

A better approach would be to hold off any UR until an accepted threshold is met based on the guideline that the insurance company uses (e.g., ODG). Prescribed care should be approved as long as it falls within the Guideline being used (otherwise, what use is the Guideline?). This just seems to be commonsense, albeit not standard practice. It also would likely improve patient care and outcomes while being a cost saving approach as well.

Not all those conducting utilization review live and practice within the state where they are licensed. Therefore, there is a greater likelihood that they are not aware of that state's practice patterns. Each state is different and thus it is important and incumbent upon those conducting utilization reviews to be conversant with the practice patterns of the state they are reviewing in. Additionally, those conducting utilization review outside of the state they live in are not available for subpoenas and depositions. This can make for an inequitable situation when their presence is needed to reconcile a conflict. There is also the legal-ethical question of practicing outside the state in which one is licensed. The simple and obvious solution is to require UR reviewers to be in the same state in which they are practicing utilization reviews. These seems to be a more rational and ethical approach.

Those conducting utilization review may deny care and have an arbitrary timeline set in which the clinician is to respond with an appeal. Having such a timeline serves no helpful purpose in the care of the patient; in fact it is to the contrary. For example, a patient may still be in treatment at the time of a denial. It is impractical then for the clinician to engage in an appeal process while still delivering care. The elegant solution to this is to prohibit appeals from having timelines. Doing so would be much fairer to patients as well as the ethical thing to do.

CONCERNS WITH INSURANCE COMPANY OPERATIONS: ONE PRACTICE'S EXPERIENCE

Silent Preferred Provider Organizations

A new problematic phenomenon has manifest more and more for contracted healthcare providers working in the workers' compensation sphere. It is known as a "stealth network" or "silent PPO."

Messinger and Welter (2003) have defined silent PPOs as "...payer arrangements that offer patients discounted provider fees without providing incentives for patients to access the providers' services. Under a silent PPO arrangement, a third party (which is usually not offering a PPO plan or policy) obtains a database of preferred provider rates from a managed care organization or a discount insurance broker. The managed care organization typically sells or rents its PPO provider network to the third party or insurance broker....In most cases of silent PPO activity, the provider is led to believe that the discount is a legitimate contractual discount. With the large number of contractual arrangements that providers have in place with health plans and the numerous products and payers included within each contract, healthcare financial managers may be confused about which discounts are justified and which are not. The American Medical Association believes silent PPO activity may be fraudulent. It has been estimate that providers nationwide have lost between $750 million and $3 billion dollars annually since silent PPOs became common (in group health plans) in the early 1990s." There have been so many abuses resultant from silent PPOs that the National Council of Insurances Legislators (NCOIL) has noted that thus far, five states (Connecticut, Colorado, Florida, Indiana and Ohio) have passed laws governing third-party network access (Berry 2009).

The clinical organization that employs the authors of this chapter experienced a very problematic situation in dealing with a silent PPO situation. (The insurance company name has been altered herein ["XYZ Corp"], all other facts are accurate.)

In 2008 XYZ Corp sent the practice organization a letter noting that the practice organization was going to be automatically enrolled into their Workers' Comp PPO Network unless the practice organization notified them that the practice organization wished to "opt-out" or put another way, the practice organization was declining participation. Consequently, the practice organization responded with a certified letter noting their desire to "opt-out." In spite of this, XYZ Corp proceeded to underpay anyway totaling $1,010,022.34 (for five states).

The practice organization received a letter stating admission of error on XYZ's part, however there had been only a partial payment after a year's time. The practice organization estimated that 50% had been recouped after 16 months, and approximately 80% at the time of publication, which is 28 months post-letter of admission. This was resultant from the practice organization continual to devotion of significant staff time to pursue collection. Additionally, the practice organization found it necessary to file a formal complaint against XYZ with the State's Insurance Commission.

Frequency of Late Payments

In spite of proper billing and a clean claims having been submitted by the practice organization, approximately half of their workers' comp accounts were not paid within the state statute's allowed time of 60 days (based on 2008 data), and of those, 50% were not paid within 90 days.

This is particularly puzzling vis-à-vis the practice organization's experience with other payors, such a BlueCross. For example, it was their experience with BlueCross to have an average range between 14 and 21 days for payment of a clean claim in 2008.

Monies Involved in Late Payments

The practice organization then conducted an analysis of 2008 dates of service for workers' compensation cases exclusively. They found that $1,162,837 was due from *partially paid* claims as of November, 2009. Furthermore, those monies only represent *partially paid* services (e.g., 45 minutes of billed services provided and properly submitted, but the practice organization was paid as if it were 15 minutes of services provided). They then conducted a further analysis of these figures and learned they represented 14,797 claims. It is important to

note that the amount of man-hours it takes our billing staff to adjudicate these claims is approximately 1447. Of course, this comes at a cost for the practice organization to bear, albeit a problem based on the payor's error.

Burden of Late Payment Calculation

In other states (e.g., Minnesota, California), late payments are to be calculated by the delinquent payor, not a burden obliged to the payee as it is in the state where the practice organization is based. It is ironic that they cannot be paid correctly in the first place, but it remains their responsibility to follow-up on unpaid billings.

Omission of Late Payment Penalty

There is a state statute that obliges an erring payor that has not promptly paid for services, properly billed for, to pay interest in the amount of 1%. However, there has not been one instance in which a clean claim has been submitted, aged over the 60 day requirement, and has been paid with the interest charge. Not one in this the practice organization's experience.

Delay in Applying Consumer Price Index Changes

The Consumer Price Index (CPI) is typically announced in September of the prior year for changes to be applied in the upcoming year, commencing on 1 January of that year. However, for January and February 2009, the practice organization was shorted $22,615.85 over the course of 1,227 dates of service during these two months as the yearly CPI change was not applied.

As a result, the practice organization had to resubmit the claims noting their error. It took their collector an additional three weeks of work to receive payment for these 1227 dates of service. Thus, adding to our operational costs and diverting staff attention from customary duties. This appears not to be a fluke, it has constantly occurred each year.

Insurance Company Misuse of the Fee Schedule

Insurance companies in the state in which the practice organization is based all work from the same, established fee schedule, statute, and rules; however, there is no uniform application of these (i.e., the State dictates the workers' compensation payment levels, while the individual insurance companies decide what they will actually reimburse; this can vary between companies, and from year-to-year). For example, a case may have a situation wherein a patient is evaluated, treated and undergoes surgery. The payor would pay for the evaluation. Another scenario may be that a patient is evaluated, treated, and then re-evaluated. That payor would then pay only for the first evaluation. This gets further convoluted as other payors would pay for both evaluations in the latter case. Summarily, one insurer may pay for iontophoresis in treatment, and another does not. Such payment decisions are done arbitrarily, without rational, and variably.

Arbitrary Procedures of Payors to Designed to Impede Solutions

This refers to the situation in which a provider, contacts, say, BlueCross' Help-Line. Contracted providers can discuss *up to* five patients per call with any BlueCross staff person, however, when it is a workers' comp case, contracted providers can only contact one-specific-adjuster, thus making it is virtually impossible for to directly connect with that one adjuster (as they are most likely on another call), and the contracted providers is routed into a voice-mailbox. Contracted providers cannot set-up an appointment to call either.

Another rule that is used is that the insurer limits the number of dates-of-service that can be discussed per call to five, even if it is for the same patient. If the provider needs to discuss more than five dates of service, he/she needs to go through the entire process again. The result will most likely be that the provider gives up due to not being able to sit on hold indefinitely. This leads to either the patient not getting his/her visits approved, the patient being seen without approval and/or the provider not getting paid for services rendered.

Delaying Care: UR's Dirty Little Secret

Another questionable practice of some utilization review firms is to go proverbially "radio-silent." That is, to neither approve nor deny care—leaving the patient and the provider in an awkward limbo. Does the provider ethically proceed to give the patient the needed services and take on the financial risk of subsequently being denied payment for lack of UR approval?

There is a general clinical dictum that the longer the length of time between the injury and treatment, the greater the likelihood of protracted rehabilitation time as well as the amount and types of services needed. These then conspire to diminish the potential of the most optimal clinical outcome. Similarly, it is believed that the longer a person is not working, the less likely he or she is to return to their prior job, or similar work at all.

This is all the more curious when compared to the average time to gain access to care is two weeks in traditional group/indemnity types of insurance coverage where as the time span in workers' compensation can be around six weeks. How does this occur? In some instances an Insurance Adjuster simple does not authorize treatment stating that he or she needs to know more info before an authorization for care can be given. The iatrogenic result often is that the patient then feels as if his employer is denying him or her needed care while he or she is in disabled, pain, not working, not getting help, and feeling scared. This then can result in the patient feeling the need to take action and decides to get his/her own doctor and treatment. In order to get this paid for, the employee gets an attorney, and off to the adversarial races they go.

CASE EXAMPLES

Patients say the Darned Things...

The following represent a small minority, but their presentation herein is meant to help provide understanding of the genesis of stereotypes.

Patients Gaming the System

In many instances upon the completion of a work conditioning/work hardening rehabilitation program, a Functional Capacity Evaluation (FCE) or Assessment (FCA) is conducted. The patient knows that his or her performance on the evaluation can make a difference as to being able to return to work. If the patient does not want to go to work he/she may claim not to be able to lift certain amounts in order to fall short of their work-related requirements.

Darned Metric System

In one situation this was exactly the case. The clinician knew what the patient was capable of, but lo-and-behold when it came time for the FCE, he clamed he could not lift certain amounts. The clinician, unbeknown to the patient, then substituted kilogram weights close to what the patient's ability to manage was, while the patient paying attention to only the numeric labels on the wrights proceeded to complete the evaluation lifting much more than what he claimed he could. Needless to say, the patient was not at all too pleased as to his successful performance.

Not So Coy, But Sure Honest

In contrast to the just noted case, some patients are quite honest in their goals. A patient completing a standardized goal sheet upon initiation into the work hardening/work condition program wrote "my goal is to get as big a workers' compensation settlement as I can." Another Honest-Abe said "I want to stay off work for as long as I can." Needless to say, in spite of the informed consent given to these patients vis-à-vis the discoverability of all clinical documents, their avarice got the better of them. Most defense attorneys really appreciate their candor and the ability to rapidly close their cases.

Jackpot! Not

It may not always be clear what an injured patient expects. Many however, may expect a windfall settlement, presuming they are indeed injured in this scenario. So, the case is settled. The patient receives X-thousand dollars. He or she is thrilled, and may have visions of new cars, houses, and toys. But, quickly reality hits. Now the person may or may not have been informed of the following, but even so, denial sets in rapidly.

First, 20% comes right off the top and goes into the person's attorney. Much of the balance then goes to surgeons and hospitals for past surgeries, medications, rehabilitation, etc., as well as paying all the debt that was racked-up while not working. Indeed, some folks, expecting a windfall, "pre-spend" what they think they will receive, leaving little for the patient in the end. This economic hardship can be further compounded by the inability to gain the same level of prior employment, and thus salary.

Who You Gonna Trust…?

Who are the smartest people in the world? Doctors and attorneys. Thus, workers' compensation patients expect that they can put their full trust in their physician (presuming him/her to be smart, ethical, trustworthy, free of conflicts of interest, holding only the patient's best interests in mind, etc.). Second, they then feel that they can trust their attorney. This person is their advocate and says so, and is also presumed to be smart, ethical, trustworthy, free of conflicts of interest, holding only the patient's best interests in mind, always on their side in opposition to the employer's attorney, etc...

Now, of course, this is often the case. Problem is, it is not always the case. If it is the latter and not the former, then the patient is in for more problems than just his or her injury. The following is an advertisement for an actual cable television program by a law firm specializing in workers' compensation cases (the name of the firm has been removed herein). The point is that some professionals will go to great lengths to communicate to potential clients that they (the professionals) are their advocates. In many cases this is the case, but *caveat emptor.*

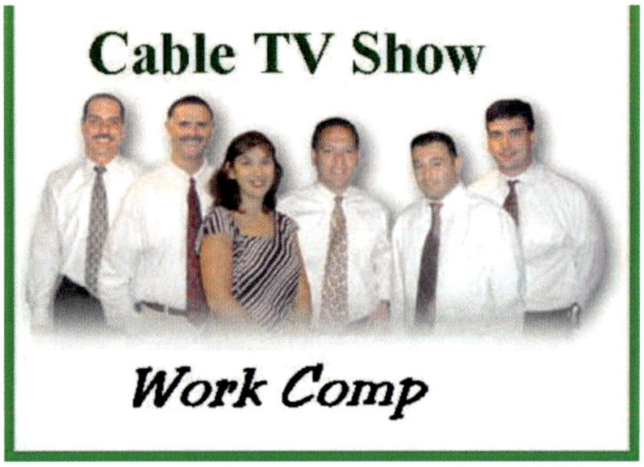

Bias Cut Both Ways

The two cases just noted can instill a mindset in some case managers or utilization reviewers that ALL workers' compensation patients are manipulative ne'er-do-wells. But of course this is not the case. Individuals who think this may unconsciously (or consciously) have a negative mindset of "gotcha" with their cases.

Bowling for No Dollars

A hypothetical scenario was presented before a group of workers' compensation nurse case manager at a workshop. The situation described was one in which a case manager learned of a workers' compensation patient going bowling; what would they do?

The majority said they would deny further care based on that evidence. Some went further to suggest that the individual should be investigated for fraud. There was definitely the "gotcha" vibe present with most of those there.

But then the case was further considered. First of all, the patient's doctor never told him that he could not bowl. In fact, he thought that it may actually be helpful for his health and condition. Certainly he felt it was helpful to is morale and psychological condition as he'd not had many positive, social activities with his friends in a long time.

The nature of his job was that he needed to lift as much as 100 pounds over his head. Lifting 100 pounds over one's head and rolling a bowling ball are biomechanically quite different, and thus, again, the patient honestly saw no negative connection between his bowling and his rehabilitation

Now, it is rare for many case managers to consider the results of their decisions concerning subsequent and long-term impact on those they deny care for. So, in a Dickensonian fashion, the speaker led the case managers through what could happen if this fellow was denied. First, he would lose his job because he would no longer have any rehabilitative servicers that would help him return to it. Ironically, without a job, he has no insurance (or settlement) to pay for the medical and rehabilitative services he needs. This results in a worsening of his physical condition, which prohibits him from seeking a new job. Not having a job, being in pain, not being able to manage physically as he could prior to the injury, he begins to additionally suffer psychological problems of clinical depression; fear that he will never work again; anxiety that he will lose his house, wife and family; anger towards his former employer, his situation, and perhaps himself; social isolation as most of his friendships centered around work and physical activities. Thus, he has lost his identity as an iron worker and thus pride as well.

Not having pharmacy benefits any longer, he turns to illicit use of pain killers to manage his increasing physical discomfort and self-medicates with alcohol to manage his emotional discomfort, both of which concern his wife and children. Additionally, he has started to smoke more and his now sedentary lifestyle has resulted in an increase of 30 pounds, so now he cannot even bowl any longer, and he pines for the time to be with those friends and the joy he had with them.

Due to his weight increase, alcohol abuse, and drug consumption, he is no longer being able to be intimate with his wife, resulting in a worsening of his self-esteem, self-respect, and motivation. His future seems to offer few options.

The moral seems to be that a rush to judgment can result in a catastrophic cascade of events—loss of one's way of life, family and perhaps home; the inability to return to the work that was so enjoyed and offered identity and social connection as well. In this story, this person could have been a productive worker and contributing husband and father, as well as taxpaying citizen. Too often insurance professionals rush to the "gotcha" moment, not taking the big picture into account. And the big picture is that there is still an injured worker out there, with a real injury, who could return to work if given the chance to finish their rehabilitation.

PHYSICIANS HAVE ISSUES TOO

The Surgery was a Success but the Patient Died

Well fortunately this is rarely the case, but the cliché does make the point of judging outcome is in the eye of the beholder. Recently on the American Academy of Orthopedic Surgeons' website (www.aaos.org) there was a discussion as to the definition of a successful surgery. From the surgeon's point of view, success may be no infection, rapid recovery time, small incision with little scaring, and no untoward events. The patient may have been expecting an immediate and full recovery back to prior functioning levels, if not better. In their example, the post-op patient expected to be able to drive, shower unassisted, etc., the surgeons' response was to simply be driven as a passenger and take baths.

In workers' compensation cases (as well as other clinical situations), if a patient is, say, post-spinal fusion and still in pain, the treatment plan would be to address the pain with more surgery, and so-on and so-on. A good surgeon does his/her work, resulting in a good functional outcome for the patient, it is "case closed." But a not-so-good physician who does a not-so-good surgery, ironically then is more likely to do more surgery. If the problem persists, then there may be a referral to a pain management physician. Then the patient's weight starts to increase due to being more sedentary, maybe he/she smokes more, and now also starts to drink more… This scenario is a sad one, and hopefully an atypical one as well.

"Lab" vs. "Life"

As noted above, many of us gain value, identity, and self-esteem from the work we do, indeed, it's typically one of the first questions strangers ask each other. In another case, a female, single parent worked for the electric company, and suffered an injury that was covered by workers' compensation. She performed very well on the Functional Capacity Evaluation. She was to very motivated to return to work, but to move up in the ranks to become a meter-reader, which offer greater prestige along with better pay.

But, her physician said "no" to her returning to work due to the nature of her clinical situation, based on imaging, not on her level of physical function. He believed he was being an advocate for her by being cautious in her recovery time and that that was in his patient's best interests. However doing so put her abilities and promotion goals in jeopardy. The rehabilitation specialist was then in the awkward position of having to "argue" with the doctor, thus feeling that he was risking their professional relationship and potential for him to get future referrals. The point is that there is often a disconnect between a person's biological/physiological state of being, their life, their work, and their needs. Similar to the case manager, physicians need to understand their patients in context of their life, goals, and abilities, not just as healing body parts alien and separate from the world.

CONCLUSION

Ethical challenges are spurred by biases as well as economic temptations, as is perhaps the case with most all ethical challenges. It does seem, however, that in the realm of workers' compensation, that there are so many involved that the complexity of anyone acting unethically can have amplified results on many. Injured workers' are typically not college educated, and certainly not educated in the inner workings of the workers' compensation system. They rely on the professionals working with them for guidance. Given the various incentives involving all parties in the workers' compensation system, it can be an uncertain path for the injured worker. It is hoped that this chapter allows for greater consideration of the end user in workers' compensation–the injured worker–and keep his/her best interests in mind.

REFERENCES

Berry, E 2009, 'Model law banning silent PPOs could serve as draft for state legislatures', *American Medical News,* 29 December, viewed 21 July 21, 2010 http://www.ama-assn.org/amednews/2008/12/29/bisa1229.htm.

Levin, DC & Rao, VM 2004, 'Turf wars in radiology: the overutilization of imaging resulting from self-referral', *Journal of the American College of Radiology*, vol. 1, no. 3, pp. 169–172.

Messinger, S & Welter, T 2003, 'Tactics for thwarting silent PPO activity - Managed Care - a discussion of silent PPO payer arrangements for the health care industry', *Healthcare Financial Management*, July, viewed 21 July 2010 http://findarticles.com/p/articles/mi_m3257/is_7_57/ai_105501126/.

Siff, MC & Verkhoshansky, YV 1998, *Supertraining: Strength Training For Sporting Excellence,* 3rd Edn, University of the Witwatersrsand, Johannesburg, South Africa.

CHAPTER 6

Comorbidities and Workers' Compensation: Responsive Approaches to Work Hardening and Conditioning

Matt Kruger, MS, CSCS, Jeff Rogers, Chris E. Stout*, PsyD and Maureen Kohl Bennington, M.S., CCM, CDMS, CPUR, CRC

ATI Physical Therapy; E-mail: Chris.stout@atipt.com

Abstract: This chapter will delve into various co-morbidities or pre-existing health/medical conditions that may negatively impact injured workers' abilities to gain appropriate rehabilitative milestones. It is surprising to see that they so often go ignored in spite of the dramatic impact they have. This chapter also looks at various ironies and then offers Bennington's (2010) wise ideas for ways to manage these problems. The chapter concludes with a description of a unique work hardening and conditioning program that has demonstrated efficacy.

INTRODUCTION: COMORBIDITIES, THE IGNORED CONUNDRUM OF WORKERS' COMPENSATION

Workers' compensation (WC) patients are complex group—especially when it comes to co-morbid conditions. Co-morbid conditions refer to concomitant illness(es) or negative "health-situations" that are present in a person along with but not, per se, directly the result of the WC injury. For example, a WC patient may have already been a smoker, or diabetic, or obese, or abusing alcohol *before* being hurt at work.

These factors conspire to negatively impact injury recovery times, diminish positive outcomes, and as a result increase costs due to more (and perhaps additional types of) care that is needed to be provided. Sometimes these comorbidities are secondary to the injury. For example, a previously fit individual with a normal Body Mass Index (BMI) may start to become obese as a result of not being able to be physically active as he/she was prior to the injury. The obesity can then result in diabetes and cardiovascular problems.

Or, prior bad habits like drug use, smoking, and/or alcohol use may increase if an injured worker attempts to "self-medicate" because these behaviors tend to increase when a person is in pain, upset, stressed, and has less structure to their day (i.e., not being at work or being productive). Also, psychological symptoms may manifest, such as clinical depression, anxiety, panic disorders, sleep disorders, secondary to having been injured. These, too, are considered to be co-morbid to the injury, albeit not directly caused by the injury. Nevertheless, if they are present, they are real and they do nothing to help the WC patient get better and back to work, they do just the opposite.

Bennington (2010) notes that injured workers' who are also diabetic "...are more likely to develop adhesive capsulitis or wound healing complications. Diabetic neuropathy makes it difficult to diagnose injuries with nerve related symptoms. Kidney failure, stroke or a heart attack are potentially fatal complications from any of these chronic diseases. The cost of the workers' compensation claim is immediately higher when an individual has any of these chronic diseases. In order to treat the industrial injury appropriately, these conditions must be stabilized. It may require treatment of the chronic disease along with the work related injury to bring resolution to the claim."

A review of 1.5 years of the most recent available data from the company where three of the coauthors of this chapter work, indicated that WC patients (N= 8405) were more likely to have more than one co-morbidity compared to non-WC patients (N= 52,946). The most frequently occurring were past surgeries, hypertension and obesity (as evidenced by a high body mass index (BMI)). Thus, it is more likely that WC patients being treated are more likely to be a more medically complex group than the general population.

Peter Rousmaniere, another contributing author in this volume, has noted that WC adjusters generally feel quite conflicted concerning what to do in such cases (2009). That is, it is hard to manage WC costs when there are causal cost-drivers that are not directly injury related. This is amplified as many surgeons will simply refuse to operate on a patient who is a smoker (due to the negative impact smoking has on healing) and they do not want to compromise their procedure or outcomes based on a variable they do not control. Similarly, obese patients generally have poorer surgical outcomes as well.

Chris E. Stout, Matt Kruger and Jeffrey Rogers, (Eds)

Julie Ferguson (2009), writing in *Workers' Compensation Insider*, notes that "Historically, the tendency has been for employers to segment potential employee health and disability issues into two discrete silos: occupational safety, prevention, and other issues related to workers' compensation are most often managed by risk managers and safety staff. General employee health issues are usually tucked under an organization's benefits and human resources department as part of group health - or under a wellness program, if one exists. But increasingly, data shows that the two are often inextricably linked and it makes good sense to address health issues with a more holistic approach." This seems to be even more so in areas where the workforce is aging and chronic health conditions have more time to manifest.

Furthermore, Rousmaniere (2009) wisely notes that workers' compensation is exempt from the Health Information Privacy and Accountability Act (HIPAA) as well as state confidentiality acts. "The(se) exemption(s) infer that occupational and nonoccupational conditions are separate or at most tangential, when in fact they are often inextricably linked through comorbidities."

Perhaps it is just easier to focus on fixing the presenting injury in workers' compensation cases than considering the complexity presented with the presence of co-morbidities, notes Roberto Cencineros in *Business Insurance*; in spite of the impact such co-morbidities have on costs and outcomes. He goes on to note that some employers are playing offence by "...collecting obesity data to help fend off future claims that may not be work-related, particularly those involving police and firefighters who must take pre-employment physicals and whose heart attacks and other ailments often are presumed to be work-related, said Glenn Backus, senior vice president for Alternative Service Concepts L.L.C., a Reno, Nev.- based claims administrator."

Conceivably a kinder-and-gentler approach would be the integration of workers' compensation professionals having a place at the proverbial healthcare table. In a NCCI Issues Report, *Wellness Comp* (Thorness, 2008), the issue of whether there is a place for health promotion programs in workers' compensation was raised. "The bottom line is that workers' compensation specialists should at least be at the table for discussions on how to make the workforce healthier. Health and productivity shifts the basic value proposition, according to Aon, into the question of 'How can [healthcare] plans be modified to incent employees to adopt healthy behaviors, moderate cost increases, and minimize absenteeism and presenteeism?'" This seems like a more proactive approach, with a potential payoff to all employees, not just injured ones, and perhaps, a realistic approach to mitigation, if not actual prevention.

THE BIGGEST CO-MORBIDITY: OBESITY

"Obesity significantly impacts the direct delivery of healthcare services and the productivity of our nation. According to the journal, *Health Affairs*, one percent of the Gross Domestic Product or $147 billion dollars a year is spent treating obesity related ailments… and… the estimated number of workdays lost to obesity related illness or injury is 40 million days per year" (Bennington, 2010). Rousmaniere (2009) reported that "the National Council on Compensation Insurance recently published a study on obesity and claims costs titled 'Reserving in the Age of Obesity.' This publication could turn out to be a landmark document. For the first time, the NCCI has marshaled its huge claims database to calculate how nonoccupational conditions (severe obesity) affect both indemnity and medical claims costs….They (found) that obesity drives up claims costs through the first 60 months of the claim." Furthermore, "obese workers' filed twice the number of workers' compensation claims, had seven times higher medical costs from those claims and lost 13 times more days of work from work injury or work illness than non-obese workers'" (Ferguson, 2009). Cencineros (2009), noted "… that workers' compensation medical claims open for one year cost three times as much when the injured employee is obese, and claims that are open for five years are five times more costly when involving an obese claimant. For smaller claims, the study will show that the cost differential can be even greater." Knowing this can act as a very helpful tool in aiding claims adjusters, managed care, and consulting firms in managing cases where obesity is the co-morbidity of concern.

It should not, however some as a great surprise. Indeed, "Duke University researchers found in 2007 that very obese workers' were more likely to incur injuries and much higher medical costs" (Rousmaniere (2009), and they were twice as likely to file a workers' compensation claim. The Duke study examined the clinical records of approximately 12,000 workers' and found that for workers' who were obese, they had (Ferguson, 2007):

- Higher medical costs, at a rate 7 times higher (averaging $51,019) per 100 employees
- 13 times the number of lost work days

- Averaged 11.65 workers' compensation claims per 100 workers' (versus an average of 5.8 claims per 100 non-obese workers'
- More slips, falls and injuries resultant from attempts to lift something

In another study, "conducted by the Medstat Group Inc. showed that moderate and severe obesity were linked to annual health care cost increases of 21% and 75%, respectively.

Moderate obesity was associated with a $670 increase in costs, and severe obesity resulted in a $2,441 increase in costs" (Ferguson, 2007).

These findings are not that different from those in a Johns Hopkins Bloomberg School of Public Health Center for Injury Research and Policy's study that was published in the *American Journal of Epidemiology* (Pollack, Sorock, Slade, Cantley, Sircar, Taiwo, and Cullen, 2007). They found that traumatic workplace injuries seem to increase as a function of obesity. Braun Consulting (2004), a consultancy focusing on labor, employee, and human resources issues, compiled the facts and statistics on the obesity problem:

- The number of Americans considered obese by the CDC in 2001 was 44 million - or approximately one in five. This is a 74 percent increase since 1991.
- Obesity is growing at two or three times GDP
- The percentage of U.S. adults classified as obese doubled between 1980 and 2000, from 15% to 31%. (1999 National Health and Nutrition Examination Survey, CDC National Center for Health Statistics).
- On average one out of every three people you know and work with could be considered obese.
- According to the Centers for Disease Control obesity has roughly the same association with chronic health conditions as 20 years of aging.
- The Surgeon General reports that more than 9 percent of the nation's health care expenditures are directly related to obesity and physical inactivity. They calculate that to cost out at about $117 billion annually and relate to 300,000 deaths per year.
- UnumProvident, a provider of disability income protection insurance, reports a tenfold increase over the past decade in short-term disability claims attributed to obesity, based on research using their disability database.

Bennington (2010) has articulated the issues associated with treating the obese workers' compensation patient and approaches to dealing with these related health complexities. Weight challenged injured workers' require specialized equipment for diagnostic procedures such as CT, MRI or ultrasound. These injured workers' simply do not fit into the scanners. The radiology industry is responding to this trend and oversized units are in development but the number of units available is limited. If the injured worker is fortunate to locate a facility with appropriate sized equipment, other issues emerge. For example, oversized equipment does not generally deliver the same quality output. Diagnostic images are frequently poor because scanning capabilities are not geared to image through layers of fat. The radiologist has difficulty reading the images due to the high level of fat obscuring the organ or skeletal structure in question. This leads to questionable diagnosis. The physician then encounters difficulty recommending a treatment plan due to the poor quality of the diagnostic image.

It may be at this point the physician chooses not to accept the injured worker as a patient. Many physicians will no longer agree to treat patients with weight challenges. The risks of surgery are disproportionately high and outcomes are poor or a total failure. Some physicians agree to treat the injured worker with the caveat that weight loss must first occur. So the physician recommends a weight loss program for the injured worker. But the carrier refuses to fund the weight loss program because the injured worker had non-industrial weight issues that preceded the injury. So the physician then refuses to perform surgery because of the risks involved without weight loss. A line is drawn in the sand and the parties addressing the industrial injury come to a stalemate. It is a no-win situation for everyone, especially the injured worker.

Injured workers' simply do not understand these challenges related to medical care. Their goal is simply to stop hurting and return to a productive life. Frustration mounts and so a second opinion is sought. The injured worker intentionally seeks a physician willing to perform surgery despite the high risks and potential for poor outcome without weight loss.

Once surgery is authorized for a weight challenged injured worker, a multitude of challenges are encountered by medical professionals providing treatment. All of the challenges translate into higher costs for employers and insurance carriers. These may include:

- **Pharmacy**: Pharmacy costs are significantly higher. Most drug dosages are determined based on weight. It takes much higher dosages to provide relief to individuals whose weight is outside of average weight brackets.
- **Anesthesia**: Intubation is difficult. Patient positioning and identifying the appropriate sized equipment and medical personnel with the expertise to properly administer anesthesia to an overweight patient is a challenge. Surgical procedures require larger amounts of anesthesia and the increased levels prolong recovery time and place the patient at risk for complications.
- **Injections**: Injections are difficult due to the size of the needle necessary to puncture or penetrate the skin. It is difficult to inject through the fatty layers and even more difficult to locate deep veins for injection.
- **Surgical Equipment and Hardware**: Special operating tables or multiple tables may be required for the patient. Additional or oversized instruments and sheer manpower is required to perform surgery on an overweight patient. Surgical hardware utilized for spinal fusion or joint replacement is easily dislodged or fails altogether because of the pressure of the weight exerted by overweight patients. The cost of the claim rises exponentially when repeat surgeries are necessary to repair these failures. Unfortunately, even with repeated procedures, the outcome is likely poor at best without significant weight loss.
- **Post Surgical Complications**: Obese patients frequently suffer from circulatory insufficiency due to decreased mobility. The possibility of pulmonary embolus or other unexplained pulmonary problems which are a risk for all surgical candidates, more easily occur with the obese surgical patient. Infection is a high probability and wound healing is problematic.
- **Durable Medical Equipment**: Post surgical Durable Medical Equipment needs are costly. Most equipment is ordered based on the patient's height and weight. It takes a longer period of time to locate or customize recommended equipment. There is a higher prevalence of breakage and repeated equipment replacement is required for overweight patients.
- **Rehabilitation**: Rehabilitation is a long arduous process. The patient was deconditioned prior to the injury. Decreased mobility due to pain exacerbates the problem and increases the length of the rehabilitation program The cost of rehabilitation is much higher due to the increased length of time it takes for the patient to regain even nominal levels of strength and range of motion.

SOLUTIONS?

Similar to the point made earlier, it is important for employers and workers' compensation professionals to collaborate and devise actionable plans *before* there is an injury. The following is a compilation for consideration (Ferguson, 2007):

- Making on-site weight loss programs available at work
- Sponsoring or subsidizing health club memberships
- Working with group health vendors to develop programs targeting obese populations
- Implementing a healthy eating campaign, including healthy options in cafeterias and vending machines
- Encouraging employees to walk outside during their lunch hour
- Seeking employee educations materials and disease management programs from health care vendors
- Providing EAPs for private counseling or community-based weight management programs
- Offering incentives, such as a discount on health care premiums.

Coppelman (2007) makes an obvious, but perhaps neglected point that it should be incumbent for employers to be concerned about obesity in their workers' in general. Doing so will most likely reduce subsequent healthcare costs across the board, not just workers' compensation. Thus, healthier workers' in safer work environments are likely a sure calculus for cost savings and improved productivity.

THE DIFFERENCE BETWEEN PHYSICAL THERAPY AND WORK CONDITIONING/WORK HARDENING

When a work related injury happens, Work Conditioning/Work Hardening (WC/WH) is often the treatment of last resort. If people can get better and back to work by other means, including physical therapy, they will do so. Sometimes an injury is ignored, minimized or denied, and in some cases it may naturally and successfully heal on its own. When this is not the case, often over-the-counter approaches are tried (e.g., hot/cold compresses, pain relievers, etc.). If the problem remains, then a visit to a general practitioner may result. This can lead to resolution or referral to physical therapy, diagnostic imaging, orthopedic consultation, etc. Depending on the outcome there could ultimately be a referral to WC/WH.

Physical therapy sessions and protocols do not focus on the return-to-work needs of injured workers' with manual occupations. The U.S. Dept. of Labor's Dictionary of Occupational Titles defines approximately 13,000 job titles. Of these, there are only 15-20% of these jobs (approx. 2000 – 2500) require a person to lift 50 lbs. or more on an occasional basis as part of their essential job tasks. Thinking logically this makes sense – society is becoming more and more automated, more and more sedentary. Thus, most people just don't have a high physical requirement or barrier to return to work. Physical therapy is focused on the acute injury, returning range of motion, decreasing pain levels, making sure the person can complete their activities of daily living (ADLs), etc. If someone can do those things, then they can most certainly return to work as a salesperson, office worker, editor of this book, etc…but they would not be physically prepared to return to work as a carpenter, ironworker, or pipe fitter. So, while physical therapy is perfectly adequate for the rehabilitation needs of 80% of the population, it is a poor fit for the 20% of people with manual labor jobs or who suffer from other physical deficits that prevent them from returning to their former occupations.

Physical Therapy	Work Conditioning/Work Hardening
Acute injury emphasis	Strength/function
2-3 x per week	5 x per week
60 to 90 min/session	4 hours per session
• 5-10 min warm-up	• 20 – 25 hrs activity/wk
• 10 – 15 min. stretching	• 40 to 60 min. cardio
• 20 min. strengthening	• 30 min. stretching
• 20 min. manual PT Modalities	• 90 min. strengthening
• 2-5 hrs activity/week	• 30 to 60 min. Work simulation
Dx specific	RTW specific

Differences between Physical Therapy and Work Conditioning/Work Hardening

The natural and understandable bias then is that physicians prescribe more and more physical therapy. The expectation is that the insurance company will pay for those services ad nauseum–when instead, those individuals would be better served by a safe and appropriate transition from physical therapy to a WC/WH program.

Obtaining prescriptions and getting approvals/reimbursement from insurance companies is difficult in WC/WH, and the patient population is more difficult to treat. As noted previously, 80% of people get better by the time they would need a WC/WH program…and those that end-up participating in WC/WH programs are likely to have experienced, or are currently injured workers' experiencing, some sort of psychological or socio-economic pressures due to the severity of the injury, and time off work.

Because of the protracted length of time a person may be off work prior to participation in a WC/WH program, they experience socio-economic problems such as loss of income, loss of reputation with family and friends, denial of injury by their employer, denial of payment by the insurance company, medical professionals (conducing an Independent Medical Evaluation [IME]) issuing reports stating there is no injury, etc. So, the WC/WH provider is in the position to treat a person who has not only an orthopedic injury, but now likely significant, comorbid psychological factors involved as well – including entrenchment beliefs against perceived "enemies" like the insurance company, work, doctor, or other involved parties.

While outpatient rehabilitation professionals however cannot control all the factors in a workers' compensation case (e.g., physicians' activities, insurance companies' role, employer decision making and behavior, etc.), ultimately better functional outcomes act to mitigate costs. This is because injured workers' need to not just heal from their injury but also return to work. WC/WH is the tool to achieve that goal.

THE CASE FOR WORK CONDITIONING/WORK HARDENING

Workers' compensation costs are a significant expense to employers. Not only is this well accepted public opinion, based on national figures, workers' compensation costs have more than doubled in the last 20 years in terms of percentage of payroll. Numerous strategies have been employed in an effort to decrease workers' compensation costs, but few have provided real cost relief to employers. One of the major problems is that few people recognize that there is a significant difference in handling patient care and cost structure under workers' compensation cases as compared to individuals with regular group insurance. In order to understand why the two are different, one must understand how costs are incurred with workers' compensation cases.

Workers' compensation differs from group health care because workers' compensation cases provide "indemnity benefits," which primarily include wage replacement and disability benefits, in addition to the regular medical costs associated with treatment. According to the state of Illinois' most recent statistics, indemnity benefits constitute 55.6% of workers' compensation costs while regular medical benefits comprise only 44.4% of the costs to employers. Within workers' compensation cases, these two costs are often interrelated. This means that any strategy to reduce medical costs must not decrease the quality of care, or the indemnity benefits will increase to compensate for the diminished care – due to wage differentials and disability benefits. Furthermore, any cost control strategy that delays return-to-work also increases the indemnity benefits by increasing the amount of wage replacement benefits paid. These factors largely explain why managed care techniques (i.e., immediate cost-containment strategies) have not provided the workers' compensation cost relief employers had hoped for. To address cost control under workers' compensation, work hardening and work conditioning programs have been developed.

THE BENEFITS OF EXERCISE

There is a certain irony that needs to be noted. While most payors are careful concerning all providers they reimburse, it seems that surgeries, pharmaceuticals, doctors' office visits, pain management specialist consultations and the like are covered at least at some level. But, the one thing that has been shown to be effective, time and time again (Gurdon, 2010) across all patient types, for decreasing weight, increasing immune system functioning, boosting morale and psychological performance, improving bone-density and strength, decreasing hypertension, diabetes onset, and damaging types of cholesterol, is exercise. And it is a trivialization of exercise to say that " a patient can just simply exercise at home so why pay for it ?", or that patients somehow will innately know what to do to improve their condition. When exercise is part of a work conditioning/work hardening program it is often "over-"managed by the payor.

ONE PROGRAM MODEL: F.I.R.S.T.™

In Illinois, cases involving Permanent Partial Disability (PPD) settlements represent only 28% of the claims filed, but account for 63% of the total workers' compensation costs. This means that the majority of costs to the workers' compensation system result from a relatively small number of challenging cases. In Illinois, the largest factor determining Permanent Partial Disability is the patient's final disability rating, which is highly dependent on the patient's functional abilities. To address this, ATI designed F.I.R.S.T.™, or Functional Integration of Rehabilitation and Strength Training, a work conditioning/hardening treatment program based in clinics in the Midwest and east coast. It is a rehabilitation program using the principles of sports performance training to improve patients' physical lifting abilities. Driven by the necessity for a far more effective option than standard rehabilitative programs, the F.I.R.S.T.™ program model was developed with input from Orthopedic Surgeons, Physical Therapists, Athletic Trainers, Exercise Physiologists, and Bio-Mechanists as to developing an optimal return to work program.

Research was conducted on F.I.R.S.T.™ to validate the theory that that improving lifting abilities mattered. In a 2002 study presented at the annual meeting of the North American Spine Society, Researchers (Kruger, Steil, Bates, Rankin, and Lorenz), found ninety-six percent of F.I.R.S.T.™ patients achieved the medium physical demand level (able to lift 50lbs occasionally) or better. Forty-five percent of F.I.R.S.T.™ patients achieved the heavy physical demand level (ability to lift 100lbs occasionally). Next, F.I.R.S.T.™ patients were assessed at both 1 year and 2 years post-program completion as to whether their improved physical abilities increased return-to-work rates. The results indicated that 97% of F.I.R.S.T.™ patients go back to work, and 50% of them back to their former occupation. Finally, re-injury rates were assessed for two years following program completion and it was found that re-injuries were rare, and occurred less frequently with greater physical abilities (Kruger, Steil, Bates, Rankin, Lorenz, and Lorenz, 2004). Taken together, these studies provide support that the F.I.R.S.T.™ program approach improves outcomes for injured workers' by increasing physical capabilities, which then improved return-to-work rates and decreased re-injury rates. Over the past 10 years the F.I.R.S.T.™ program has successfully returned over 5,000 post-therapy patients back to work.

The referral path for an injured worker to become a candidate for the F.I.R.S.T.™ program typically follows treatment in physical therapy if he/she has:

1. Reached a plateau in physical therapy,
2. Has strength/tolerance deficits (vis-à-vis his/her prior level of function), and
3. Has remaining occupational deficits (PDL).

F.I.R.S.T.™ is not just for "healthy" individuals, but is also used with people of all ages and all levels of function. The F.I.R.S.T.™ program is an individualized program based primarily around the client's current level of function, with an identified return-to-work end-goal in mind.

SCHEDULING

Scheduling is actually an important aspect of the program, demonstrating its attention to the details of how most "work" actually works. Thus, the F.I.R.S.T.™ program is designed to be a "morning" program. The majority of F.I.R.S.T.™ clients are scheduled between 7 am – 1 pm. There are various reasons for this:

1. **Psychologically:** Typical F.I.R.S.T.™ program clients are off work while attending the program. The argument of "this is your work, until you get back to work" needs to be made. Clients feel better when they get-up, get moving and get back in the habit of a daily routine. F.I.R.S.T.™ helps to break the cycle of non-activity.
2. **Physiologically:** The body is fresher and physically ready in the morning. The injured population generally gets a better workout first thing in the morning, and as a result, they then have more energy throughout the balance of the day. Physicians typically don't want their patients lying around. They send them to the F.I.R.S.T.™ program to "get functional," not to sleep until noon.
3. Insurance companies aren't paying for injured workers' to sleep-in. In Illinois, insurance companies are paying injured workers' 66% of their salary while they are off work to attend the program like it is their job, so they want them there first thing in the morning.

Time-wise, F.I.R.S.T.™ is also similar to the commitment one has to a job—4 to 5 hours a day, 5 days a week. And like a job, being on time, committing to do the work appropriately, having accountability for one's performance, and accomplishing goals and expectations, are all part of the program as well.

F.I.R.S.T.™ STRENGTH AND CONDITIONING PHILOSOPHY

F.I.R.S.T.™ clients have compensatory injuries, and this is where the "art" of strength and conditioning comes in. The volume and strength progressions of the F.I.R.S.T.™ program is an approach simply that has not been done before.

The focus is on returning to work, and improving physical attributes that allow for a successful return to work. Work is generally defined by repeated, sub-maximal efforts over the course of a 6-12 hour day. Therefore, the F.I.R.S.T.™ program was designed to improve primarily muscular endurance, with secondary concerns of strength and flexibility. While the F.I.R.S.T.™ program has a proprietary algorithm as to its schedule and type of exercise and activities, the following aspects are publicly available:

1. **Exercise Volume:** This is a very important component of the F.I.R.S.T.™ program. Most strength and conditioning experts, as well as the literature, indicate that muscular endurance is best improved by increasing the DENSITY of the workout. This means increased exercise volume over time. In short, the F.I.R.S.T.™ program is designed to increase the amount of activity over the same 4-5 hour period. This is a very objective way of measuring progress in the program, and has been underutilized as an industry metric.
2. **Progressions in Exercise Volume Expectations:** Published Lumbar Fusion Outcomes indicate a starting daily exercise volume of 10-15,000 lbs. per day during the client's first week and progressing to 30-40,000 lbs. per day by Week 6 is optimal for most conditions. Shoulder/Upper extremity diagnoses have more varied Volume Expectations that co-vary depending on the client (generally, Week 1 volumes of 5 – 15,000 lbs. per day progressing to Week 6 at 25 -40,000 lbs. per day).

This is an important part of the F.I.R.S.T.™ program's success. The F.I.R.S.T.™ program is a 4-5 hour program by design. Many referral sources are traditionally used to less time, because they are more so used to ineffective work conditioning/hardening programs where clients are not as active. The difference in outcomes between traditional programs and the F.I.R.S.T.™ program lies in the objective progress from approx. 3-5 TONS per day to 15 – 20 TONS per day of activity. It is this increase in daily muscular preparedness that leads to successful return-to-work outcomes. The remainder of the day is needed for muscle recovery and consolidation. F.I.R.S.T.™ program research has indicated that most people get the best results in a 4-6 week timeline, with 4-5 hour sessions per day. However, some patients' injuries may require modifications to be made. For example, severe surgical cases may require longer duration, light duty concerns may need shorter sessions, and so on.

GROUP PSYCHOLOGY IN THE F.I.R.S.T.™ PROGRAM

The F.I.R.S.T.™ program is a group program. It is conducted with multiple people attending the program simultaneously, and as such has a "group ethic." A F.I.R.S.T.™ provider has to understand what motivates each and every patient. Some clients are truly motivated by their injury to gain prior levels of functioning and they are motivated to return to work. But other clients are upset, tired, and frustrated. Perhaps these patients haven't received proper medical attention and by the time they get into the F.I.R.S.T.™ program they may be motivated by:

1. anger towards the insurance company,
2. love/anger toward their attorney,
3. anger/love towards their physician,
4. a desire to return to work,
5. lifestyle considerations.

Regardless of the motivations of the patients in the F.I.R.S.T.™ program, providers need to know what "buttons to push" in order to help all the patients reach their maximum potential. F.I.R.S.T.™ is the LAST stop of the workers' compensation system for them.

There exists a small percentage of the stereotypical "Work Comp Con Artists," that is, clients who have no intention of getting better or ever returning to work. A F.I.R.S.T.™ program provider needs to know how to manage those who try to manipulate the system. Injured workers' carry with them a certain stigma of "faking" or fraud. For F.I.R.S.T.™ clients, about 50% are honest people who want to get back to work with no ulterior motives, 30% are legitimately injured but are confused with what to do next or do not want to perform exercise, 15% are being misled in some way (e.g., getting bad advice from their attorney, MD, spouse, or another outside source, and temporarily not putting full effort into rehabilitation), they may also harbor bad feelings toward work, their life, etc.. It is truly a small percentage of injured workers' that try to manipulate the system (approximately 5%).

The success of the F.I.R.S.T.™ Program depends on what the provider can do with the "bottom 50%." The bottom 50% is where the F.I.R.S.T.™ Program provider takes a sub-optimal outcome – the kind that typically gets lost in the workers' compensation system– and transforms it into a positive. A large portion of this success comes from treating the injured worker as a person—with dignity and respect. The reason this works is that, as mentioned above, most injured workers' have legitimate injuries and intend to return to work.

WORKERS' COMPENSATION SYSTEM COORDINATION

The F.I.R.S.T.™ program provider needs to help their clients navigate the Workers' compensation system, which can be frustrating, disconnected, and sometimes antagonistic. The F.I.R.S.T.™ provider spends approximately 20 hours per week with his/her patient, and as a result, the F.I.R.S.T.™ provider has a remarkably good perspective as to how things are going with each patient. F.I.R.S.T.™ providers must also function as active and clear communicators with all parties involved in the case. These can include contacts and/or documentation dealing with:

a) Occupational requirements
b) Primary physician
c) Surgeon
d) Insurance Company/Adjuster
e) Nurse Case Manager
f) Patient's Attorney
g) Employer's Attorney
h) Injury/Diagnosis
i) Likelihood of full duty RTW
j) Likelihood of RTW in general
k) Length of time since surgery
l) Length of time in PT
m) Length of time in FIRST
n) Length of time total off work
o) Personality
p) Where is this case going in your professional judgment?

The ability of the F.I.R.S.T.™ provider to navigate the idiosyncrasies of the workers' compensation system is an underrated key to achieving good outcomes.

The results of the F.I.R.S.T.™ Program have been studied for the past 10 years, resulting in publications or presentation at the North American Spine Society (NASS), American College of Sports Medicine (ACSM), National Strength and Conditioning Association (NSCA), World Spine I, II, and III, and many others. A full list can be found in the Appendix D. As everyone involved in workers' compensation knows, and this book certainly illustrates, workers' compensation is not a world of black-and-white clarity. However, the essence of the approach of the F.I.R.S.T.™ Program down is based on solid science. The following is the F.I.R.S.T.™ Outcomes Comparison: Maximum Medical Improvement.

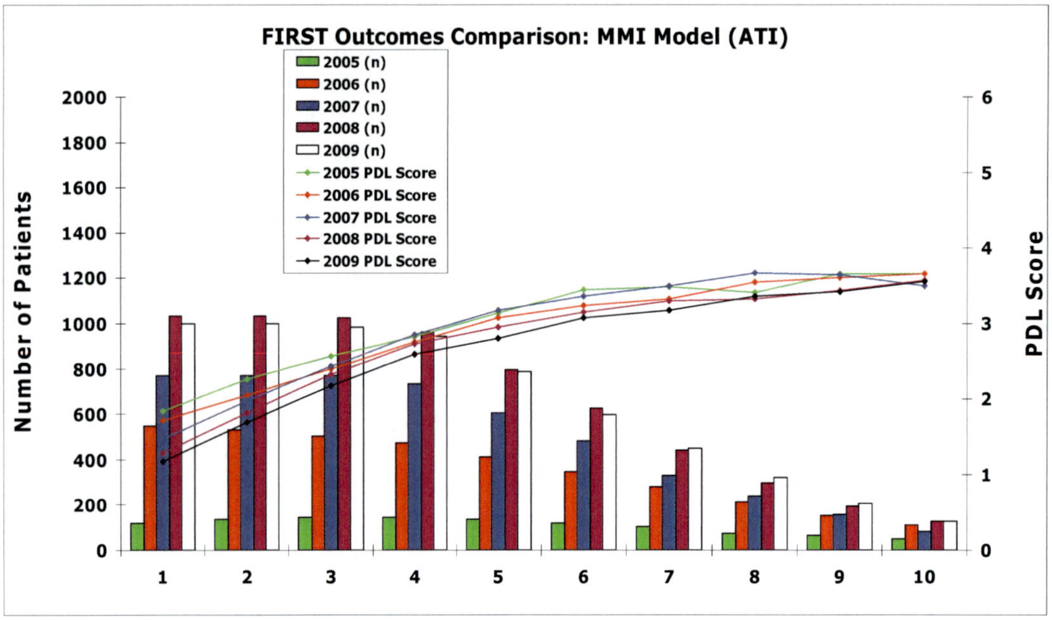

Legend: Horizontal axis = number of weeks in the F.I.R.S.T.™ program, far right is the Department of Labor's Physical Demand Level (PDL) scoring, 0 = Sedentary Work (Requires the occasional lifting of 10lbs or less); 1 = Light Work (Requires lifting a maximum of 20lbs), 2 = Light/Medium work; 3 = Medium Work (Requires lifting a maximum of 50lbs, but with frequent lifting of up to 25lbs); 4 = Medium/Heavy Work; 5 = Heavy Work (Requires lifting a maximum of 100lbs); 6 = Very Heavy Work (Requires lifting in excess of 100lbs, with frequent lifting of 5lbs or more).

This graph depicts the number of patients in the F.I.R.S.T.™ program for each year from 2005 to 2009 (5 years inclusive). Noting Week 6 on the horizontal axis, one sees that most patients attend a WC/WH program for 6 weeks or less. More than 6 weeks tends to be true "outliers," such as those having had multiple surgeries, Very Heavy Occupations, multiple co-morbid conditions, etc. Additionally, at this same point, the lines tend to "plateau" around 6 weeks. They represent the functional outcome level achieved during the time the patient was in the program. As the weeks progress from 1 to 2 to 3, etc., there is a concomitant increase in function (indicated along the far right axis). It is interesting to see a consistent rise in function for the first 4 weeks in particular, but also up to 6 weeks across all 5 years in the program. Looking to the right of 6 weeks, there does not seem to be a significant improvement in function on average. This finding is consistent with what is seen in the F.I.R.S.T.™ clinics and the outlier population that would be prescribed more than 6 weeks in the F.I.R.S.T.™ Program. People may improve occasionally past 6 weeks, but generally that occurs less frequently.

Overall – injured workers' make progress from the LIGHT or LIGHT-to-Medium (1 or 2) to the MEDIUM or MEDIUM-to-HEAVY Physical Demand Levels (3 or 4) over the course of their 4-6 week F.I.R.S.T.™ Program, on average. This means if the F.I.R.S.T.™ protocol is followed, good results will follow – despite all the "noise" and competing incentives in the workers' compensation system. It proves that injured workers' really aren't all that different from other people in terms of response to exercise, if managed in an intelligent approach.

IMPORTANCE OF INFORMED CONSENT

While informed consent is the *sine que non* to all medical and healthcare procedures by insuring patient understanding and choice, it holds an additional and significant import in workers' compensation care. First of all, it is critically important in establishing clear and specific expectations for the patient. For example, most patients will feel muscular soreness during the first week of participation in the F.I.R.S.T.™ program. They are told to expect this. Simply doing this mitigates their anxiety and fear that they may have re-injured themselves, when indeed this is a positive indication of strengthening formerly weakened or atrophied muscle groups. This then acts to minimize the impulse of the patient to drop out precipitously from the program, bolstering compliance and thus positive outcome.

In workers' compensation, informed consent also serves to demystify the upcoming therapeutic process by clearly describing what will occur, what the expectations will be of the patient, what the patient can expect in terms of process and outcome, and establishes a "baseline" of open dialog between the clinician and the patient. Indeed, this is the start of a very intimate, while relationship that blends clinical skills, demand on the patient, and psychological support balancing coaching, pushing through difficult demands, and dealing with all of the additional aspects of the case that manifest.

Furthermore, many workers' compensation patients may be confused with their situation and treatment options. There are still many physicians that recommend their own services more so than discussing all the treatment options available. This is understandable, and not always an issue of ethics. For example, it is unreasonable to expect that a general practitioner could fully discuss the risks and benefits of treatment options of other specialties such as orthopedic surgeons, pain management physicians, physical therapists, and so forth.

Indeed, it is frequently unclear whose responsibility it really is to serve as an advocate or ombudsman for the WC patient. Logic could suggest it is the patient's attorney, but he or she may not have one. If they do, the attorney may not feel it is his/her place to do more than recommend a physician or practice or clinic that they trust. The patient may not feel comfortable or competent to question the attorney's recommendation regardless if they feel comfortable with the referral of not.

Rehabilitation specialists may be misunderstood when they tell a patient that they can go back to work based on their performance on a Functional Capacity Examination, while their physician feels that they should not go back to work (more on this in the chapter on ethics). This can be mistranslated to "XYZ rehab talks people out of surgery all the time..."

The initially evaluation may or may not feel on-point for the case if a specialist is called upon. Likewise, that specialist may or may not feel in the driver's seat of patient care, understanding, and advocacy. Thus, often by fiat or default the case management and conduit between the patient and all other involved professionals and medical specialists may be with the rehabilitation processional working with the patient. This level of responsibility makes it incumbent on this provider to ensure all is going as it should with all peripheral parties, as well as properly managing the rehabilitation aspects of their own case. Sometimes this is a smooth and collaborative process, and other times is can be a frustrating and time consuming process filled with non-reimbursable time spent in behalf of the patient, and ironically, often invisible to the patient who may be presuming their doctor or attorney is managing everything in their behalf.

CONCLUSION

The medical complexities of injured workers' can be manifold and Byzantine—both before and after the injury. Obesity is a ubiquitous problem for the general population however often ignored in workers' compensation cases wherein it exacerbates treatments and procedures and thus diminishes rapid or complete clinical outcomes. For some the response is to simply focus on fixing the presenting injury rather than deal with any co-morbidities, which results in an iatrogenic approach to care. Others take a more reasonable and humane approach that actually addresses all presenting issues.

Many professionals that work with workers' compensation cases actually do not understand the differences between physical therapy and work hardening/work conditioning. The authors have worked to clarify this confusion, as well as demonstrate an effective model of treatment. Ironically, the various and powerful benefits of exercise play a critical role in rehabilitation as well as general health functioning (e.g., decrease morbidity in heart disease, hypertension, diabetes, etc.).

REFERENCES

Alder, SC, Gren, LH, Hegmann, KT, Lyon, JL, Wendelboe, AM, White, GL 2004, 'Associations Between Body-Mass Index and Surgery for Rotator Cuff Tendinitis', *The Journal of Bone & Joint Surgery (American)*, vol. 86, pp. 743-747.

American Obesity Association 2005, *AOA Fact Sheets*, viewed 14 March 2010, http://obesity1.tempdomainname.com/subs/fastfacts/Health Effects.shtml, www.obesity.org/.

Asher, A 2009, *Does Obesity Affect the Results of Back Surgery?*, viewed 14 March 2010, http://backandneck.about.com/od/medication/f/obesitybacksurg.htm.

Bates, D, Kruger, M, Lorenz, MA, Lorenz, P, Rankin, S, Steil, G 2004, 'Does functional capability in a Sports Performance based Work Conditioning/Hardening Program correlate with RTW capabilities at 1-yr follow-up with worker's compensation subjects s/p lumbar fusion? [Abstract]', *NASS 19th Annual Meeting,* North American Spine Society, Chicago, IL, 26-30 October, 2004.

Bates, D, Kruger, M, Lorenz, MA, Rankin, S, Steil, G 2002, 'Sports performance-based work conditioning/hardening with subjects' status after lumbar fusion: an outcome based study', *NASS 17th Annual Meeting,* North American Spine Society, Montreal, Quebec, 29 October– 2 November, 2002.

Bennington, MK 2010, *The Impact of Obesity on the Resolution of Workers' Compensation Claims,* viewed 13 July 2010, http://www.lexisnexis.com/Community/workers'compensationlaw/blogs/workers'compensationlawblog/archive/2010/03/27/the-impact-of-obesity-on-the-resolution-of-workers'-compensation-claims.aspx.

Braun Consulting Group 2004, 'Obesity In The Workplace', *Braun Consulting News,* vol. 7, no. 5, viewed 13 July 2010, http://www.braunconsulting.com/bcg/newsletters/summer2004/summer20043.html.

Cantley, L, Cullen, MR, Pollack, KM, Sircar, K, Slade, MD, Sorock, GS, Taiwo, O 2007, 'Association between Body Mass Index and Acute Traumatic Workplace Injury in Hourly Manufacturing Employees', *American Journal of Epidemiology,* vol. 166, no. 2, pp. 204-211.

Cohen, JW, Dietz, W, Finkelstein, EA, Trogdon, JG 2009, 'Annual Medical Spending Attributable to Obesity: Payer and Service-Specific Estimates', *Health Affairs,* vol. 28, no. 5, pp. 822-831.

Coppelman, J 2007, *Obesity in Workers' Comp: Duke Sounds the Alarm*, viewed 13 July 2010, http://www.workers'compinsider.com/archives/000670.html

Ferguson, J 2009, *The effect of obesity and other comorbidities on workers' comp*, viewed 13 July 13, 2010, http://www.workers'compinsider.com/2009/03/the-effect-of-o.html.

Ferguson, J 2007, *Weighty matters: the high cost of obesity in the workplace*, viewed 13 July 2010, http://www.workers'compinsider.com/archives/000693.html.

Gurdon, MC 2010, 'More, please', *Wall Street Journal*, 10 May, Page A15.

Hays, D 2009, 'Obese Workers' Comp Claims Far Exceed Slimmer Employee Costs', *P&C National Underwriter News* viewed 19 March 2010, www.property-casualty.com/news/2009/9/pages/Obese-Workers'-Comp-Claims-Far-Exceed-Slim.

Kowalczyk, L 2006, 'Obesity if Fueling a Rise in Joint-Replacement Surgeries', *The Boston Globe,* viewed 14 March 2010, http://www.boston.com/news/local/articles/2006/07/18/obesity_is_fueling_a_rise_in_joint_replacement.

Rousmaniere, P, 2009, The elephant in the room. *Risk & Insurance.* http://findarticles.com/p/articles/mi_m0BJK/is_14_20/ai_n42125308/

Seaman, J 2010, *Obesity and Knee Surgery Recovery*, viewed 14 March 2010, http://orthopedickneesurgery.net/obesity-and-knee-surgery-recovery.

Tom, PA 2009, 'Workers' Compensation Industry Worried About Obesity Claims', *Insurance Journal National News,* viewed 19 March 2010, www.insurancejournal.com/news/national/2009/06/09/101211.htm?print=1.

Trimble, T 2001/2008, *Oversize Patients – A Big Nursing Challenge! Emergency Nursing World*, viewed 14 March 2010, http://ENW.org/Obese.htm.

CHAPTER 7

Report of International Workers' Compensation Survey

Matt Kruger, Jeff Rogers, Chris E. Stout, Hema Burra and Jillian Richardson

ATI Physical Therapy; E-mail: Chris.stout@atipt.com

Abstract: This chapter will discuss the results from a new, online survey that is a bit unique in its scope and design that canvassed all providers involved in workers' compensation cases. The survey's anonymity seems to have fostered very frank responses for many respondents. Summary tables of aggregated data are provided and augmented by categorized, verbatim responses of various professionals—many of which are very eyeopening.

INTRODUCTION

The authors were interested in canvassing the opinions and experiences of various professionals involved in the field of workers' compensation. To that end, a survey questionnaire was developed and publicly posted online for interested individuals to be able to complete and submit electronically. The survey, in its entirety, appears in Appendix B herein. (Additionally, it is currently planned to leave the survey live online for interested individuals to subsequently complete it and send in to the authors. The plan is to annually compile the findings and post on the same website. The hope is that overtime the number of respondents will grow and the tabulated results will become more interesting to all.) The survey appears at: http://www.atipt.com/Webpages/Research/Workers'CompensationSurvey.aspx

Initially, the instrument was sent along to various clinical and non-clinical professionals working with workers' compensation cases. The authors then asked those they had given it to, to also feel free to send it out to their colleagues and contacts that would be appropriate. In at least one instance, one of the contributing authors made its availability known to conference meeting attendees. It was recommended by a colleague that it could be fitting to utilize 'LinkedIn' as a vehicle to get the word out via workers' compensation groups therein. There were about half-a-dozen such groups that were appropriate for the survey, and the group moderators were very kind and open in allowing a descriptive post and a link to the survey website to be uploaded.

Individuals going to the website were told the book's title and editors, and were thanked for their participation in the project. The authors requested respondents to "...feel free to be completely honest, gloves-off, and even provocative if you so wish in your responses....We are looking to gather your opinions, stories, perspectives and wisdom." They also offered differing levels of anonymity to those completing the survey and they could choose to have their name associated with their comments or to be completely anonymous, depending on what they felt comfortable with. The survey was available on line for approximately two months, and another month prior to that it was sent directly to some. So, at this time the total respondent number is 46. While this is a bit disappointingly small in consideration of the various venues it has appeared, it nevertheless is a start. Of course, any broad generalizations are limited; however, of the responses received, there are definitely some interesting findings. It would seem that many took to heart our request to be frank in their answers.

The authors were pleased with spontaneous, and unsolicited feedback about the survey itself, for example: "you got it all- very comprehensive survey." However, another seemed to think our questions were somewhat politically stilted or biased (readers can judge for themselves by reviewing the survey in its entirety in Appendix B). He or she said: "From your questions, I suspect you will tout the praises of a hard working, professionally run bureaucratic system, with the weight of the country on its shoulders, and doing all it can to help the little people. That is too bad, the WC system needs to be blown out of the water." Sounds like we hit a raw nerve... Another respondent offered an interesting forecast: "The future of workers' compensation in the U.S. will be driven in large measure by success or failure of insurers and employers to apply better medical intelligence in working with the medical community."

With Special Thanks to: Jillian Richardson and Hema Burra

Chris E. Stout, Matt Kruger and Jeffrey Rogers, (Eds)

The following will be a presentation of the findings in this inaugural survey. First we will provide a description of the respondents themselves for readers to gain a grasp of who-is-saying-what. We present this information in various ways to facilitate understanding and comprehend the results. The balance of the chapter will present verbatim responses clustered and identified.

SUMMARY OF DATA

Profession (N=46)

Respondents were first asked to identify their profession. Mainly, most professions were noted in a check-box list, and additionally there was a free-text area to write in another profession if it was not one of the default options provided. If more than one profession was noted, the authors made a judgment call as to the most appropriate single category. The results are as follow:

- 2% - Adjuster (1)
- 20% - Athletic Trainer (9)
- 15% - Case Manager (7)
- 2% - Employer (1)
- 7% - Employer Attorney (3)

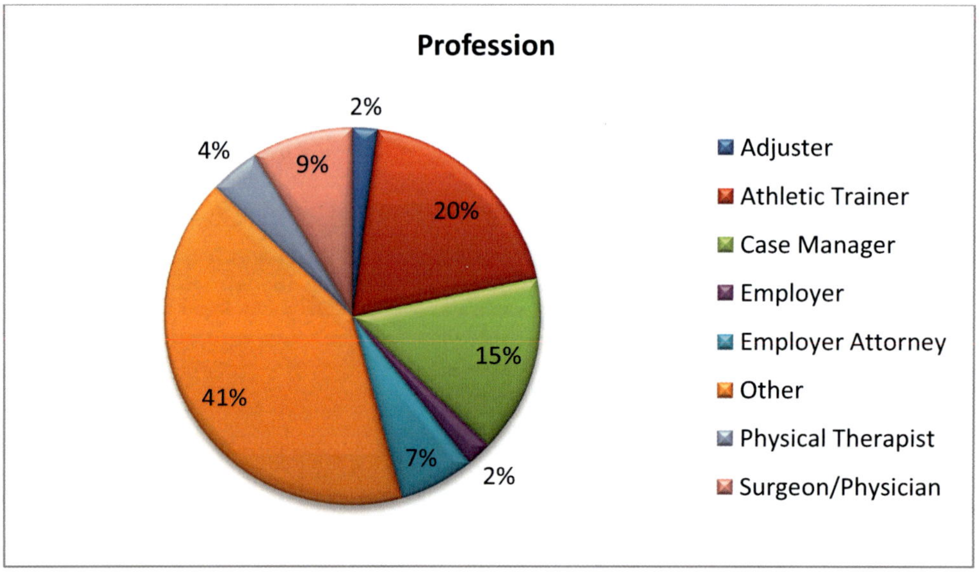

- 41% - Other (19)
  - 6% - Advocate
  - 5% - Associate Vice President – Claims
  - 5% - Community Advocate
  - 21% - Consultant (4)
  - 11% - Exercise Physiologist (2)
  - 27% - Insurance (5)
  - 5% - Insurance Agent
  - 5% - Network Sales Rep
  - 5% - Non-Attorney Advocate
  - 5% - Physician's Assistant

- 5% - Registered Nurse
- 4% - Physical Therapist (2)
- 9% - Surgeon/Physician – Occupational Medicine (4)

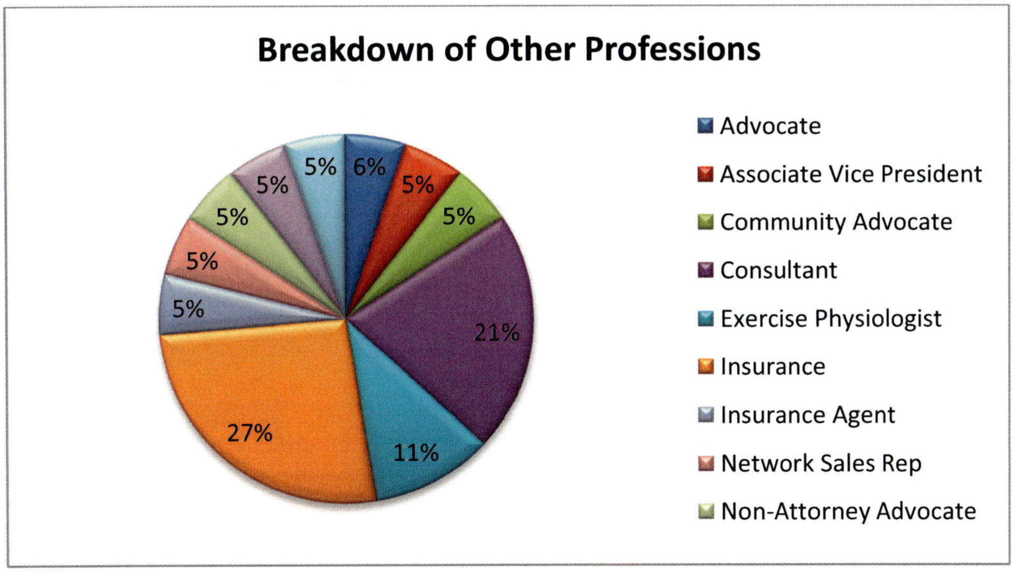

Respondents were then asked to describe the nature of their work vis-à-vis workers' compensation. The following are verbatim responses with the exception of some limited editing for grammar, spelling, and punctuation. They provide a fine-grain picture of the heterogeneity of the group:

- I manage workers' compensation claims.
- I perform the same services as an attorney for injured workers'. State law does not permit me to be paid for my services.
- I do injury evaluation, treatment and post-rehabilitation.
- I oversee staff of ATs and PTs that provide care to WC injuries for 12,000 airline workers' in 2 different divisions: 6000 bag handlers, gate agents and ticket agents; 6000 mechanics.
- My position provides injury care and management for the 2,100 employees working for a city government (i.e., police, fire, transit, executive, utility, and public works).
- I am an Athletic Trainer Physician Extender in an orthopedic surgeon's office. I am involved in all aspects of care in the office as well as communicating with adjusters, case managers, utilization review, and marketing to work comp providers.
- I assist with initial injury reports which directly go to the TPA; I receive daily injury reports for the entire department and follow-up on them for treatment, clinical evals, rehabilitation, etc. I speak directly to TPA and physicians daily, I work in concert with WC physicians on the care and return to duty for employees.
- I direct Work Conditioning/Hardening program for Injury Workers' allowing them to return to their prior level of function/PDL following injury.
- I am the director of the Work Conditioning/Hardening Program in a PT Clinic.
- I do hands on quality assurance of work comp rehab programs.
- I am a FIRST Director.
  - This is a difficult question to answer. My role in an injured workers' life is to try to unscramble the situation that they are in. That could be- just read and explain the letters that they receive showing alternative work situations, so as the injured worker can return to work in a supported manner.

  - Attend medical and case conference appointments to provide food relief parcels.
  - Attend legal hearings
  - Work with the injured worker and the employer to reach a common ground, so as the injured worker can make a successful return to work..
  - Each injured worker needs something different.So my role is very flexible.
- I give training sessions to claims agents so as the case managers get to know what it is like being an injured worker -I am an injured worker-
- I give training session to groups of injured workers' to encourage them to find ways to return to work.
- I do work in the areas of return to work, workplace accommodation, and work comp case management for a large technology company.
- I conduct utilization review, initial clinical review and I also worked as case- manager for Work Comp self insured company.
- I have many fingers in many WC pies. I like working across multiple aspects of the industry, to gain multiple perspectives.
- I am a Field Nurse Case Manager. Manage simple to catastrophic cases while attempting to obtain RTW full duty/MMI.
- I am a Medical Case Manager.
- I build rapport with injured worker, advocate for work comp services, collaborate, coordinate, and monitor medical progress.
- I advise employers and insurers on work injury risks, primarily to improve post injury response.
- Helping public entities manage their worker's compensation claims.
- I am the person who financially pays for this program (regardless of culpability). The other true stakeholder is the employee who physically/emotionally pays for this program. Everyone else, on your list (save the medical folks) is feeding off this program.
- Defend employers and insurers at the hearing and appellate levels. Advise employers regarding workers' compensation policies.
- I have been a WC attorney for 8 years, and for 7 of those years as a respondent's attorney. In the last couple of years I have worked as a legal consultant in the area of workers' compensation.
- I am a former UPS HR supervisor who went to law school intending to return to the sport industry as an attorney. I now work with small businesses and a few high-deductible insured, defending them in their workers' compensation claims and facilitating resolution of a variety of conflicts. I am a trained mediator and therefore carefully selected by my clients to seek quick, fair resolution. Despite my approach, I find that New York Judges are often "claimant-friendly" and therefore lack the required impartiality. I believe these judges must be removed and all parties in the process be given a fair opportunity to present their cases. However, New York characterizes the parties as "claimants" and "carriers," unless an employer is self-insured or uninsured. Although this structure conflicts with the Code of Professional Responsibility, which refuses to recognize any such tri-partite relationship in personal injury or workers' compensation cases, the practices and attitudes persist. Additionally, the bias and unfair practices persist. Employers are not always sent notices of the hearings in the cases against them. The Board refuses to place "carrier attorneys" on notice, so they do not receive them, either. Notices go to the carrier, which is merely a payor--not a party--and often the Board does not have the proper carrier on notice. So, cases can go on for years before the proper parties learn of them. By then, cases and sites of injury have been established, and awards have been made (effectively in default). I spend a lot of my time just trying to get the Board to review cases on their merits and correcting the errors.
- I perform functional capacity evaluations.
  - Develop commercially-available FCE system.
  - Conduct research (published) on the topics of assessing function and validity of effort.

- Provide litigation support to attorneys (petitioner and defense) on the issue of functional assessments.
- Provide CUE and CLE classes to comp professionals.

- We sell workers' compensation insurance to employers and work closely with our clients to provide loss control and claim management services. We interact with claim adjusters, injured employees, employers, plaintiff and defense attorneys, medical treatment providers, and others on all aspects of workers' compensation insurance coverage, underwriting, claims and loss prevention activities.
- I am a risk professional for a large multi-state, privately held, Franchise Corporation.
- I am the Associate Vice President of a workers' compensation claim department. We insure a niche market of nursing homes in the Midwest. We see claims mainly for back injuries and slip & fall injuries.
- I create medical cost containment programs for workers' compensation carriers, third party administrators, and self insured employers.
- I treat and manage workers'.
- I am the medical director for WC insurance carrier; oversee network development and education; utilization management; medical bill review; disability prevention; pharmacy services.
- I initially evaluate the case and if it has merits) I send them out. I then follow up the case trying to coordinate services and get them back to work. I also serve as liaison for benefits that they may be entitled to. I also respond to management's questions and sit on a committee to assess what happened and what can be done to prevent further incidents.
- As an Occ Med physician I assess employees' complaints for causation (work relatedness) and communicate with employers, insurers and occasionally provide depositions or testimony before WC Commission representatives. I perform Independent Medical Examinations, often I am requested to assist in causality determination. As a Family physician I treat patients with work-related illness and injury.
- I evaluate, treat and manage all aspects of Orthopaedic work comp injuries.
- I provide the same services as a plaintiff attorney at the agency level.
- I'm involved in evaluating, and treating WC patients, measure PDLs, and transfer patients to work conditioning.
- I provide physical therapy.
- I do Work Conditioning/Hardening & I am a FCE provider & supervisor.

The authors also inquired about the range of years the respondents were involved with workers' compensation cases (46 responses). The break down is:

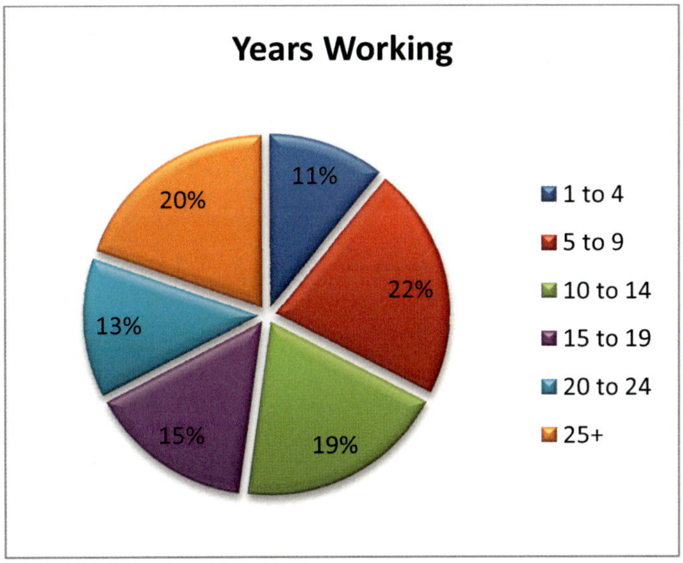

- 11% - 1 to 4 (5)
- 22% - 5 to 9 (10)
- 19% - 10 to 14 (9)
- 15% - 15 to 19 (7)
- 13% - 20 to 24 (6)
- 20% - 25+ (9)

When looking at the amount of time working with workers' compensation cases, by profession, the authors found:

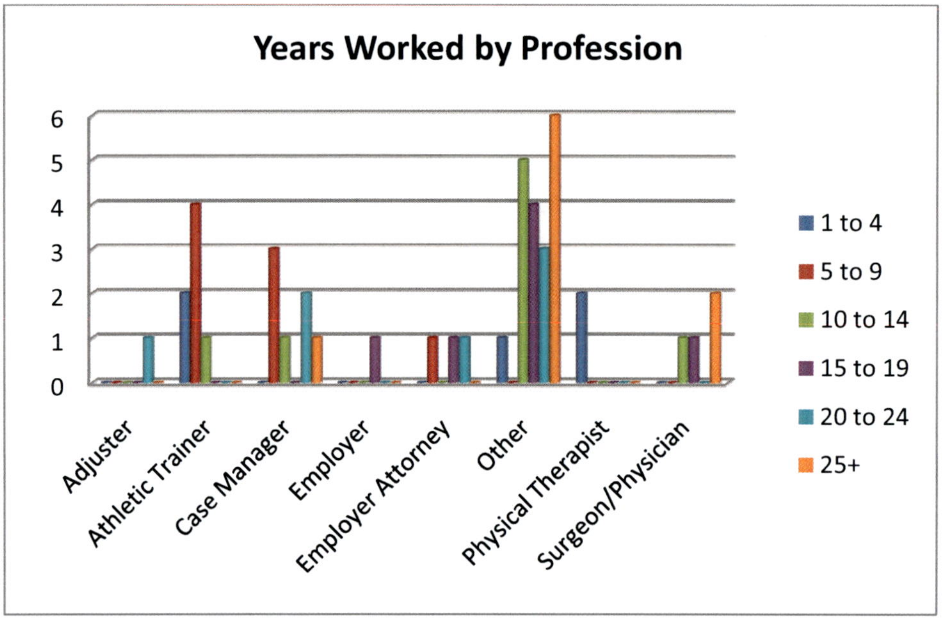

Forty-four subjects responded to the question of on an average, annual basis, how many workers' compensation cases did he/she manage, treat, represent, review, adjudicate, etc. The mean average was 793 a year (SD $\pm$ 2366), however there was an outlier (Network Sale Representative) who noted an average of 15,000/year. Also, three occupational medicine physicians noted that they saw 5000, 2800, and 2000 patients annually. When running the data without these three subjects the mean annual average was 251 (SD $\pm$ 302).

Only forty three subjects responded to the question concerning annual income. There is a question that the authors have concern with, and that is the >$500,000. While there is an n=4, one is an attorney and one is an insurance manager, which both seem reasonable; however the other two are both athletic trainers, and one of those is 24 years old having 1 – 4 years of experience, so perhaps this latter, if not both respondents may have made an error in completing this part of the survey. The breakdown is as follows:

- 5% - < $25,000 (2)
- 16% - $25,000 - $49,999 (6)
- 15% - $50,000 - $74,999 (6)
- 26% - $75,000 - $99,999 (10)
- 18% - $100,000 - $199,999 (7)
- 10% - $200,000 - $349,999 (4)
- 0% - $350,000 - $499,999 (0)
- 10% - >$500,000 (4)

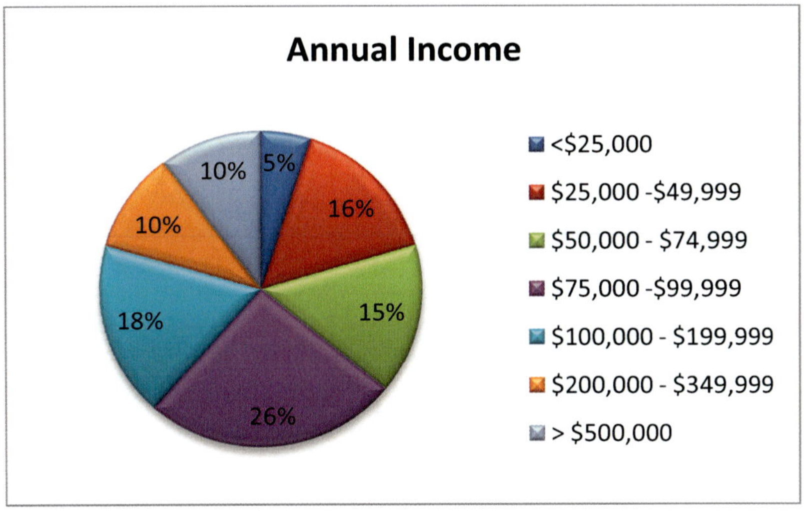

When broken out by profession, income parsed out as follows:

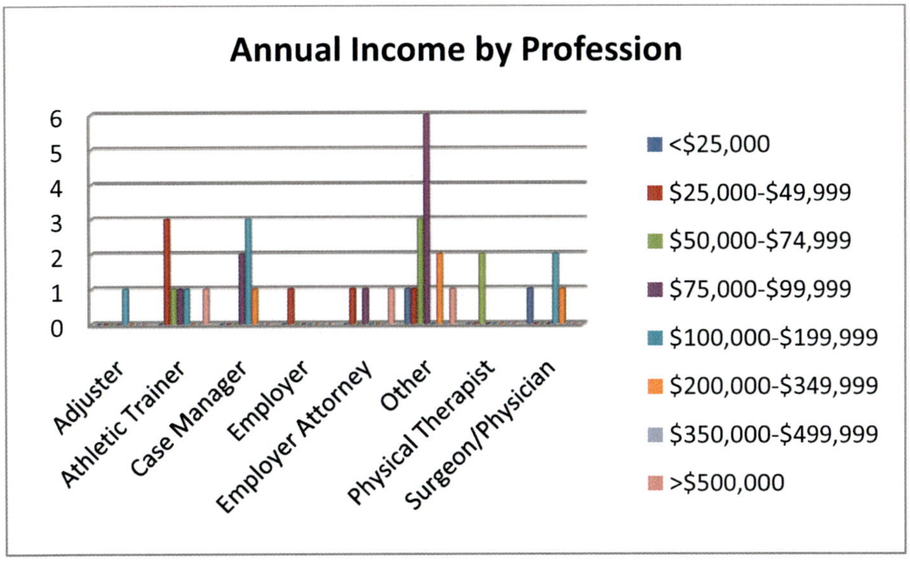

While understanding that not all income of the respondents may come from workers' compensation activities, we also queried what percentage of their total income was borne from workers' compensation. Thirty-nine subjects noted the following:

- 13% - <25% (5)
- 2% - About 25% (1)
- 13% - 25% to 49% (5)
- 3% - About 50% (1)
- 0% - 50% to 74% (0)
- 5% -About 75% (2)
- 20% - 75% to 99% (8)
- 40% - 100% (17)

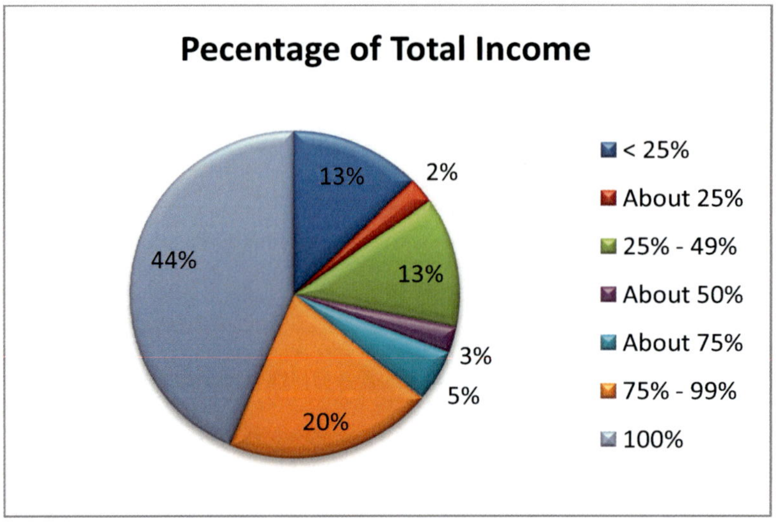

The authors also looked at this by profession and found the following:

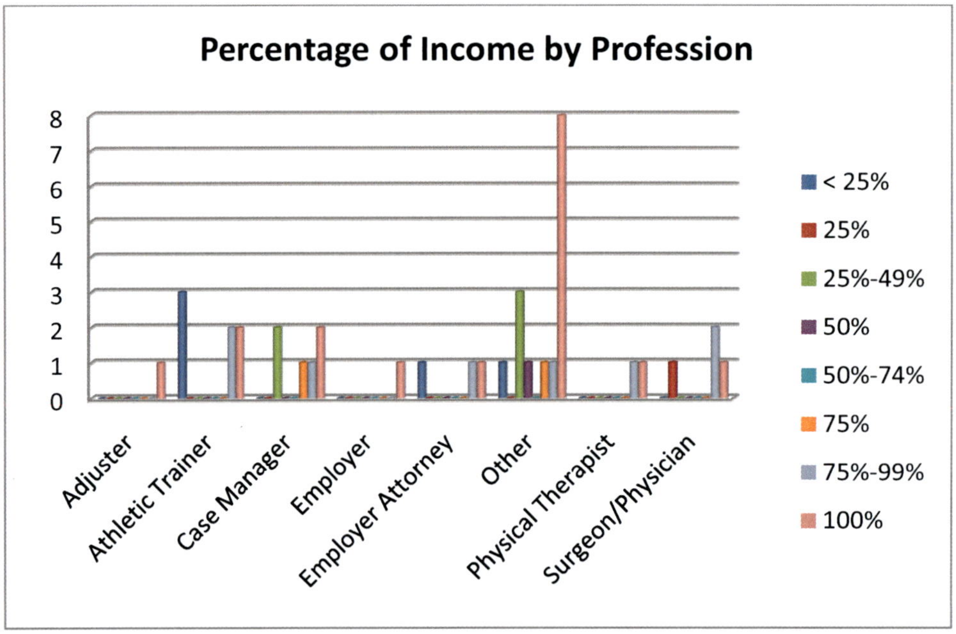

The authors were curious to know what drew the respondents to work in the filed of workers' compensation in the first place. The answers were somewhat surprising (again, verbatim responses with the exception of some editing for grammar, spelling, and punctuation are provided):

- Looking for a job.
- Shortage of attorneys willing to represent injured workers'.
- I was not drawn to them; it is just part of my job.
- Good fit for Athletic Training model of health care deliver.
- On-site management has been shown to the most effective administration of care. I saw an opportunity to start a full-time position at the city.
- I enjoy working with these patients to assist in the diagnosis and treatment of musculoskeletal conditions.
- Part of the job when I was a County employee.

- An interest in high level aggressive rehabilitation and exercise.
- It fell in my lap, but has worked out since.
- I enjoy getting individuals back to a Functional level to return to work.
- I became an injured worker in '94, the system made no sense to me, so after learning as much as I could about the system, I decided that the only way to have any form of social justice within the system was to build the programme that was needed for my self as it just was not there. So I have spent 16 years in the WorkCover system, the first 3 as a drug dependant injured worker, the next 2 as an injured worker trying to get out of the system but for almost all of the 16 years building the process I now have in place.
- I fell into the field accidentally through a master's degree internship and no other jobs were available for nurses who are hoping for clinical positions but California overregulated for those of us who want to be clinical but have been behind a desk...
- I fell into WC by accident. Thought I wanted to be a School Counselor but after I graduated with a degree in Educational Psychology and travelled the world, I needed to work and found a job as a vocational evaluator for injured workers'. The rest is a long history in WC!
- As an occupational health nurse it was part of my job description as well as the Wellness Program and the Safety Program. However, it makes sense as these areas dove tail each other. Later I was offered a position strictly dealing with WC individuals and being the person to communicate with the injured worker, the employer, the physician, the insurance company and anyone else related to the claim. When someone says "work comp" it's often followed with an "ugh!" But I believe there is purpose why WC was developed...to protect the worker AND the company. And I believe education is essential when working in the WC area, because safety and wellness are critical to a good outcome and prevention of further injuries/conditions. WC is more than treating the injury/condition. It's treating the whole individual. When these all come together: the injured worker is healed and returned to a safe environment and has taken initiatives in a healthier lifestyle, then that is success.
- Opportunity to assist injured worker with return to gainful employment.
- I do not work on individual cases; rather I work on systems of managing the entire portfolio of cases.
- Default. Was a risk manager for years, and I ended up managing self-insured program, large deductible program, monopolistic (retro) program, and state fund program.
- Had no choice.
- I came across a job at a claimant's side workers' comp. firm in my search after law school, and when I took the job, found that I had an interest and an aptitude for the subject.
- I kind of fell into it. The more WC cases I handled the more I enjoyed this field of law.
- Workers' compensation chose me. I clerked with a leader in this practice area while I was in law school, but I declined to post-graduation job offer because I was still working as a minor league hockey agent and the firm would not allow me to do anything but WC defense. I came to NYC to get a few years of experience in a major metropolitan area with a plan to move to a smaller market and eventually start my own practice. Instead, I took a job at a litigation firm in the Wall-Street district so I could get some courtroom experience and I ended up running the WC department in my first few days at the firm. When the firm began having financial problems, I looked for other work but could not find it. My family, friends, colleagues, and a few co-workers' encouraged me to leave and try starting my own firm here. Now, I compete with the firms that weren't interested in hiring me. LOL.
- No two cases are ever the same. I realized soon after getting into this field that validity of effort testing was being done very poorly.
- Employers need direction and assistance to control their workers' compensation costs. Getting involved in the management of workers' compensation cases is an integral part of the process.
- A part of my many risk management responsibilities.
- My background is in health education and wellness. I enjoy the medical aspect of workers' compensation cases. I love the business side of the insurance industry.

- At the time...a growing industry.
- I needed to work in OM field and WC has most jobs available.
- Interesting, varied cases, the ability to impact people's lives medically, psychologically, socially, economically.
- Part of my job as the medical director of our employee health services.
- Rewarding.
- High percentage of patients in locality of clinic.
- It was completely by accident. Started working with WC cases in a search for employment and opportunity.

As workers' compensation laws differ from state-to-state, the authors queried respondents as to in which state(s) they work and if they work in more than one area, what state, region, and/or city did they find the most challenging cases and why. Here is what was noted:

- Illinois and California, because the plaintiff's bar rules those states.
- Texas, Oklahoma, Florida.
- California WC laws have scared my client from expanding to LAX (airport), and NY comp laws combined with union/mob work has scared them from moving program to JFK (airport).
- We work in Missouri, but we also see patients from Illinois. Both states have different WC laws regarding the specifics of causality and ability of patients to choose their medical providers.
- I am never sure as to what is the most challenging; sometimes the hardest part of my work is to help injured workers' to understand that case managers really do not have a voodoo doll that they stick poison pins into. The lack of knowledge that injured workers' have about the WorkCover process frustrates me, because the system expects that at point of impact the injured worker also gained a degree in WorkCover not just a broken body. I am also frustrated by the lack of knowledge that case managers have in regard to injured workers', for instance the needs of a rural or regional based injured worker are different from metro based injured workers'. Transport is a major concern to rural and regional based injured workers'. Case managers do not seem to understand that public transport does not exist, and that if there is a bus service it is once a day not every 15 minutes. Case managers do not understand that for some injured workers' the nearest chemist may be over an hour's drive away, or that the local doctor only comes once a week. Case managers also lack industry knowledge, for instance the transport industry has many different components to it -short-medium-long haul- means different things in each component of the transport industry :for a courier driver a short haul may be from one suburb to the next for as transport driver a short haul may be 200kms and for a transport company a short haul may be 500kms: the case managers need to have some basic industry information so as they can help the injured worker return to pre-injury employment, not just say that there is medical clearance to return to work and therefore the injured worker can now go back driving.
- I don't see much difference between regions. They are equally challenging.
- States in which it is difficult to direct medical care to appropriate physicians and physical therapist, i.e., IL, AZ.
- California is the most challenging.
- Rhode Island- because it has its own worker's comp court which seems to be full employment for plaintiff lawyers and the judges! I could not make much progress at all closing claims that seemed to be of workers' who found a great system and didn't want to return to work even with light duty. California was challenging in the earlier days.
- Arkansas. The standard for compensability in Arkansas gives the employee the benefit of the doubt, as though it was the employer who has the burden of proof.
- Illinois and California, as both states are so overly pro-labor that the statutory advantages that workers' have over their employers makes workers' compensation a major cost item for all businesses.

- California, Florida, and Illinois.
- Oklahoma and Illinois:

    Spinal fusion surgeries are more prevalent in these states vs. other Midwest states

    Physicians seem to be less likely to follow the Occupational treatment guidelines

    Demographically, the employees seem less motivated to return to gainful employment and there seems to be an underlying culture of disability.

    We see a lot more injured workers' who are approved for SSDI in these 2 States

    The injured employees by culture seem to be more litigious.

- OH - Monopolistic state for workers' compensation.
- Los Angeles
- NJ - lack of fee schedule, doctors do not practice (or understand) evidence based medicine, resulting in higher disability and costs
- Illinois, due to the litigious nature of the state and entrenchment on all sides Numerically, the numbers look like this for the areas in which respondents work. The authors realized that those responding to our survey were "international" in the venues of
- their work, going beyond the United States, but also working with clients in Canada, Australia, and Puerto Rico:
- All (1)
- Canada
- Australia (2)
- Puerto Rico
- Individual States

    Arizona (2)

    California (5)

    Delaware (2)

    Florida (2)

    Illinois (14)

    Indiana (6)

    Michigan

    Missouri (2)

    Nebraska (2)

    New York (2)

    Oklahoma

    Pennsylvania (2)

    Texas

    Wisconsin (9)

The mean average of the 44 who responded to the question of their age was 47 years ($\pm$ 11).

Graphically, the age spread looks as follows:

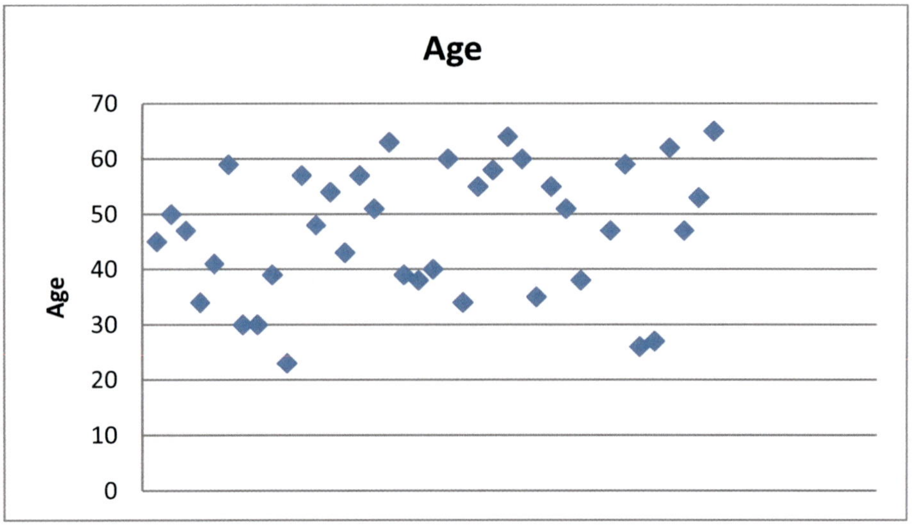

The composition of respondents by gender was:

- 65% Males (30)
- 35% Females (16)

When looking at gender breakout by profession, we found:

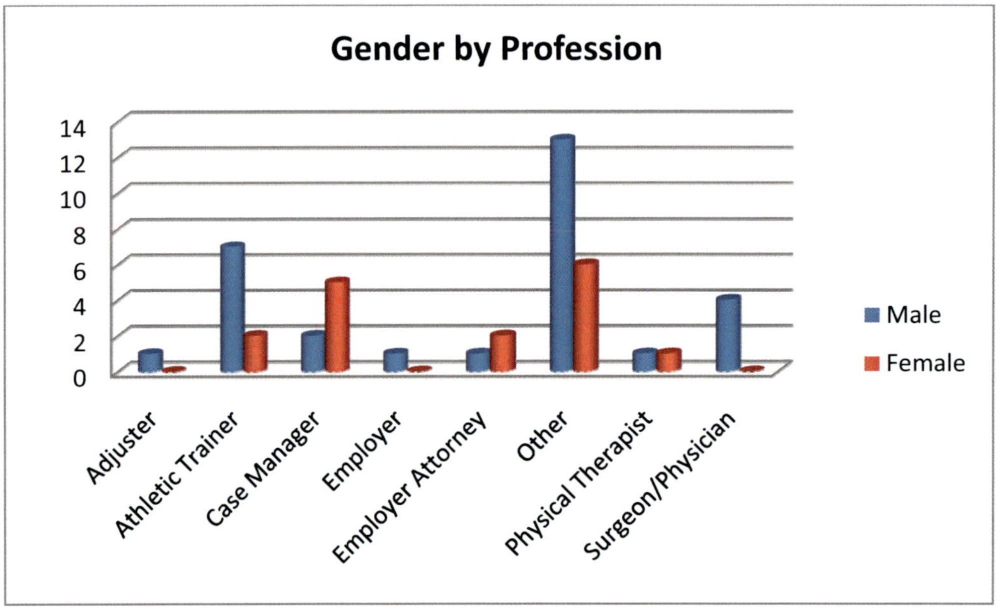

OPINIONS AND PERSPECTIVES

Readers should have a clear picture of those responding to the survey. The following is a verbatim listing (with only stylistic edits) of the perspectives of the various individuals categorized by their profession, but responding to the same questions, along with observations from the authors.

IT'S THE SYSTEM, STUPID

First it was inquired about whether the subject felt that spine/hand/shoulder/knee or whatever type of surgery performed on a workers' compensation patient was generally cost effective.

Of the physicians responding, it was learned that they were generally not too keen on spine procedures:

- From the perspective of a heavy labor industry with few opportunities for restricted duty, some procedures have higher rate of recovery while others rarely allow an employee to return to their prior job. Nature of a specific job has an impact as well. For example, rotator cuff repair may be helpful in returning a laboratory technician or an engineer to work, but not for a log handler. Union contract limitations regarding job reassignments often thwart attempts in appropriate job placement. Knee surgery, even replacement, generally allows a worker to return to adequate function, while spinal fusion seldom does.
- No. Too much spinal surgery in patients who do not require it and who cannot give informed consent. The majority of shoulder injuries are deemed by providers to be work related when, we know, most RCTs are degenerative in nature and the result of aging, not a specific injury.
- Yes, except spine. Usually the hand/shoulder/knee conditions are of a nature that surgery resolves and /or improves function. Back is unfortunately a poor responder to surgery, better for physical therapy. Getting them back to work faster or just getting them back to work makes it cost effective.

This is likewise with adjusters and employers:

- No. Based on numerous studies that have been done, the surgical outcomes in workers' compensation are significantly worse than non workers' comp patients. This is because too many unnecessary, or ill-advised, surgeries are done.
- No. People in the system (less stakeholders - employers/employees/medical) are paid to sustain the system not mitigate the problems.

Such feelings were also generally shared by insurers, but with some exceptions :

- Spine surgery definitely does not seem to be an effective treatment in workers' compensation cases. There is an underlying mentality among injured employees of disability and oftentimes there is an underlying psych component that rears its ugly head once the employee undergoes spinal surgery. The majority of back cases could be treated non-surgically, but that onset of acute pain is scary to most employees and the physicians do not do a good job of reassuring employees that the acute pain is temporary and will resolve. Physicians also do not appear to either be comfortable with the topic or invested enough to deal with the underlying health issues of obesity, deconditioning, smoking, etc. It doesn't make sense to perform surgery on someone who is already sedentary and whose back pain would likely greatly improve with a little lifestyle change. To protect themselves legally, physicians often keep spinal surgery patients off - work for extremely long periods of time. There are many published studies that document that as the amount of time off work increases, the likelihood of ever returning to gainful employment decreases. There would probably be much better treatment outcomes if physicians were willing to rehabilitate patients by returning them to work in modified capacities as early as possible. The psychological and physical benefits are extraordinary.
- Totally depends on the injury, the employee and the treating physician. It is amazing how many surgical procedures do not resolve the problem, end up with complications or require additional surgical procedures.
- 32 years managing WC leads me to feel that spine and shoulder surgeries are not generally cost effective.
- Yes. With out this treatment fewer injured workers' would be able return to work.
- It really depends on the injury. There are some situations where surgery is necessary, such as torn meniscus or rotator cuff tears. In those cases, I would consider surgery cost effective. That being said, I believe physical therapy is a more cost effective form of treatment for most injuries.
- While surgery may be appropriate treatment for some injuries, I feel that often in the WC area it is treatment of first resort rather than under group health where more often is considered as treatment of last resort.
- I also feel that surgery can be cost effective, however; follow up and release need to be consistent and consideration for the person as a whole is important when making surgical intervention determinations.

- No.

Case managers, were a bit more mixed in their opinions:

- Surgery is cost effective in the hands of a good diagnostician and surgeon. Properly diagnosed conditions of the spine/hand/shoulder/knee with appropriate treatment, given in a timely manner offer the best opportunity for full recovery and RTW.
- Not without specific proof of need as verified by an MRI. Most procedures I find do no better than 6 months of light-duty work.
- Yes. I do. Especially for older full time or committed part time older workers', who represent a good investment in the workplace due to their sense of loyalty and their accumulated skills which can include management. More so because it can return them to the workplace and this is a benefit for the employer.
- In the case of younger individuals, save for traumatic injury, no. This can represent a lengthy cost to the employer that may never end especially if the individual does not tend to want to work.
- Spine surgery rarely seemed to benefit injured workers', unless it was a laminectomy.
- Knee surgery generally was successful, if arthroscopic. Hand surgery outcomes were very variable. Carpal Tunnel releases seemed to be 75% beneficial. Shoulders were notorious for not responding well to surgery, especially for rotator cuff repair. Fusions of any type, anywhere, seemed to create more problems than the original issue. Ankle fusion was the worst.
- If the diagnosis is correct and there is something surgically that can be done to remedy the symptoms, then surgery is answer. Having said that, surgery is still surgery...opening your body and that alone comes with risks even before you fix, remove or reconstruct anything.
- It depends on the diagnostic testing results & symptoms that a patient is experiencing. The bottom line is that if it is not necessary, the patient doesn't get better and it is certainly not cost effective. If it is medically necessary, the patient should "get better' and have a better RTW (even if it is with restrictions) & MMI.
- Surgery is cost effective in the hands of a good diagnostician and surgeon. Properly diagnosed conditions of the spine/hand/shoulder/knee with appropriate treatment, given in a timely manner offer the best opportunity for full recovery and RTW.
- If it is indicated! I heard an old physician from Texas put it this way: The less the indication for surgery the more the complications post operatively.

Athletic trainers are more optimistic, but still mixed:

- Yes when warranted. Because it works.
- On one hand I find that WC patients are quicker to receive MRI and surgery compared to off-the-job injured patients. On the other hand, I find that conservative treatment is sometimes hastened.
- Yes, but only after proper conservative care has failed. This includes injections, medications, physical therapy, and work modifications.
- It can be, depending upon the surgeon and the effective care and rehabilitation following. Athletic trainers are super with case management of these post-surgeries in rehab and constant communication with surgeon, injured employee and managing the return to full job skill status.
- Depends on the nature of the injury. Sometimes surgery is needed and sometimes it is more cost effective to have an aggressive course of physical therapy and work conditioning/hardening.
- Spine, less so than knee or shoulder but that **very** much depends on the surgeon, but shoulder and knee, definitely. With hands I have limited experience but my experience has been "no" because it made little or no difference for their RTW capabilities.
- No, I feel in many instances insurance companies for workers' compensation want to cut corners and get the individual back to soon. They will try and get something done before it needs to be and end up having to back track anyway.

And physical therapists were more in favor, but with caveats:

- If it allows the patient to return to their previous employment and make it a successful case then it is worthwhile. At times it seems that the delay of having surgery does not benefit the case.
- It depends on diagnosis. If there is no other option of treatment, then yes.

Employer attorneys generally saw pros and cons:

- I think surgery can be effective, but not in every case. I have seen surgery make established conditions worse and add to them when doctors do not fully review the claimant's medical history. Many WC physicians (on both sides) are in this for the perceived easy money and forget their ethics. We need to be as careful authorizing surgery for claimants as we would be a family member.
- Yes and no. The essential question, on a case by case basis, is whether this particular claimant needs the surgery proposed by the doctor. There are cases where the claimant doesn't get care quickly enough, and that is just as bad for an employer as the case where there is a rush to do an unnecessary surgery that makes things worse for both employer and employee. In particular, spinal fusion surgeries concern me. There are so many factors that go into the success or failure of a fusion, and a claimant who won't lose weight, quit smoking and participate actively in PT after surgery is NOT going to improve. In my experience knees, hands and shoulders can all present great cases for surgery and can present great cases to avoid surgery as well.
- It depends on the particular case. In some cases, surgery is completely unnecessary and unfortunately it is prescribed by some doctors who lacked any kind of concern for their patients. On the other hand, in some cases, surgery may be the best or only way to get the injured employee back to where he was before his injury. It is really case by case.

Consultants were more split:

- Absolutely not. Any time you cut on a back, there are major issues. I hate to send anyone to an orthopedic surgeon for a back. You get an employee with greatly reduced mobility.
- I do not have a strong opinion, other than I expect that surgery must always be considered an option.
- I feel it depends on the patient. If the Patient has not had previous surgeries, it may be effective. However, if it shows that the claimant has not responded well after an initial surgery, additional surgeries are probably not worth while
- Sometimes - results vary greatly. Much depends on the claimant's age, job, and the general motivation to get back into the work force and be productive.

Advocates view surgery as a necessary evil:

- When conservative treatment fails, surgery is the only alternative other than palliative care. Not all surgery is successful, but the rate of success has increased as research provides more information. Quality of surgical treatment is the most significant factor.
- If there is to be surgery then it should be completed as quickly as is possible, with the understanding that some injuries may require several surgeries to happen. I am always guided by the treating specialists as they are the ones who will be doing all that they can to ease the burden of the injury for the injured worker. I never totally disregard the Independent Medical Reports, but I am aware that the Independent Reports favor no surgery as the cost of surgery is high. I am of the belief that if a highly trained medical person is indicating surgery then they are doing so based on many years of medical training and practice. I am also of the belief that post surgery exercise and treatments are required if the injured worker is to make a full return to well-being. I am also aware that case managers will do all that they can to reduce the amount of money spent on the injured worker so as to reduce the cost of the claim regardless of the impact of the cost reduction on the long term health benefit for the injured worker.

Exercise physiologists were much more mindful of the associated complexities:

- I feel that WC related surgeries have a tendency to get abused on either side -- either by the "pro surgery side" of things or the "anti surgery-side" of things. Pro-surgery side can be something as simple as a surgeon motivated by WC reimbursement levels, to as complex as misleading a case or diagnosis for personal profit -- either by the MD, attorney involved, or patient himself. Anti-surgery side would be flat out denial of treatment regardless of merit. Both scenarios lead to poor outcomes, and lowers the cost effectiveness of treatment. So, I guess that's a long way of saying "not really" to the cost-effectiveness question.

- There are only two broad categories of information that can provide any meaningful information pertaining to the treatment of the comp patient: The medical and the behavioral. Of these two categories, only the medical is currently capable of being addressed objectively. The category of behavior is comprised of a long list of independent variables summarized here: social, financial and psychological. Of these, social and financial factors cannot be accurately quantified and the impact of financial factors can only be a matter of speculation. The psychological category is, in turn, subdivided into factors that include personality and motivation. The most commonly-used instruments to classify both of these factors are themselves the subject of debate, e.g. there is legitimate debate as to the appropriateness of the MMPI and similar instruments to assess the compensation patient. The field of industrial rehabilitation has attempted to address the issue of motivation with the use of various tests for validity of effort. The protocols are also said to classify function. The hope, presumably, has been to fill a void by providing information in the context of the claimant's diagnosis. Then, by combining what is known of the medical condition with the information from the FCE, it has been hoped (and promoted) that the FCE provides information on function and motivation (or behavior, etc.) that will move the case forward. The flaw in this thinking, however, is that function cannot be quantified unless something is definitively known regarding whether or not the claimant cooperated during the test. Unfortunately, attempts by the field to classify function and validity of effort have been largely based on plausible theories that simply do not work in the "real world." Examples: 1) Activities assessed in FCE protocols include range of motion testing, manual strength testing, assessments of tolerance for maintaining static postures, assessments of ability to take part in job simulation, and a variety of orthopedic assessments. Of these activities, there should be significant doubt that any of them can be used to add meaningful information to the picture---because they are almost completely under the control of the claimant and there is no objective method of verifying or disputing the results. 2) Two studies accepted for publication show definitively that static testing neither accurately quantifies function or validity of effort. 2) The most commonly-administered hand strength assessments for validity (the Bell Curve "analysis," the COV and Rapid Exchange Grip testing) have been called into serious doubt in at least 25 published studies in the past 20 years. 3) The most widely-used method of classifying levels of exertion and effort during a lifting assessment is based on the use of the so-called "visual estimation of effort." This concept, on its face, is not science. The application of "operational definitions" to classify either the level of exertion or cooperation is nothing more than guesswork. 4) In a study that has been conditionally-accepted for publication, the visual estimation of effort was shown to be accurate at a level that is slightly higher than chance and that lay subjects' estimations are as accurate as trained and experienced therapists. 5) Alternatives to the standard assessments of effort for hand strength testing and for the visual estimation of effort have been described in accepted-for-publication studies. The FCE provides a unique and one-time look at what is obviously a seminal moment in the administration of a compensation case. The potential importance of the event is not lost on the claimant. In effect, this is the juncture which all factors, medical and behavioral (which encompasses all of the aforementioned sub-categories) converge at one point in time. It is submitted that when objective data regarding the claimant's medical condition is combined with what can be objectively determined about behavior, these two axes of information can be combined to make better decisions related to case management. A simple matrix system can be used for this purpose, making the case management decision-making process more uniform, not arbitrary or capricious. Decisions made in this manner can be used to make rational decisions related to the need for additional diagnostic testing, the need for treatment or surgery, and whether the claimant is able (or should be able) to return to work in any capacity. With this answer in hand, the decision making process is based on objective information and becomes less a matter of attempting to control the outcome by changing various processes without reference to the two most important categories of information in the administration of compensation cases.

As a follow-up question, the subjects were asked whether they felt that **surgery affects patient outcomes.**

Occupational medicine specialists felt that:

- There are many variables, including patient's attitude and expectations, whether claim is readily accepted or challenged, surgeon's skill, patient's conditioning and commitment to rehab, supportive nature of employer, availability of work hardening, employee's job satisfaction, and supervisor's support. I have seen patients with median neuropathy (carpal tunnel syndrome), for example, improve and flourish having decided to avoid surgery, and others not improve after surgery and regret the intervention.
- Yes. We know that in many operations, patients in WC do worse than the general population.

Case managers are more mixed:

- Yes, surgery affects a patient's outcome, especially in work comp cases. Injured workers' tend to take longer to recover after surgery but outcomes can be managed. Using the Official Disability Guidelines (ODG) or the Medical Disability Advisor (MDA) provides guidelines for recovery.
- Maybe 50% of the time there is a positive result. If the case is litigated that drops to 10%. Back surgery is the least effective, carpal tunnel release seems to be the most successful.
- Surgery is individual. Patient outcomes for the older patient who hopes to return to work can be affected because there is a more reasonable expectation on the part of the patient. If the patient sees a physician for whom the surgery only represents a business number on the resume or more money in the pocket, then the care is not going to be useful for the patient outcome, only the MD.
- Patients placed so much faith in surgery; but were often disillusioned. They were so looking forward to cure. A lot of time/money was spent in helping to support/address their disappointment when things didn't work. And often, cases were closed by the insurer, before the workers' had reconciled to their fate.
- It depends on the surgery and circumstances. As the workforce ages, I feel that some workers' see surgery as a fix to all their problems. Certainly some things can be fixed, some things are beyond repair and some things are a result of aging and the best might not be what the injured worker sees as the best outcome.

Advocates were more concerned about the surgeon's skill and post-op care:

- Again, quality of surgical treatment is the most significant factor. There are far too many poor to bad surgeons practicing.
- Surgery is a small component of the outcome, it is a pivotal point where a major medical treatment is done, however if the follow up treatments are not done or are cut due to cost restraints that is where the real issues lie. If an injured worker needs 13 weeks of physio or hydro as recommended by the treating medical specialists then there should be no interference on the part of the case manager. If another 6 weeks of physio or hydro is recommended then that too should be agreed to. Case managers do not have medical degrees nor do they ever medically examine the injured worker, nor do they read the treatment notes or plans. So to my way of thinking case managers have no role in the medical component of an injured worker. I have seen very important surgeries fail because the case manager has not approved the cost of shower chairs, toilet chairs or high chairs for injured workers' to be in place when they return home, so weeks of surgery and post surgery care is undone due to want of a few hundred dollars of home care assistance.

Consultants seem to consider the complexity of the patient a more significant factor:

- It affects outcomes adversely. Many times those that seek surgery are bad candidates in the first place (i.e., overweight, diabetic, smoke etc).
- The results are bifurcated: some patients experience great relief and return to work. Others, for primarily psycho-social reasons, remain disabled. I do not believe that failure to recover is driven by surgical errors, but it is driven in part by poor patient selection (not attending to the psycho-social issues).

- My experience is that surgery is effective in about 50% of the cases. In most cases, it should be considered as the last alternative in treating an injury.
- Yes. It generally helps.

Employer attorneys consider that a necessary and well performed procedure does act to optimize positive patient outcome:

- Surgery can certainly affect patient outcome, but I do not understand the presumption that surgery makes a disability rating higher. Isn't the purpose of a medically necessary surgical procedure to improve the claimant's condition? If so many procedures are being authorized and performed without a successful outcome, doesn't that suggest that my comments above are accurate? If surgery is not improving conditions, is it really necessary? Are we over-prescribing it because we don't want to slow down and use our common sense? At times, **everyone** in the system is guilty of forgetting that the injured worker is a person. Although surgery is less invasive than in years past, it should still be considered carefully, and when it does not improve a patient's condition, we should be considering why rather than giving a blanket monetary award.
- Absolutely. A good surgery, timely delivered (particularly for spinal surgery) can spare a claimant unnecessary pain and hasten recovery time. When a surgery is done that should not have been done (particularly for spinal surgery) the result is almost always to make the claimant worse, extend disability, increase permanent injury and create an injury that requires much more medical care over time.
- Absolutely. If the surgery is a success and the person is recovering well his/her attitude will be much different than that of a person who was not a true surgical candidate and still went ahead with a surgery. A good surgical outcome also depends on the patient's determination and desire to recover. If you have someone who just wants to feel sorry for himself/herself, no amount of treatment is going to make a difference.

Exercise physiologists take a generally more positive view:

- Yes. Surgery either fixes legitimate orthopedic concerns or leads to better outcomes, or surgery is performed for a variety of WC related factors and leads to low-to-moderate outcomes. That's my experience. Most of the nebulous outcomes come from unrealistic patient expectations, poor direction/advice to patients from WC professionals, entrenched behaviors, stereo-typed opinions and view points -- all these factors and more lead to lower patient outcomes.
- Surgery will help---but only if it is indicated (the medical axis) and if the patient is motivated (the behavioral axis). Professionals in the field are reasonably competent on the first of these, but patient selection is the weak link in this two-link chain.

As do physical therapists:

- At times surgery is necessary due to the traumatic nature of some injuries. I believe that surgery should be performed as early on as possible in WC cases to allow for proper rehab potential.
- Depends if surgery is needed.

And, perhaps surprisingly, so do most insurers:

- Yes, generally for the positive, but the number of surgical procedures that do not resolve the problem is surprising. I do not know if sometimes treating physicians "over promise" and get the injured workers' expectations too high that surgery will "fix the problem" or if the surgical treatments are not successful due to error.
- It does, usually positively, though frequently not in a positive way.
- Yes, I believe it often provides patient ability to return to full duty.
- Majority of injured workers' have mind set of getting back to work quickly. However,a small percentage malinger and put forth less effort.

- Depends on the person and the surgery being considered. If the patient has a realistic expectation of the outcome of surgery quite often there are no problems. If the patient undergoes surgery without fully understanding limitations following I do not feel the outcome is positive
- Yes. It can assist with healing and/or bringing them back to a condition as close as possible to their condition before an injury.
- Yes.

Adjusters think that is affects outcomes, but...

- Of course it does. Once you alter a body part surgically, it is never the same as its original state.
- ...not necessarily for the better, just different.

At least one employer holds a more sardonic perspective:

- Absolutely. Using just one "workplace" injury as an example: Predictive probability of CTS diagnosis is (according to AMA) at 48% and the efficacy of CTS release surgery is 45% - why are you asking this question? The WC system finds that quite adequate (flipping a coin is more accurate) and there are a lot of people in the food chain drawing from the system - fixing the problem is not the objective of the WC system.

The majority of athletic trainers think so, and in a positive direction:

- Yes, if surgery is indicated; because if they need it they need it
- Yes, it can fix a structural problem, but also cause additional "perceived" complications/complaints from the patient.
- Of course. The intent is to correct the "disabling" condition.
- Yes, following surgery a patient never returns to 100% of their PLOF.
- Absolutely. With shoulder and knee you often (if not always) regain some degree of function and can improve with skilled therapy beyond that.
- No, if surgery is performed correctly and following an appropriate rehabilitation program an individual would be able to have the same outcomes as an individual with a group insurance.

The authors then moved on to cost estimates. Knowing that perspectives would vary as a function of one's position they thought they would gain some interesting responses to the question **"what they thought should spine/hand/shoulder/knee surgery procedures should cost".**

Occupational medicine physicians said:

- Less! Rates for Workers' Compensation are 100% guaranteed in this state (in comparison to 80% or less for other insurers), so physicians are incentivized (a) to declare a problem work related, and (b) to provide maximum interventions (including surgery).
- Surgeries in general are costlier than they should be (generalist speaking), I think we need more prevention (mother is 97, father 100) and surgeons should earn their keep but less. How much, I leave it up to society and medicine as a whole to decide.

Advocates noted that:

- Even in countries with socialized medicine, fee-for-treatment medical care is available. Fees charged by U.S. surgeons are the highest in the world. Insurance company exemption from RICO laws are one of the reasons this problem exists.
- I can not comment on this as cost would vary from hospital to hospital and surgeon to surgeon. I much prefer to look for the outcome of quality surgery rather than the cost in dollar terms of doing or not doing the surgery. I have never met a surgeon who has operated without due cause.

Consultants noted that it was more a matter of true medical necessity that was important, but another also wagered an amount:

- It is not the cost; it is the surgery that is done that shouldn't be.
- This is an impossible question to answer simply, but as a very rough estimate I would way 150-175% of Medicare rates,

Employer attorneys, physical therapists, and exercise physiologists felt they could not legitimately say a specific amount, but they had opinions:

- No idea. The only thing I know for sure is that they should cost more than Medicare reimburses.
- The price should be market-based. In other words, the price should be whatever the market will bear. If it is allowed to be market-based, good practitioners will rise to the top----if they make good decisions related to patient selection. Here again, behavior has to be quantified.

An adjuster thought that it should be:

- The same as it is for group health and Medicare.

Most athletic trainers did not offer an amount or opinion, but for those that did, they said:

- Cost plus 15%
- I think it should be similar to usual and customary charges of reimbursement similar to other major medical plans. I do not think it needs to pay much above that due to my beliefs in cost containment.
- Medical treatment costs are way too high anyway. I think surgical procedures should cost about 90% LESS than what they do now.

One case manager got down to dollars and cents while another looked at the context of the market and context of the individual, and another in the context of other third party payors:

- Spine surgery: $15,000, hand: $5,000, Shoulder: $5,500, Knee: $4,500
- Two things: look at comparative costs AND what is the value of that surgery to the injured worker.
- I think the cost of surgery in workers' comp should be somewhat related to the amount paid through private health insurance. If a work comp surgery pays the surgeon and hospital 200% more than group health, the pressure will always be to do more and questionable surgeries.

Insurers opined:

- I think this has been adequately addressed in the states that either have fee schedules or UCR databases. The fee reductions in those cases are quite high.
- Interesting question. I'm far less concerned with the pricing than the lack of consistent positive outcome, especially in the WC arena. I have better outcomes in the group health arena.
- Not sure, but would like to see more equality amongst w/c, group health, and private pay.
- Unsure - would depend on the surgery involved. Would like to see most surgeries be consistent with group health costs
- For the best corrective action possible for the client.

Our smart employer representative took a different tact and said:

- Efforts should be made to fix the problem, not sustain the system. Why are we measuring in only financial costs - if we fix the problem there are no continuing/residual costs. Bottom line: The system encourages disability not mitigation.

It would seem that our occupational medicine specialists are, as a group, not to be pleased with their orthopedic surgeon cousins. When we asked the question about their feelings as to **the data that suggest that spine surgeries have not improved patient outcomes but have nevertheless increased in frequency**, they said some pretty strong stuff:

- Not surprised. While I have seen some successes after back surgery, e.g. return to work without restriction, they are usually minimally invasive procedures, e.g. microdiskectomy. Many more patients are permanently maimed and/or analgesic (and Social Security) dependent.
- It's sickening. Until malpractice cases against surgeons are brought (on the basis of lack of informed consent) the system will be unlikely to change.
- I have that experience.

Employer attorneys tend to agree:

- I am not surprised. My personal and professional experiences have led me to similar conclusions.
- I reject the idea that this is true across the board. However, for the most part, fusion surgeries have that reputation, and I have seen many cases of failed fusion surgeries in which the result was bad for everyone (except the claimant's attorney and the doctor). Diskectomies seem to work, sometimes, and it is my experience that they either work, or don't work, but seldom make a claimant worse.
- I would agree. Again, there are many outstanding surgeons out there who will only perform necessary surgeries. However, there are several doctors who treat workers' compensation patients who prescribe surgeries like candy.
- Consultants seem to share a similar perspective, but are concerned with patient co-morbidities:
- You pay doctors for procedures, you get surgery. Let's have more "Biggest Loser" help for these overweight, out of condition folks who have medicated themselves with food and narcotics.
- I agree. There are two problems with spinal surgeries. One is not providing sufficient conservative care -- such as physical therapy / graded exercise -- before to see if that resolves the pain issue. The other is poor patient selection, with surgeons not attending to co-morbidities such as obesity, smoking, and mental conditions.
- I think surgery is often treated as the initial treatment option and not the FINAL option (as it should be in my opinion)
- Not surprising.

And exercise physiologists seem to consider such factors as well, along with the skill of the surgeon:

- It's hard to sift through all the contributing factors in such a question, but spinal surgeries have improved over the years -- I'm just not sure patient selection has kept up with innovation. Is that fair?
- Review the care providers' records. Find out what is going on. Surgeons who have poor outcomes are either taking on more seriously injured patients----or do not select their patients properly. (They could also simply be bad surgeons with the ability to talk people into having a surgery.

Advocates seemed a bit more forgiving, saying:

- Improved patient outcome depends on the type of procedure utilized and the point in the disease process at which time the surgery is performed. Many surgeons are very slow to adopt new technologies. In workers' compensation there is a bias centering on media fed beliefs of malingering and fraud.
- Spinal surgery is never an exact art; the variables are as much to do with the injured worker as to the skills of the surgeon. I have seen many injured workers' have spinal fusions over the years, some have returned to work within the expected time frame and others have not. The variable is the injured worker and the attitude that they have, the skill of the surgeon can only repair the damage to the spine.

Physical therapists are a bit more mixed, again, weighing the role of the patient, while another has had a generally positive experience with patients, thus contradicting the literature:

- I am a strong believer in core stability of the spine and mechanical diagnosis and treatment. If you do not modify the pt's habits then a surgery will not be successful.
- Surprised because the patients that had surgeries had overall good outcomes.

Athletic trainers as a group seem to have seen a great deal, and thus have varied opinions from one another as a group:

- An aging workforce and co-morbidities have more to do with **that** data than the type of surgery or the type of injury.....that study was incomplete.
- An efficacy study should be done and reported to W/C administrators. I note that W/C patients are more demanding of surgery and other expensive treatments than off-the-job injured patients.
- If you send a patient to a surgeon, they are going to think in surgical terms. That is their training and perhaps even so far as to say their job.
- I don't find that necessarily true in my local area; our spine surgeries have specific causes and specific strategies to have positive patient outcomes.
- That is the nature of the spine. Often times “rest” or “do not use” are large parts of post surgical procedures/protocols and that is impossible with a spine surgery. Everything you do, including breathing, eating and going to the bathroom put stress on the spine. Watch a surgery! You have to brutalize someone's insides just to fix their back. Many people think surgery is the cure-all and will find a surgery to cut on them, despite the potential for a good outcome.
- Surgery is only one aspect of treating the injury. The surgery may not have improved the patient outcome, but that is dependant on therapy received pre and post surgery, patient demographics, lifestyle...
- That I have had several individuals go through a work conditioning / work hardening program complaining of several problems. Although by the time they leave they may still have pain but they are functioning at a higher level then before the injury.

It was found that case managers’ perspectives reflect an abundant amount of experience:

- New techniques have advanced the field but matching the appropriate surgery to the patient's medical condition if often lacking.
- Actually since beginning in 1976 I have seen a dramatic drop in back surgery, but a higher success rate with better result in those cases that did have surgery. I attribute this to micro surgery techniques and earlier ambulation.
- The frequency of creation of MD offices that are specialized in this area causes an increase in surgeries for the financial benefit of providers but patient outcomes are not improved because the motivation for the care is displaced.
- Not at all surprised. People want to believe someone will 'fix' them...and while that is the case, there will always people who step up to try to fix them...even if the evidence is clear that surgical fixes do not lead to improved patient outcomes.
- Some people will risk the surgery and not look at other issues that can be worsening their symptoms. Smoking, obesity, lack of physical activity, poor attention to nutrition and mental/health well-being. People want a "quick fix" and sometimes that is the answer if there is the severity of symptoms to coincide.
- Because the general public will have a “non-perfect” MRI secondary to the aging process, I believe that patients want a “quick fix” and they also know that they get much more in the way of a settlement when they have had surgery.
- Claimants are too willing to undergo surgery immediately, very few are patient and willing to try conservative treatment, as a result too many spine surgeries are performed without positive outcomes.

- I think the data also suggests that the frequency of back surgery is related to only one meaningful factor: the number of back surgeons in the area. It is like asking a carpenter what he sees when he walks into a room. He sees nails that need to be pounded. Surgeons are no different.

Insurers were a bit more mixed:

- I think that physicians are put in a difficult position oftentimes, likely because of malpractice concerns. In certain geographic areas, employees are more likely to **demand** surgery, to have exaggerated pain complaints and to wallow in their disability mentality. The physician then has to decide whether to take a hard line position and make a judgment call about the validity of their patient's complaints, or after exhausting all other treatment options, they proceed with surgery. Then they have operated on someone who likely has underlying psych issues that complicate their recovery, they are unmotivated to return to work and now have a difficulty recovery which will prevent a quick return to work and they will likely become dependent upon narcotic pain medications. It is definitely a vicious cycle.
- I would agree with that statement, that is our observation as well.
- This is a known-known with business for years.
- Surprised...I didn't realize.
- I don't find it surprising. It seems that surgery becomes the fall back plan of action when a patient continues to have problems and conservative care has not provided improvement.
- I agree, however; I think this is true in both wc claims and group health issues.
- Extremely disappointing and concerning for people who advise and perform back surgery.

Our physician's assistant offered a helpful perspective on outcome studies:

- More individuals are performing these surgeries as instrumentation and techniques have become 'easier' to master. Some individuals perform surgery on patients who might otherwise improve/heal with other less invasive measures - this causes significant alterations in outcome data.

The next survey question sounds almost like a psychological projective test item. The authors wanted to know, **when they think of work related injuries, they think…"**

Our physician respondents said:

- …of how much better a "no fault" system of care would be, eliminating the need to establish causation, especially in areas of uncertainty (e.g. carpal tunnel syndrome, degenerative joint "disease", etc.), removing much of the legal and bureaucratic entanglement and costs.
- For workers' who need to work in order to make a living and to be fulfilled in life, I think about a biopsychosocial construct that requires expert handling to prevent disability. I see too much cynicism on the part of many claims adjusters and too much greed on the part of some medical providers and most attorneys, leaving the majority of injured workers' worse off than they should.
- …of strains/sprains related to poor posture and bad work habits, many that could be prevented by management/employee working together to identify and correct adverse work situations.

Advocates thought of sad situations:

- …media-driven bias against the injured worker. In two recent cases, the injured workers' each underwent three surgeries. The third surgery proved, without doubt, that the fist two were not performed correctly. The horror comes with the fact the individuals waited 4 to 5 years for the final surgery, having to first prove eligibility for Social Security and Medicare. Even sadder is the fact that these cases came to me after their attorneys had withdrawn.
- Confusion, frustration, fear, loss, legal, medical, jargon. Injured workers' are in pain, they find themselves in an insurance system that they have no understanding off, they have professional

strangers talking at them about all that needs to be done, paperwork to fill in and send off, they have no time to think about the process that they are entering.

Consultants thought of the worker as a victim or as a co-conspirator to the injury, or a function of poor design.

- I think of an impairment which triggers a psychological, social, and economic predicament for the patient. Whether the impairment is temporary or permanent, the predicament must be addressed constructively and directly by the patient, her or his medical providers, the employer, and the workers' compensation insurer.
- Of someone who has not taken care of themselves with appropriate diet and exercise. I also see some middle age employees who have not performed their jobs safely over a number of years. In addition, I see someone who most likely has a pre-existing condition but attributes all their pain to the current injury.
- I think of poor loss prevention efforts; including employee training, disregard for established safety procedures and employer indifference of a safe workplace.

Employer attorneys looked to the law to shape their views:

- ...we should remember the purpose of the WC laws. This is not a retirement system or a supplemental unemployment benefit. The law was intended to compensate injured workers' for lost earnings while expediting their access to reasonable and necessary treatment. Yes, it's a no-fault system, but this does not mean it is an automated system. The Judges are there to bring reason and common sense to disputes and to resolve them fairly. At least in New York, it seems most merely want to collect a state pension and play Robin Hood with insurance carriers (who they still believe are the parties to the action). They can't seem to comprehend that employers of all sizes and in all industries have employees who occasionally get hurt while working; not all employers are corporate giants out to screw the little guy.
- For the most part, I think of hard working employees who suffered legitimate injuries and need to be protected by the law.

Exercise physiologists and physical therapists focus empathically on the injured employee:

- …of injured workers' who are not prepared for A.) the injury itself, B.) the WC system and C.) all the social and economic upheaval they will experience. With good advice and good behavior, they will get good outcomes. If they encounter poor advice, behave poorly, or let things cloud the end result, they will likely be unsatisfied with the outcome.
- … of a group of people who may or may not be getting appropriate care. Most of the time, the clinical paths are ill-defined and haphazard because behavior is not being measured properly.
- People involved in a very physical and demanding job that are usually struggling to make a living.
- …getting them back to work through PT and WC/H

While one may think that athletic trainers may hold a similar perspective as exercise physiologists and physical therapists, they are a bit more divided:

- …a person is hurt, it will cost my client, and it is an honor to manage the two interests.
- These injuries could be prevented if greater caution taken at work and if the employee would take better physical care/wellness of his/herself.
- I become frustrated with pre-existing conditions that become "aggravated" by their work injury. If someone has knee osteoarthritis and they slip, of course their knee is going to hurt. And they end up with an MRI to discover they have a meniscal tear. The surgeon offers a knee arthroscopy and work comp agrees to it. While an MRI many times cannot determine whether a meniscal tear is new or degenerative, I think that WC should not have to pay for the scope to find out.
- Falls, sprains, strains, repetitive syndromes, poor computer workstation ergonomics.

- Malingering patients.
- Lack of safety, lack of education. So incredibly many of the injuries I have seen could have **should** have been prevented with proper safety precautions and education on how to use equipment properly, including safety equipment.
- Acute injuries - falling at work site. Chronic injuries - overuse, repetitious activities over a long period of time.
- Spine, Knee, Overuse.
- that professional athletes sustain different kind of work-related injuries and that athletic trainers and their team physician are best suited to care for them.

Case managers look empathically at the injured workers' situation, but also causal (and presumably) factors in the work environment:

- Not only is the individual injured but she/he has been impacted by a decrease in income.
- …of lack of good ergonomics, employer commitment to safety, poor risk management, overall carelessness.
- Companies do not prevent injury sufficiently and many large companies are not training staff adequately. Also companies that want to tighten the belt often do not repair pallet jacks and other large equipment, using older manual equipment that is a strain on the worker even if he/she is not injured. I think more can be done to protect our workers'.
- ...does the injured worker like his/her job?...does the employer truly value the injured worker? The answers to these two questions are the most influential drivers of case outcome.
- Keep walking backwards and asking "why" until you find the direct cause of the injury or symptoms.
- Let's get them better by providing the best medical care, the best physical therapy and let's close this case.
- Excellent benefits and resources for the patient and a lot of potential headache and difficulty for the employer.

Insurers offer interesting and varied points:

- At least 25% are questionable as to compensability, either the result of fraud from not occurring in the workplace, or are grossly exaggerated as to the severity by the injured worker resulting in longer than needed lost time and cost.
- Difficulty for an expedited return to work.
- 90% of all claims are without question and the other 10% cause more concern. With that being said, if a claim is not handled appropriately in the beginning even the 90% become more costly and litigated
- Insurance costs could go up.
- It could have been prevented.

The Employer minces no words as he/she thinks only two things when thinking of workers' comp:

- Bureaucracy and fraud.

Now, at the Individual Level

It was learned that survey subjects aren't shy about sharing their thoughts or being vague or cryptic—which is great. The next set of questions, the authors were curious about, dealt with the 'people-aspect' more so than "systems" of workers' compensation. To start things off, subjects were asked to **describe the ideal workers' compensation patient.**

The occupational medicine physicians described them as:

- An employee with a tangible (e.g., fracture) injury with readily identifiable on-the-job mechanism of injury, who responds to treatment with full recovery.
- Good job; good premorbid state; supportive employer and family. Non-smoker, non-obese.
- Employee who has a real work related condition, who has a keen interest in getting well, who listens to the medical advice given and not to the neighbors advice as to how to get an early pension, and who takes his treatment in stride.

Advocates see the ideal injured worker as:

- A person who seeks legal assistance and advice immediately. (Once even an innocent infraction of law has taken place, the claim becomes a nightmare.)
- For me the best WorkCover claim would be a claim that I was involved with from day one so as I could put control steps in place and each person involved was informed continuously as to the progress being made by the injured worker at key intervals. The injured worker would be involved in the entire process instead of what happens now is that the injured worker almost becomes a by-product of their own claim.

Consultants aren't too dissimilar, but their fear of manipulation manifests somewhat:

- Someone who is motivated to get well, doesn't have alternative agendas (like staying home with their kids because they suddenly don't have any childcare expense), and who is willing to rehabilitate themselves; Some one who is willing to do light duty; Someone who does not watch daytime TV with ads about attorneys telling them how awful their employer is.
- Someone who regardless of the severity of injury or illness, is highly self-effective and thereby can work with all involved parties to recover functioning as much as possible.
- Someone whose primary goal is to return to the workplace in a modified....and then <u>full</u> duty capacity as soon as possible (reasonable and practicable).
- Someone who was legitimately injured on the job, and is motivated to get proper treatment and return to work.

Employers' attorneys would be happy if:

- The ideal workers' compensation patient gives a consistent history of the accident and fully discloses all prior injuries to the same body part. Authorizations for release of medical records are signed without requiring judicial intervention. Appointments are kept. Recommendations are followed. There is cooperation with attempts to accommodate work restrictions, and the injured worker returns to work. If restrictions cannot be accommodated, vocational rehabilitation is welcomed. Upon completion of the program, there is a return to work.
- Motivated to return to health, and to work. Understands the need to participate in his/her care, and to do the work that will enable recovery.
- Someone who truly wants to go back to work. If you have an injured employee who doesn't like the employer, doesn't want to go back to work, feels he won the lottery by getting injured, etc. successful medical treatment will be almost impossible.

Exercise physiologists are by this point our most existential of the professions responding; here are some more examples:

- A person who never intended to get injured, has a legitimate injury, and understands that he/she can never retire off of a WC claim—so their entire goal and mindset is to return to work and provide for themselves and their family.

- Regardless as to the type of injury, the ideal patient is one who is fortunate to have a job that he/she likes and a job for which there is security. This person will also have good self esteem and be motivated to have the best possible outcome.

Of course, physical therapists want to get down to business:

- A patient who is motivated to return to work, whether it is to achieve overtime or because he/she truly enjoys their profession. They are excited and prepared for PT.
- Motivated, good HEP compliance, good attendance.

Adjusters, who seem to be pragmatic, albeit a wee bit pessimistic, said:

- Someone who is motivated to get back to work and does not focus on their pain and disability. Someone who wants to get better, but understands that sometimes you never get back to baseline. Someone who will adapt to their current situation and make the best of it.

Athletic trainers were broader:

- Health (other than the injury of course), compliant, motivated.
- The ideal W/C pt is one that is motivated to return to work. One that doesn't treat W/C like an entitlement program. A W/C pt would act more like my off-the-job injury patients.
- Ideal? Patients who are realistic about their injury and they understand that they should not be seeing dollar signs. They should be concerned with getting better and not the monetary aspect.
- Motivated to get back to work, attends rehab sessions, completes home program as assigned, continues with whole body wellness while rehabbing the injured body part, and is up-front with health care professional on difficulties or successes in performing tasks relating to injury care.
- One who is motivated to return to work and do what it takes to improve their condition.
- Great attitude. Legitimately wants to get back to work and is willing to work hard at it but at the same time listen to their clinician. Minimal pain. Shows weekly progress. They are happening to be here, appreciative of the work we/I put in to their program.
- Motivated to get better and re-enter the workforce - whether at old job or new job.
- An individual motivated to get back to work, but at the same time take the necessary precautions to control their rehabilitation instead of becoming too aggressive. They would also have an insurance company that would allow the therapist and MD to decide the appropriate treatment needed for the individual instead of a case manager who does not see the individual on a regular basis.

Case managers, who by this point seem to be the most ecumenical, said:

- Accepts responsibility for their participation in the treatment plan.
- Goal is to return to work as soon as possible.
- One who is committed to rehabilitating and getting back to work - no matter what.
- The ideal patient asks a lot of questions, seeks second opinions, goes to appointments, values the physical therapists and pharmacists as sources of information (since the physicians do not have time to explain to patients) and the patient will have a direct dialogue with the nurse case manager regarding expectations, often because the adjuster is not available to talk with the patient or avoids being readily available.
- Someone who doesn't perceive himself/herself as a victim and rather sees themselves as temporarily delayed but soon to get back in the swing of 'normal' life.
- Ideal? Appreciative of their job/employer, good attitude of life/family in general, responsible individual, follows the physicians orders and suggestions, doesn't see himself as "sick" but just not

100% right now but getting better, willing to learn from the experience and pull something positive from what has happened.

- Compliant and puts forth an effort.
- A person without baggage when injured. A person who possesses insight and who understands that to become whole again they must accept their injury, rehab and return to their normal life as soon as possible.
- Understands her/his injury and need for appropriate treatment.
- Accepts responsibility for their participation in the treatment plan.
- Goal is to return to work as soon as possible.
- Someone I can work with early in the case to ensure that long term rehabilitation goals are being addressed from that point. You will then generally have a person, despite severity of injury, etc who will maintain future focus on work and career. Once that focus is lost (sometime between 6 and 12 months) you start to develop long term chronic pain problems that are very difficult to treat effectively.

Insurers seem to blend the employer with the employee:

- It all starts with a positive relationship with their employer. If the employee likes their job and likes their employer, the work comp claim is going to have a dramatically different outcome than a claim from someone who is disgruntled about their job. An early return to work has so many positive psychological and physical rehabilitation benefits, so an employee is willing to return to work and an employer who is willing to accommodate modified work is essential. The patient must also have a reasonably stable home environment with no underlying psych issues or drug dependency issues.
- An employee that is self-motivated to return to work in a reasonable period and accepts responsibility to follow treatment protocols including physical therapy. The ideal patient would also acknowledge if their negligence in following work procedures, instructions or common sense was the cause of their injury.
- One whose interest is returning to work but not in accruing the largest payout.
- Someone who is motivated to get better, and is compliant with Dr's orders, Therapist direction, etc.
- The ideal workers' comp patient is someone who works with their doctors, therapists and employer in order to reach the end goal of healing and returning to work.
- Understanding that healing is as much mental as physical - someone who asks questions and responsive
- One who is legitimately injured at work and wants to be treated and return to work as soon as possible.
- One who is informed about everything regarding the safety, claims and medical management policy of their employer before ever entering the medical facility. How much their employer cares about them and their welfare.

And, similarly, physicians' assistants see patients as:

- Suffering from an acute injury, anxious to return to occupation. Motivated to rehab, follow restrictions and precautions.

Professionals Involved

The next set of questions involved getting into areas where there was the potential for some biases to show as well as egos. The authors structured a series of questions asking respondents to opine on the role of MDs, Surgeons, Pain Medicine Physicians, Case Managers, Adjusters, Vocational Counselors, Patients, Employers, Plaintiff Attorneys, Employer Attorneys, Judges, Arbitrators, Physical Therapists, Athletic Trainers, Psychologists/Psychiatrists and Chiropractors, and occasionally some respondents additionally chose to offer their opinions as well.

The formatting for this section of questions is based more so on the role of the professional and a notation of the profession of the person responding.

Role of the Physician in Workers' Compensation Cases

A) From the Case Manager's Perspective

- Assess if treatment plan is working, Address work status at every appointment, Refer to specialist in a timely manner
- ...the MD should be committed to returning function, minimizing pain and establishing RTW criteria at as early a date as possible
- MDs can be educated as far as workers' compensation regulations and reporting requirements, and they have a better chance of behaving in a collaborative way if they are not the older doctors who still resist providing information since they remember the days prior to Work Comp reform during which they could prescribe unending treatments. Those with a proper attitude (and they need to recognize that about 30% of health care in this country right now is industrial related injuries, therefore the patients bring them the work they need) will embrace the chance to teach the patient and be proactive in prevention of injury.
- Traditionally MDs tend to "medical-ize" non-medical issues - but I work with a large number of them now -and promote the message summarized by Dr Jennifer Christain (Webility) and her work with ACOEM re: time off work if MEDICALLY necessary; with a view to preventing needless disability in the workplace. This concept is slowly making inroads with MDs who treat work-related injuries.
- Their role is one of listening to the Injured worker, getting as many facts about what happened or what the Injured worker does at work and away from work, get the correct diagnosis as soon as possible with attention to the cause and to explain his role in assisting the worker to continue his routine of work etc, with some minor set backs or restrictions. He is to evaluate the worker on what he feels they are capable of performing.
- It depends who the MD is. If he is a good, reputable MD then he is the driving force who provides excellent medical and/or surgical care. If he is not reputable, then he is a barrier to the patient & to the work comp industry as a whole by increasing costs with unnecessary tests, treatments, therapy etc.
- Properly diagnose injury, Create treatment plan within ODG, Implement treatment plan, Assess if treatment plan is working, Address work status at every appointment, Refer to specialist in a timely manner.
- In other words, differential diagnosis, appropriate treatment and goodbye.

B) From the Athletic Trainer's Perspective

- The MD is top of the food chain. The client gets to choose who is on their WC panel. I balance patient interest and company interest. Injured workers' have to trust company is not out to screw them. The company has to trust injured worker is not out to screw them. We balance each perception and drive for a low cost positive outcome.
- They are the key to making sure the patient understands their care and that the surgery may or may not make them better. Perception of improvement should be discussed.
- Involved, supportive, responds to healthcare provider phone messages, emails, fax, etc.
- Overall direct the care of workers' comp cases.
- Very important. They can set the stage by telling the client "you will never _______ again" and have some crazy restricting protocol or they can give the client a boost when they need it, hold their hand when the need it and listen to the people that work with them day to day. Ultimately, I can't do my job if they don't.
- Should be the ultimate gate keeper - educating the pt. on injury, treatment options and then steering them down the right path.
- I believe the MD should be the actually Orthopaedic Surgeon. That way they can receive the same care throughout the entire process.

C) From the Adjuster's Perspective

- They are the engine that drives the entire system. Approx 60% of all WC dollars are medical.

D) From the Physical Therapist's Perspective

- They serve as the gatekeeper in providing the pt. with the appropriate care.

E) From the Occupational Medicine Specialist's Perspective

- Central, but often misused or misappropriated.
- Crucial. The doctor should understand the injury, the job functions of the worker, the psychological and social issues that could influence the recovery, he/she should have a functional mindset, he/she should be an educator and a great communicator since he has to deal with so many stakeholders. BTW, these skills and behaviors should be rewarded above and beyond physicians dealing with the same injuries in the general population.
- Keeps in touch with the employee, has a keen interest in the employees well being and acts as a coordinator to make sure that the services are being offered as needed.

F) From the Exercise Physiologists' Perspective

- They are the quarterback of the team. They set the tone and it all starts from there.
- The MD has a critical role. They need to be competent in their clinical skills and their ability to solve complex problems. They need to always put the patient's interest first---whether that means to do additional testing or provide another service, or to give that person a therapeutic boot in the ass.

G) From the Insurance Professional's Perspective

- A physician who has the ability to reassure patients regarding their symptoms, expected recovery and is willing to lean towards conservative treatment is helpful. I think that physicians are put in a difficult position oftentimes, likely because of malpractice concerns. In certain geographic areas, employees are more likely to **demand** surgery, to have exaggerated pain complaints and to wallow in their disability mentality. The physician then has to decide whether to take a hard line position and make a judgment call about the validity of their patient's complaints, or after exhausting all other treatment options, they proceed with surgery. Then they have operated on someone who likely has underlying psych issues that complicate their recovery, they are unmotivated to return to work and now have a difficulty recovery which will prevent a quick return to work and they will likely become dependent upon narcotic pain medications. It is definitely a vicious cycle.
- Most MD's do an excellent job treating injured workers' and attempt to maintain a fair and open-minded position as to what is in the best interest of the patient and employer. Some however, are not objective and honor any and every request by their patient to prolong time off of work or light duty restrictions when in fact the employee should be able to return to their jobs. I'm sure this is the doctor not wanting to upset their patient or open themselves up to malpractice concerns.
- Critical yet very frequently disappointing.
- To provide patient with best options for treatment, and assist with making these difficult decisions.
- Doctors are extremely important in workers' comp cases. They are on the frontline, so to speak, and it is their findings and actions that can make or break a claim.
- The primary factor in release from treatment and ability to return to work or normal activities of daily living
- The party who is directing the medical treatment.
- Some are extremely good, proactive, and consultative, respect their employer and try to get people back to work within their job restrictions.

H) From the Employer's Attorney's Perspective

- The MD is there to make money. This, however, is not the ideal. The ideal MD will take a complete history of the accident and questions details that do not make sense. Tests and treatment are requested as truly necessary, not merely because the MD can perform them in an attached or affiliated office. Records are well-maintained and produced according to Board rules. The MD remembers the goal is to return the injured worker to an occupation and self-sufficiency whenever possible.

- Two roles: First to give the employee reasonable medical care, with the aim of achieving healing and return to function; Second to provide opinions and explanations so that the parties to the workers' compensation claim can all understand what is occurring on the claim.
- The role of a doctor in a WC case is of the outmost importance for all parties involved. A good doctor will guide his patient through the very difficult process of recovering from his injury until he can go back to work. If you don't have a good doctor, your case will linger forever and the injured employee will suffer greatly.

I) From Consultant's perspective

- They should be independent with the goal of returning their patient to work. Many times, these folks are enablers. In addition, I have seen physicians overuse pain relievers because they don't know what else to do. Not a solution.
- The MD is essential as providing a central provider / medical home for the patient. The treating MD is the most important party in ensuring that the patient is well educated on treatment and in ensuring that all clinical and non-clinical (such as modified duty) approaches are taken into consideration.
- To be on the same page as the employer in trying to return the worker to the workplace as soon as practicable.
- Helpful - recommends proper treatment - but must be monitored.

J) From Employer's perspective

- Just below the employer and employee as stakeholders. Everybody else feeds on the system.

K) From Advocate's perspective

- The physician must be an advocate for his or her patient. The patient's medical needs must be the only factors relevant to the doctor's decision making. Too often, the insurer directs the care provided. Frequently, the physician lacks even minimal knowledge of workers' compensation law. More importantly, experts for hire must be outlawed. An IME exam becomes a haven for those who find they cannot practice medicine.
- The most important person within each claim next to the injured worker is the attending doctor, the attending doctor builds the framework of return to pre-injury health around the injured worker, yet the case managers appear to over ride the medical training of the attending doctor with the belief that the legislation is far better than the medical training of a highly skilled doctor.

2. Role of the Surgeon in Workers' Compensation Cases

A) From the Case Manager's Perspective

- Examination of injured worker, mechanism of injury and diagnostic testing should correspond. Explain expectation of outcome in percentage. Confirm injured worker understands time frame expectation for RTW post-operatively. Provide firm RTW plan.
- Generally as unnecessary. They should do the deed and return care back to the PTP.
- Surgeons, if they are legitimate and caring can be very useful. They do not have a great track record in terms of sharing information but we cannot live without them.
- They are distant, remote; tend to focus only on the physical aspect of surgery rather than the holistic individual aspect.
- Again, it depends on the surgeon. Dr. Alex Ghanayem, Dr. John Fernandez, Dr. Simon Lee, Dr. Merck, Dr. David Burt --- awesome. You can be very confident that they did the absolute best job in the world. Umm, I won't name the other surgeons. Then you just know you have a "mess on your hands"!

- Examination of injured worker, mechanism of injury and diagnostic testing should correspond. Explain expectation of outcome in percentage. Confirm injured worker understands time frame expectation for RTW post operatively. Provide firm RTW plan.
- Technical skill is crucial but judgment is a very, very close second.

B) From the Athletic Trainer's Perspective

- Overall direct the care of workers' comp cases.

C) From the Adjuster's Perspective

- They do surgery, nothing else. If you refer someone to a surgeon, they will probably have surgery.

D) From the Physical Therapist's perspective

- They seem to play almost a secondary role in performing the surgery to allow for the supervising physician to progress their care.
- Important, but should be more conservative initially.

E) From the Occupational Medicine Specialist's Perspective

- Consultant to the primary physician caretaker of the employee.
- Limited. Provides an informed opinion as to the necessity of surgery; if indicated, fully informs the patient on the risks and rewards of any procedure, as well as the other available options.
- Depends on the condition. Last resort in many, first resort in obvious correctible cases (broken bones, torn ligaments, burns, etc.).

F) From the Exercise Physiologist's Perspective

- The surgeon becomes the quarterback in surgical cases. Other MDs fall to support roles.

G) From the Insurance Professional's Perspective

- Even more critical and even more disappointing.
- To provide patient with best options, as well as, alternatives to surgery.
- Surgeons are important to workers' comp cases because, like the treating physicians, their actions can greatly affect the outcome of a claim.
- If surgery becomes apparent I feel the surgeon should take on primary care of the injured worker
- The party who is assessing the need for and performing the surgery.
- Oftentimes like Darth Vader...

H) From the Employer's Attorney's Perspective

- No different from any other medical provider. Each must exhibit the highest possible ethics and processes to ensure that the injured worker receives competent care that will improve the injury or condition.
- If there is a need for surgery, a surgeon then is extremely important. Not all cases will require a surgeon's involvement though.

I) From Consultants' Perspective

- Should be extremely conservative in their treatment. Surgery should be the absolute last resort.
- The surgeon is a specialist who must learn how to approach the patient with knowledge of all possible ways to addressing the patient's impairment, not just the surgical approach.
- To perform quality intervention on injured workers' where evasive medical involvement is really the last and only option.
- An expert. Performs procedures, and recommend recovery.

J) From an Advocate's Perspective

- Surgeons come in for a short space in time, and then they do their craft and then exit all within a short space in time of the over all claim. The surgeons know only what went wrong and how to fix it then how to give directions of post-operative care. After that surgeons have no role within the injured workers' claim.

3. Role of the Pain Medicine Specialist in Workers' Compensation Cases

A) From Case Managers' Perspective

- Provide adequate pain relief but allow for injured worker to function in his personal and work life.
- I assume you refer to a physiatrist, in which case very positively. They tend to work best at returning function, managing pain and returning the employee back to work quickly.
- Pain medication clinics are becoming more prevalent, but the pain med doc who is dedicated to keeping the patient from addictions and is a good treater/teacher has a strong future role.
- For many years I snidely looked sideways at pain management practitioners, viewing their efforts similar to teaching pigs to sing; it frustrated both the teacher and the pigs. A harsh view, I realize. However, with recent, more subtle application of CBT techniques and pain control methodologies, I have changed my tune and have seen some constructive outcomes with the most hardened 45yr+ truck drivers and construction workers' developing self-control in managing chronic pain.
- The pain may or may not be something that will go away completely. In the meantime, how can the physician make the person most comfortable and most functional.
- I do not trust any of them in the Chicagoland area with the exception of Dr. Samir Sharma. They bill like crazy and create addicts by not recognizing the "secondary gain" issues and the addiction issues.
- Provide adequate pain relief but allow for injured worker to function in his personal and work life.
- Pain medicine is usually the dumping ground for chronic pain patients. They treat the patients who have lost future focus on work and career. Many times the only model that they offer is pharmacology with no demonstrated or documented outcomes. **There is a need for pain treatment outside of this model.**

B) From Athletic Trainers' Perspective

- As the guy who handles chronic pain management cases.
- Often, pain management physicians are slow to return a patient to full duty. The un-motivated patient can "milk" the system more easily under a pain management physician as opposed to the others.
- It should be limited in that the patient has to take a certain amount of responsibility for their pain.
- Assist surgeon/MD and prescribe pain meds/injections to decrease patients' pain.
- If they see one, very important.
- Last option in treatment (in regard to MD's).

C) From an Adjuster's Perspective

- It depends. A good pain management physician can help the injured worker return to a functional state. They should be minimizing narcotic pain medication and focusing on coping skills. Unfortunately, there are too few good pain management physicians out there and lots of bad ones that hand out narcotics like jelly beans.

D) From an Adjuster's Perspective

- I believe that pain medicine physicians usually prescribe meds too soon and that these meds interfere with PT interventions at times. Patients then become too dependent on a passive way to treat their pain. These meds interfere with driving and daily activities.
- They should wean themselves off when no longer needed ASAP.

E) From Occupational Medicine Specialists' Perspective

- Consultant to the primary physician caretaker of the employee. Often resorted to when no other treatment is available or effective.
- Pain medicine today generally means (1) lifetime opioids and (2) lucrative injections and procedures; none of these generally help the patient with chronic pain, although they may be useful in the acute period. A biopsychosocial, functionally restorative approach does work, however. I have never (?) seen a chronic pain WC patient graduate from a pain management program.

Important if they offer physical therapy and alternatives to work in a rehabilitative phase. What I see mostly is an attempt to alleviate pain but nothing else. This leaves the patient with less pain but fear of its recurrence and of losing their job.

F) From Exercise Physiologists' Perspective

- A last ditch effort for cases that have not gotten better through conventional means.
- Limited role. Too much use of methods that do not work.

G) From Insurance Professionals' Perspective

- Unfortunately, I have not had any real positive outcomes as the result of treatment with a pain management physician. The amount and cost of medications prescribed seems to increase when treatment begins with a pain management physician. I wish their role was to identify areas in which patients could be tapered off of certain medications, and possibly all medications over a period of time. Instead, the mentality seems to be that once you are on these pain management medications, you will need to continue taking them for your life expectancy.
- Pain management is a new yet critical dynamic that the US needs to further develop. There have been some intriguing advances in other parts of the world with pain management specialties.
- In my experience, very necessary. However, often over utilized.
- Questionable and feel that measures need to be taken to confirm usage of medications as well as potential for addiction
- The party who is assessing the need for it and monitoring it's effectiveness.
- Oftentimes like Voodoo...

H) From Employer's Attorneys' Perspective

- Pain management should be a last resort; after all other treatment has failed. The risk of addiction and destruction of internal processes due to long-term pharmaceutical use is too great.
- At the end of the line, after curative treatments have failed, a good pain management physician can help to maximize a claimant's function while minimizing the pain he or she experiences.
- Not all injured employees require this type of care. That being said, pain management can be the difference between a decent recovery or someone who will abuse medications.

I) From Consultants' Perspective

- Pain medication can play a proper role. Too often, it is misused.
- The pain medicine specialist similar to the surgeon delivers one of several complementary or alternative solutions to the patient's pain issues and much understand all the various approaches. Generally speaking, most pain management specialists are ignorant of the other solutions and/or discount them.
- To issue prudently RX that gradually and consistently return the injured employee to their drug free pre-injury status. They need to make firm and medically prudent decisions and should NOT serve as an enabler for the injured employee to remain on narcotics long term.
- Support role to assist in recovery.

J) From Advocates' Perspective

- A patient's medical needs must be the only factors relevant to the doctor's decision making. Human beings should not be allowed to suffer needlessly. Superior pain management permits successful rehabilitation. The treating physician must write adequate, timely reports which comply with legal requirements. The legally required forms must be filled on time.
- The attending medical doctor should understand that medication is a control component of the injured workers' claim. I would like to see much more information given to injured workers' in regard to the side effects of medication, especially pain medication. I would like to see nutritionist being involved so as the injured worker can understand the need to eat foods that will ease the passage of the medication throughout the body. Far too many injured workers' take pain medication and end up constipated because they do not increase the amount of fiber or water in their diet to enable to body to expel the medication before constipation sets in. I would also like to see an increase in natural medications used instead of the chemical based medications. I know that the process takes longer, however the side effects are far less and the damage to the injured workers' system is not great.

4. Role of the Case Manager in Workers' Compensation Cases

A) From their own Perspective

- advocate, coordinate, facilitate, educate
- Absolutely crucial. They keep the medical people on task, they make sure the employee is getting all that they need and on a timely basis and they keep the employee moving forward, connected to work and thinking only of RTW.
- Nurse case managers have a great role in supporting communication between the patient, the therapist, and the adjuster. Nurses must teach the patient how to communicate with physicians and adjusters. Patients have need for someone to listen. The therapist and the nurse are two individuals who can provide these important supports.
- Case Managers can be highly influential and supportive, but too often Case Managers are restricted by legislation and corporate rules. The best Case Manager tell injured workers' on Day One that they have a limited time to maximize recovery and then encourage/assist the worker to optimize available benefits (on a broad level) to recover.
- To educate, listen, assist in getting the injured worker back to his pre-injury state, and to help keep the focus on recovery.
- They can impact a case in a very positive or very negative way. It depends on the nurse case manager!
- I view the Case Manager role as an advocate for the injured worker, physician and insurance company. The Case Manager understands the positions of the injured worker, physician and insurance company. Case Managers frequently get involved in a case long after there have been numerous misunderstandings which have resulted in delay of treatment, non compliance and increased cost. They are experienced at resolving these issues and moving the treatment/rehab toward closure.
- Most of the time, they are empathetic and caring and can have a huge impact on helping the injured worker in the acute phase of injury. They can also be passive and intimidated and not effective in helping the injured worker maximize his recovery including return to work at an appropriate level. I often see cases where a Case Manager has worked on the file for years, yet the outcome was disastrous anyway. That should never happen.

B) From Athletic Trainers' Perspective

- My best friend to help manage the cases.
- Vital! They are the gate keeper, they round up all of the information from various sources, and they can be huge with regards to problem people.
- The athletic trainer is the case manager and follows the injured employee from traumatic event until return to full duty. It is a comprehensive roll -- not unlike that of the athletic trainer in a collegiate/university setting.

- Link between the Adjuster, MD, Attorney, Patient, and Rehabilitation.
- Important. They are the link between us and what is going on outside of the clinic. The more they understand that, are willing to work with us and listen to what we see/here/want the easier the case runs.
- The Case Manager should be involved to help the pt; handle the decisions involved with their work comp case - my check didn't arrive, can you help track it down for me; I need to set up physical therapy, can you help schedule my appointment. The Case Manager should not be involved with determining the case outcome directly.
- I feel that some Case Managers are individuals that try to cut corners for a work comp injury and eventually cause more damage to the individual in the long run.

C) From an Adjuster's Perspective

- Advocate for both the injured worker and the employer. They are supposed to keep things moving in the right direction.

D) From Physical Therapists' Perspective

- They allow for quicker referrals, imaging, and overall treatment in these cases.
- Important means of communication, all WC cases should have a Nurse Case Manager.

E) From Occupational Medicine Specialists' Perspective

- Supplementary to the managing physician. Often an unnecessary step/expense that insurers defer to, when an effective primary physician should provide same or more extensive services.
- Limited; should only be used in catastrophic cases to assist the family and insurance company to provide the best care and to educate.
- Very helpful. They take a load off the physician, dedicated to the service. I personally have one.

F) From Exercise Physiologists' Perspective

- If a Case Manager is a professional and works with the true intention of getting the patient appropriate medical care and RTW is the end goal -- they are a value add. If not, then an unnecessary hurdle to the system.
- Critical. Just as important as the treating physician. Should be the person who has a bird's eye view of the entire case.

G) From Insurance Professionals' Perspective

- Reassure the patient regarding symptoms, treatment plans, and treatment options. Communicate modified return to work options to the physician. Work with the employers to devise appropriate modified job responsibilities for injured employees.
- Generally they have good instincts but their effectiveness has diminished in recent years due to patient confidentiality requirements and certain state imposed limitations as to what carriers and employers may impose on injured workers'. Case Managers do not have the same access to medical information on injured workers' as they did in past years. This lack of informational access has diminished their ability to be as effective as in the past.
- Can be a valuable asset to achieve cost effective case closure but is entirely dependent on their dedication and ability to create a rapport with the claimant.
- Very beneficial with coordinating care amongst providers, doctors, etc.
- Case managers can be an extremely important member of the claim team. They can be vital in ensuring that a claimant is following through on the treatment plan outlined by the doctor, which in the long run, can help keep down the ultimate cost of the claim.
- Should be very positive - however; case manager (if you are referring to medical case manager) must remember he/she is there to assist the patient first & the carrier/employer second.

- The party who is coordinating the overall treatment of the patient to assist in expediting the injured persons recovery and return to work.
- Extremely helpful if they are a high level professional.

H) From Employer's Attorneys' Perspective

- To monitor the treatment, keep the employer apprised of developments and serve as intermediary between the claimant, the employer and the treating physicians.
- Not all cases require a case manager.

I) From Consultants' Perspective

- Nurse case managers are invaluable.
- The case manager's role is partly patient education, and partly to serve as an advocate to help the patient navigate through a complex medical maze.
- An active link in working with Employers and Medical providers to return injured workers' back to the workplace. (Initially in a modified and then Normal position) They need to be an employer advocate with the medical professional showing the willingness of the employer to provide alternative working accommodations.
- Good resource to assist in communication and aid in getting an appropriate return to work - and assure that injured workers' are compliant with care.

J) From an Employer's Perspective

- They are a "crumb" offered by the WC system to show the "people that they care about the injured."

K) From Advocates' Perspective

- Case manager services in workers' compensation would be an advantage for both employer and employee -- if they were not influenced and paid by the insurer/employer. The primary responsibility should be to prevent duplication of services, and to insurer the plan of care is followed.
- **Badly.** I have very little trust in the current system of case management.

  Case management should be about making sure that the injured worker is the center of the claim at all times, not about cost reduction, not about removal of rights, not about intimidation, but about the best possible outcome for injured workers'.

5. Role of the Adjuster in Workers' Compensation Cases

A) From their own Perspective

- The adjuster should be working to ensure that the benefits are paid timely, that the injured worker receives appropriate medical care, and that the case progresses towards resolution. They should be the driver of the bus.

B) From Case Managers' Perspective

- Monitor total cost of claim, apply work comp laws.
- The adjuster should be working with the employer to maximize effective medical treatment, minimize costs, educate the employer on how to proceed and to make positive decisions and to promote early RTW. They should always remember that they work **for** the employer.
- Adjusters are overworked and undereducated about treating people with respect. Since they are so busy supporting the bottom line of the insurer, they have to sacrifice skills which portray them as sensitive. They must be cutthroat, thus the roles of nurses and physical therapists are critical.
- The adjuster can make or break a workers' motivation to recover. A supportive, clear, focused adjuster can significantly influence positive recovery outcomes. Unfortunately, industry turnover is high and

the lack of experienced adjusters perpetuates negativity in the industry. A higher level of professionalism, training and career development would encourage adjusters to remain in the industry.

- Explaining the benefits/payments of WC, keeping contact with the injured worker so that they don't feel ignored. These people are KEY as they hold the money.
- The adjuster is the key in the whole process. The adjuster needs to be very knowledgeable in specific state work comp laws and know what to authorize and what not to authorize.
- As a group, they are increasingly untrained and overworked. When you have a good one who works well on the "team" they are priceless.

C) From Athletic Trainers' Perspective

- A pain in the rear.
- Supportive of the athletic trainer, communicates with athletic trainer, AT given access to database to monitor patient progress notes from physician and provide accuracy.
- Authorize payments in workers' comp cases.
- Approve it or not, at our company we approve treatment if the MD wants. The problem is that this one person, this one medically uneducated individual, can dictate very much of what I said is so important of what the MD/Surgeon does, how the patient progresses and what their attitude is.
- Keep track of the expenses and make sure things are getting done from the comp insurance side of things.
- The adjuster is one who does not have the knowledge of the health field and just authorizes or denies based on the case manager rather then the necessity of treatment.

D) From Physical Therapist's Perspective

- They usually are not in touch with PT. They are purely a financial director for resources. They do not have enough medical background to provide opinions about the case.

E) From Occupational Medicine Specialists' Perspective

- Supplementary to the managing physician. Often an unnecessary step/expense that insurers defer to, when an effective primary physician should provide same or more extensive services.
- Should ensure that laws are being followed, clients' interests are protected, disability payments (if due) go out on time, medical care is expedited.

F) From Exercise Physiologists' Perspective

- If an Adjuster is a professional, looks at cases individually, and works with the intention of getting the patient appropriate medical care and RTW is the end goal -- they are a value add. If not, then can obviously hinder treatment, outcomes, RTW, etc.
- Same as the Case Manager----but only if there is no Case Manager.

G) From Insurance Professionals' Perspective

- Ensure timely and accurate benefit payment for the injured employee; Provide reassuring information about the availability of benefits; Assist in directing medical care; Reassure the injured employee about the anticipated outcome and promote the expectation of a full duty return to work; Facilitate second opinions when necessary Mediate legal disputes; Coordinate all involved parties (employer, employee, RN, MD, attorney, etc) in the resolution of the claim.
- Despite the evolution of technology and IT systems that offer improved tracking and benchmarking of injuries, the number of case files of adjusters today has also diminished their ability to aggressively manage claim files. As insurance agents, we find our role to intercede more frequently on behalf of our clients to hold adjusters more accountable in managing their case files. Claims take forever to close these days, most adjusters have too many files to manage and not enough support to do the job as effectively as in years past.

- Less critical each year but an excellent adjustor is worth their weight in gold.
- Role of adjuster should be to assist patient with getting proper treatment, and ensuring they understand their benefits as a workers' compensation recipient.
- Adjusters are the line of first defense in a claim. How they handle the claimant and his/her claim can be the difference between a smooth running claim that benefits all involved or an incredibly complicated process that does not end well.
- The front line individual in the claim
- The party that manages the claim from "cradle to grave" on behalf of an insurer to third party administrator.
- Extremely helpful if they are a high level professional.

H) From Employer's Attorneys' Perspective

- The Adjuster and Defense Counsel should work fluidly as a team. They should coordinate and implement the checks and balances to ensure the injured worker gets appropriate care without abusing the system or committing fraud. The Adjuster, if assigned by the insurance carrier, should only function as the payor and part of the employer's administrative team. If the Adjuster, however, works for a third-party administrator, he/she might have a different role and function more as a direct agent of the employer (which should **not** be contacted by the claimant's attorney without approval from the employer's attorney).
- Besides the patient, the claim's adjuster is probably the only other person who truly knows and understands the claim better than anybody else. I was lucky enough to work with many outstanding adjusters who made my job so much easier by doing a fantastic job on every claim. However, there are some adjusters who are clueless as to looking at the big picture and that will lead to many problems.

I) From Consultants' Perspective

- The adjuster should move a case to resolution. Too many times in this current climate, the insurance companies and third party adjuster companies (TPAs) are just not making the investment to train their workers'. Thus, you get mediocre claims handling. It is costing employers twice what it should.
- The adjuster's primary roles are to determine compensability and to address the non-medical issues associated with the claim.
- Serving as the "Floor General" to assure that all parties are working in concert with the goal of mitigating the overall cost of the injury. (including medial treatments, WC benefits and ultimate case resolution settlements)
- Important - helps manage the entire process - assure action plans are followed up as outlined.

J) From an Employer's Perspective

- A group of people that found a way to the feeding trough.

K) From Advocates' Perspective

- The role of adjuster should be limited to processing claims data. Their communication with medical provider offices should be limited to that function. Too often they provide "legal advice" about claims to physician's office staff -- not always truthful, not always correct. For example, day before yesterday, an adjuster informed a client's doctor's office that a controversy had been issued because the ordered physical therapy exceeded the regulatory frequency limits -- that there was nothing the doctor could do to resolve the issue. In reality, the frequency limits had been exceeded three months previously -- no controversy was issued because the employer physician had expressed a treatment plan which included extended treatment. The workers' compensation regulatory agency can, and does order extended treatment. The treating doctor's reports and recommendations play an important role in that legal action.
- Adjustors work for the system not for the injured worker.

6. Role of the Vocational Counselor in Workers' Compensation Cases

A) From Case Managers' Perspective

- Hope for the severely impaired injured worker.
- I'm in California, and we don't have them any more.
- Vocational counseling is a dying art in workers' comp. So many schemes have cut this aspect away. No wonder claim durations are longer, despite lower injury numbers!
- There is little or no funding **early in the piece** for workers' who are obviously injured to the extent that they won't return to work with their existing employer. Voc rehab should kick in the second day after injury for these people! Also, the lack of insurer funding for decent retraining is a problem. Similarly, lack of funding for comprehensive job search/placement activities protracts the return- to-work process.
- They focus on what the person is capable of performing and helping the injured worker find the right job for the person.
- Necessary when there are permanent restrictions. They can bring closure if they're good, or they can be a waste of money if they aren't good.
- Most misunderstood aspect of the work comp claim. Most of the time it is an afterthought 3 years after injury. It should be an intricate part of the claim from the beginning. The Illinois law (section 7110.10) actually calls for voc rehab after 120 days of disability or when it is "reasonably determined" that the IW won't be able to return to work, which ever first occurs.

B) From Athletic Trainers' Perspective

- A non-factor.
- Not used as athletic trainer assumes that role.
- Help them move on. Work with them to help them find something in their lives to get back to, move on to, and figure out that they are worth something and can move on to a "normal" life.
- Should be an early intervention when it is determined that Voc. retaining may be needed. Voc. counselor should meet with the pt. and map out course for reentry into workforce - starting classes before all rehab is finished.

C) From an Adjusters' Perspective

- Find a job for the injured worker and complete vocational assessments.

D) From Occupational Medicine Specialists' Perspective

- Helpful once return to work at prior job is clearly not an option.
- Veeeery important. I think that this is the crux of the matter. People seem to believe that because I have an operated shoulder I can no longer work. Yet we see people with out legs, arms, etc. working and being productive (sometimes more than those who are whole). We need to change the mind set of those who have an injury to realize that there are alternatives.

E) From Exercise Physiologists' Perspective

- Necessary for those persons who cannot return to work at their former occupation and do not have many transferrable job skills. But, Vocational Counselors that simply throw the newspaper classifieds in front of people are certainly not helpful.
- Over used. More speculative than current FCE methodology.

F) From Insurance Professionals' Perspective

- Useless.
- I have personally not seen a great deal of success with Vocational Counselors, but I do believe in theory and purpose behind their role.

- Positively
- The party to assist in finding a vocation for an injured person.
- Extremely helpful if they are a high level professional.

G) From Employer's Attorneys' Perspective

- A vocational counselor would be very useful in New York. The 2007 reforms implied VR would be a vital part of the process, but we're still waiting on the new Medical Guidelines that were due in December 2007!
- The vocational counselor needs to be reputable and know what he is doing. This person also needs to understand the WC system in the state where he is located. Furthermore, a good counselor needs to look at the person as a whole with honesty if he is going to be helpful in helping the employee find a job.

H) From Consultants' Perspective

- If they are involved early, they can be a big help. However, I have seen voc counselor's want to advocate for much longer training than necessary.
- The role of the voc counselor is to find long term solutions to the patient's search for economic and societal security post injury.
- In those rare situations where the injured worker will NOT be able to return to their pre-injury job, they need to provide creative suggestions that utilize the injured workers' educational, avocations and personal passions in finding some appropriate employment possibilities.
- Useful in getting claimant back to workforce - reduce claim costs.

I) From Advocates' Perspective

- Injury is a life sentence, without parole. The Vocational Counselor's job is to help the injured worker obtain the skills that permit him/her to continue to be a contributing member of society, a bread-winner for family, and have security for eventual retirement.
- The sad part of vocational assessment is that the process has not really altered since it was established in the early 1900s. Questions are asked in a set process to give the impression that this is the way "it is" for all time. The questions do not take into account that the person answering the questions may be strung out on medication so not clearly understand the concepts. The person may have left school 3 or 4 decades back therefore have no understanding of spatial concepts or what figure is closest to or what number goes next. The person may be so stressed from needing to attend the appointment that they can not answer the questions clearly. None of the vocational questions clearly reflect the truth within the injured worker, not do the questions reflect the physical capability of the injured worker. So even if the vocational assessment comes back that the injured worker has the perfect aptitude to do a particular line of work but the physical capacity is no longer in place, the outline in front of the vocational counselor is of little to no help. Case in point. An injured master painter that I did some work with did a vocational assessment, the results came back that his best vocation was in house painting, next was sign writing, next was building repair. The vocational assessment did not show up that the injured worker had over many years developed an intolerance to the dyes used in paints and to the solvents used in cleaning the walls and brushes or that the injured worker needed to be on oxygen for 30 minutes every 3 hours 24 hours a day. The vocational counselor told the injured worker that the best he could hope for was a redemption pay out of his workers' compensation claim. This injured worker now works from his own studio where he makes small hand blown glass objects using natural dyes and colorings. The vocational assessment did indicate that the injured worker should pursue an art based career, but it was discarded because there was no immediate benefit or cost reduction for the Work Cover scheme.

7. Role of the Employer in Workers' Compensation Cases

A) From an Employer's Own Perspective

- They are the bill payer and the second of two stakeholders.

B) From Case Managers' Perspective

- Provide safe work place for employees. Offer a modified duty work plan.
- They are responsible to the employee to provide a full work comp benefit, make certain that they are treated well, fully and timely. They are most responsible to provide a reasonable and appropriate RTW situation as soon as the employee is ready to return to work.
- The employer needs to provide training for prevention of injury. Without the workers', the employer is nothing. Valuing the people working for a company is key, and keeping those people safe, if not happy, is what the employer is supposed to do.
- Employers are pivotal in workers' comp. The relationship prior to injury was strictly between the employer and the worker. This is often forgotten once a work-related injury occurs. Other stakeholders can blur communication between the employer and worker. The employer's support or lack thereof significantly influences recovery outcome.
- To assure the injured worker that he will get the care he deserves—is first and foremost.
- A key component in the process of obtaining RTW. Very important to address restrictions etc & encourage them to accept accommodated work.
- Very critical in creating their own destiny in work comp. They can learn to manage their workers' comp costs by integrating a successful team including, MD, atty, case manager, in-house managers, and insurance adjuster. Or they can leave it all up to a claims adjuster to handle.

C) From Athletic Trainers' Perspective

- They trust me to turn the key.
- Unfortunately, they get stuck in the middle and also get stuck with the bills. Sometimes that is not fair.
- Supportive of injured employee, upfront with Worker's Comp requirements so no surprises as to what is covered and what is not, supportive of the athletic trainer and treating physicians; not likely to expedite return to duty.
- In many cases the worker got hurt (yes, I only get one side of the story) because something at the job was "wrong." Uninformed, uneducated, understaffed, pushed too hard, work too fast, cutting safety corners. SO, work with them to get better. Let them go to their therapy and their conditioning, but ask for proof they were there. Communicate and respect.
- Should be supportive of their employee - establish return to work programs, establish preventative measures to decrease rate of injuries, hold job for injured employee so as not to pressure pt. to return before they are deemed ready.

D) From an Adjuster's Perspective

- The employer must stay involved with the claim. They should stay in contact with the injured worker, offer modified duty, and keep the worker feeling part of the team.

E) From a Physical Therapist's Perspective

- It's important that they fax over job description, open communication with patients.

F) From Occupational Medicine Specialists' Perspective

- Critical, but too often not supportive. With a suspicious or unsupportive attitude, may set the stage for employee resentment and delayed recovery.
- Must not punish the injured worker; must make every effort to bring the patient back to work in a full or transitional (modified) capacity. Should keep in close communication with the employee.
- Must have the view that the employee wants to return to work and be active in helping the employee in returning to work.

G) From Exercise Physiologists' Perspective

- Employer is the responsible party and should have a vested interest in developments of each case.
- Somewhat less important than the Case Manager. If they can be shown objective information related to the claimant's medical condition and behavior (same old theme), most will be reasonable people who will help resolve issues and produce the best possible outcome. Those who are not reasonable must be dealt with by using the objective medical and behavioral data as a blunt instrument.

H) From Insurance Professionals' Perspective

- Employers play an important role in the psychological impact of a work injury. It all starts with a positive relationship with their employer. If the employee likes his job and likes his employer, the work comp claim is going to have a dramatically different outcome than a claim from someone who is disgruntled about his job. An early return to work has so many positive psychological and physical rehabilitation benefits, so an employee is willing to return to work and an employer who is willing to accommodate modified work is essential.
- Most employers want their legitimately injured employees to obtain the best treatment possible and to receive full compensation for the extent of their injuries. Most employers are frustrated due to the fact that many state workers' compensation systems encourage employees to attempt to get rich quick due to the pro-labor, liberal bent that most arbitrators have against employers.
- An employer must be willing to accommodate the claimant when restrictions are available and must be understanding that the re-entry after an injury is not an easy transition.
- When possible, employers should help workers' return to work as soon as possible, i.e., light duty, etc. I believe the longer injured worker is off work (in any capacity) the harder it becomes to re-assimilate to work environment.
- The employer's role is very important. Keeping in touch with the claimant, helping to get him/her back to work and generally making the claimant feel that he is an important part of their operations can drastically reduce complications and the ultimate cost of the claim.
- A true partner in the claim process.
- The party who is ultimately paying the bill and the most affected by the loss of the injured party's employment.
- Extremely helpful if they are a high level professional.

I) From Employer's Attorneys' Perspective

- Employers are the respondents. They are the parties against whom actions are taken and who have superior knowledge regarding the accident, the injured worker as an employee and person, the opportunities to accommodate work restrictions, terms of bargaining unit contracts, etc. Employers must remain involved in every step of the WC process.
- The employer not only needs to abide by the WC Act, but also needs to be fair with the injured employee. An employer should treat an injured employee the way he would like to be treated if he was the injured party.

J) From Consultants' Perspective

- They need to become adjusters in their own right if they are going to influence the resolution of this claim. They have abdicated their responsibility for getting these claims cleaned up for too long. They also need to be sure they have good light duty return to work programs available for **all** employees.
- The employer expedites post injury response, from the moment of injury through return to work.
- Someone who is fair in acknowledging legitimate injuries and someone who is willing to make accommodations to get employees back into the workplace
- Should work well with all other aspects of the claim (adjuster, patient, case manager, etc..) - be proactive.

K) From Advocates' Perspective

- Let us be specific here -- while the employer and insurer may be united legally, in reality they are not. Too often, especially with large organizations, the employer simply turns the case over to the insurer and terminates all involvement with the case -- even when the injured worker has worked for the company for many years. Small businesses, where owner/management know and value employees do much better. Simply expressing caring is important. A company that puts together puts a part-time, light duty position -- even if initially just a few hours per day -- has a much better chance of retaining an experienced worker. The worker who believes his company actually cares about him retains significant motivation to recover.
- The employer is very important and should be involved at every step, the employer needs to know and to understand that the incident happened at work and they need to ensure as much as possible that there can be no re-occurrence of the incident. Blame and anger have no part in the workers' compensation process/system, so the employer must accept that the incident happened, do not look for a way to reduce the accountability of the workplace rather work towards removing the ability of the incident happening again. Also the employer must encourage the co-workers' of the injured worker to be a part of the return to work process. it is important that all the co-workers' know what are the medical restrictions in place for the injured worker and not to allow that belief that the injured worker is doing anything wrong by only returning to work for a limited number of hours per day over an extended time frame. A buddy system could be used to ensure that the injured worker is eased back into the work place. The injured worker should be encouraged to attend such things as workplace events or even attend at lunch time so as not to lose touch with the day to day events of the workplace. Even if there is no medical capacity the employer should be encouraging the injured worker to remain "in place" so that when the injured worker is able to make a partial of full return to work the process is as seamless as possible.

Role of the Injured Employee in Workers' Compensation Cases

A) From Case Managers' Perspective

- Commit to recuperation and RTW.
- If you mean the employee, they are responsible for cooperating and committing to getting better. They need to remain focused on return to work and to do so as soon as practical.
- The patient has a difficult role, but the patient needs to be diligent to care for himself/herself, and this can be tough. The patient first must be taught to ask questions and advocate for himself/herself. The patient needs to be determined to return to work. If not, the patient can lose track and become depressed and this leads to lower functioning.
- Can vary. Especially with a tenuous workforce, I see a lot of fear right now. In general, the injured worker needs to play the active role in his work comp care.
- My livelihood.
- Commit to recuperation and RTW.
- They have access to great benefits, but also face a gauntlet of professionals who make their income off of their case which can lead to overtreatment, medicalization and disability.

B) From Athletic Trainers' Perspective

- The key.
- They have to be realistic - if they perform a physically laborious job, they have to expect to get hurt sometime; with that, overuse injuries should not be the responsibility of the employer to pay for care.
- Compliant with paperwork, with appointment time, with home care program. Even though in pain or discomfort gives best effort in rehab activities.
- Getting better is now your job. It sucks, but that is your role. Have a bad day, but don't make everyone else's day bad and know it's ok to have bad days as long as you bounce back (referring mentally, physically takes care of itself). Be compliant, communicate but be respectful, put the effort in...Your role is to get yourself better.

- They are the ultimate decision maker - do I have symptoms or not, do I work hard at getting better or not, do I plan on returning to same job...
- Patient needs to be a motivated individual to return to work. They are just victims of keeping pace with a company's policy to avoid being terminated in most cases. Or they get injured from improper lifting techniques from not being educated properly with ergonomics. Then there are the few that just have the accident.

C) From an Adjuster's Perspective

- It's their job to focus on rehabilitation. They are getting paid to heal. I don't view them as a victim, but instead they are the main participants in the system. They had an unfortunate accident and all parties need to be focused on getting them back as close to baseline as possible.

D) From Physical Therapists' Perspective

- I believe that the patient has a different perspective depending on whether they are being pigeon-holed or not. If they get off to a poor start due to improper care, it may lengthen their case and lead to unwanted outcomes.
- They need to get back to work.

E) From Occupational Medicine Specialists' Perspective

- Clearly central, but may be misguided by advice from family, coworkers', and uninformed health care providers.
- Must take responsibility for recovery; must not be passive.
- They need to have the desire to get well and return to work. Then they must be active in getting treatment and complying with it.

F) From Exercise Physiologists' Perspective

- The patient is the person we should all be serving. The patient is also the person that has the most to win/lose with the professional decisions being made. Patient has the responsibility to work as hard as possible to rehabilitate and RTW.
- The key to the whole puzzle. They are usually either motivated and go back to work, have motivational issues or are perfectly innocent people who get chewed up in big impersonal systems. In the latter case, their medical information is probably either disputed, inadequate/inappropriate or objective and being ignored because the carrier "questions" the claimant's motivation. (Alternatively, these same carriers simply deny, delay or don't pay.)

G) From Insurance professionals' Perspective

- Patients really have a responsibility to mitigate their own losses. This responsibility isn't communicated to them enough and they certainly aren't held to any expectations. The patient has the responsibility to participate fully in their medical treatment, to participate in rehabilitation whether it be in active physical therapy, modified work or a home exercise program. It frustrates me when the mentality of the patient is that of an innocent bystander who is passively "along for the ride". They should be thinking about what outcome they would like, depending on the severity of the injury and they should be doing everything in their power to work towards that goal.
- The number of injured workers' that have learned to game the system these days is outrageous. So many injuries are over exaggerated and / or fraudulent in nature, and so many state workers' compensation systems are so tilted in favor of the injured worker it is outrageous.
- The patient is the case so their role is more critical than any other.
- Once the patient decides on plan of treatment with Dr, therapist, adjuster, etc. They should do everything necessary to be compliant with treatment, i.e., do not miss appointments, etc.
- The patient is the key factor in a claim. If they are not willing to cooperate with their physicians, therapists, adjusters and the myriad of other individuals that may be involved in their claim, the whole process can become painful and expensive.

- Generally worried and needing assurance from either the Dr, Case Manager, or adjuster
- As the injured party.
- Extremely helpful if they are a high level professional.

H) From an Employer Attorney's Perspective

- He is the center of the case. His actions are going to determine most of the outcome of the case. It's really that simple.

I) From Consultants' Perspective

- Their role is to recover and return to work.
- The patient is the principle party with regard to selection of recovery options, including medical care but also including return to work.
- Someone who is striving to return to their pre injury work status
- Need to be motivated to get well & return to work.

J) From an Employer's Perspective

- They are paying with their health, their vocation, their life. They are the principle stakeholder in this debacle.

K) From Advocates' Perspective

- To recover to the extent that is possible. To be as emotionally strong as possible and to seek professional emotional help when it is needed.
- The injured worker for me is the central point of the entire claims process, anything less than that and there is room for litigation and cross-purpose comes into play. Each injured worker for me is the centre of their own claim, I work to ensure that the injured worker is informed and is focused on moving forward within their own claim. That does not always suit the professional strangers within the claims process, and to be honest sometimes it doesn't suit the injured worker either. However if the injured worker is not in the centre of the claim then all is out of balance and the process is harder to resolve.

Role of the Plaintiff Attorney in Workers' Compensation Cases

A) From Case Managers' Perspective

- Assure injured worker's rights per law are provided.
- Unnecessary and derisive.
- The plaintiff attorney should have a balanced role in supporting communication between the adjuster and the patient. The plaintiff attorney needs to encourage the patient not to expect the attorney to do all of the thinking, and the attorney must concentrate on doing what is right for the patient.
- Often misinformed, sometimes obstructive - generally looking for a fight rather than a solution.
- Protector of the injured party.
- Again, it depends. Sometimes they help keep the patient on track & focused. They usually want to close the file quickly so they get paid. They can be complete PIA.
- Assure injured worker's rights per law are provided.
- Their role can be summed up very simply: They profit from bad rehabilitation outcomes for their clients. If they have ethics they know this and do not try to manipulate the outcomes. If they know this and try to manipulate outcomes (negatively), they should be in prison.

B) From Athletic Trainers' Perspective

- Most of them know when their client is FOS, if they don't we will prove it. The ones that are honorable take on honorable clients. Honorable clients have a good case and seek fairness.

- Watch their client's back. Make sure they get a fair shake and only a fair shake. Accidents happen all the time, that doesn't mean someone needs to get rich off it. Encourage your client to participate **fully** in getting better and don't encourage them to get away with something.
- The patient's advocate - fighting for the rights of the injured worker.
- Individual that looks over the best interest of the patient

C) From an Adjuster's Perspective

- They are leeches that suck the money out of the system and make everything cost more.

D) From a Physical Therapist's Perspective

- The attorney can be a valued resource for PT if the pt. is not being compliant with their attendance. They seem to be necessary when the patient is working for a large corporation and does not know their rights.

E) From an Occupational Medicine Specialist's Perspective

- Usually a narrow orientation, seeking maximum financial return. Unfortunately their incentive is to encourage the employee's disabled role, rather than supporting recovery.

F) From Exercise Physiologists' Perspective

- In good times, a plaintiff attorney represents injured workers' and makes sure they have fair treatment throughout the WC system. In bad times, a plaintiff attorney is combative and works for their commission. Can be very helpful in tough cases, but can make things more difficult than necessary with routine injuries.
- A necessary evil, most of the time, otherwise, when they advocate for their claimants in good faith, they are needed professionals.

G) From Insurance Professionals' Perspective

- Most over exaggerate what they can obtain for their clients and attempt to push for settlements that are not in line with the extent of injury suffered by their client. If attorneys would focus their efforts to fight harder for the severe cases and be more reasonable on demands for basic simple cases, everyone would be better served.
- Useless and very frequently an obstacle to conclusion and rarely in the best interests of the claimant.
- To ensure their client is receiving proper care by all parties.
- Plaintiff attorneys can be a blessing or a curse depending on the claim situation. They are blessings when the claimant is extremely unreasonable in their demands because they get the claimant out of the middle of the situation. They can be a curse when they foster unrealistic expectations regarding the final settlement amount of the claim.
- Often difficult to work with
- Most of the time as friction on the process that adds costs.
- Extremely wasteful and not even needed in the WC system. They take (30%) money out of injured workers' pockets they would have already received.

H) From Employer's Attorneys' Perspective

- Assuming you are referring to the attorney for the injured worker in the actual WC case (not a related civil action), the attorney is typically the magician. In New York, I've seen them cleanse sets of medical records and produce only those that support their case. I've seen them write letters to doctors and direct care...
- First of all, the plaintiff's attorney needs to know his case well. If the attorney doesn't know the case this will turn into a nightmare for everybody. In my years of practice I have dealt with one too many

attorneys who didn't know when the employee had surgery or whether the employee was still being treated or not for example. Attorneys need to know their cases.

I) From Consultants' Perspective

- They get in the way. Why are they even needed? All they do is take 30% of the claimant's award. I have seen very few get more than what the claimant would have been awarded anyway.
- The plaintiff attorney protects the legal rights of the injured worker.
- Trying to Maximize any potential ultimate settlement award the claimant can obtain. In my opinion is NOT usually looking after getting the best (and appropriate) medical treatment for his client.
- Hopefully they are reasonable and responsive. Should be (but aren't always) looking out for injured workers' best interest.

J) From an Employer's Perspective

- A shark in a suit.

K) From Advocates' Perspective

- My first and foremost duty as an advocate is that of teacher. It is my job to insure my client fully understands their duties and responsibilities under the law. Second, it is my duty to take all reasonable action to insure my client's rights under the law are fully protected. Thirdly, I must insure communications between the parties and the administrative agency continues. I am soldier, referee, priest/confessor and cheering section -- and whatever else is needed to bring the claim to a satisfactory conclusion. What most plaintiff attorneys forget is that for the injured worker and his/her family, an injury is a capital case, which depending on the seriousness of the injury, may end with a life sentence without parole.
- I view the legal profession as a required nuisance within the workers' compensation system and should be involved as little as possible rather than the first or second phone call by the injured worker or the system.

Role of the Employer Attorney in Workers' Compensation Cases

A) From an Employer Attorney's Perspective

- The job of a respondent's attorney should never be to deny an injured employee's rights under the law. The job or role of a good respondent's attorney is to know the facts of the case inside and out and to determine what the case is worth based on the medical treatment and the facts of the case. The "I don't like the guy" defense does not exist, so we should move away from that. Fairness is key. That being said, as a respondent's attorney my job is to protect my client and make sure that we don't overpay or let someone abuse the system. And yes, there are employees out there who truly want to retire of a simple injury, let's not kid ourselves.

B) From Case Managers' Perspective

- Assure employer's rights per law are provided.
- Occasionally helpful, ideally unnecessary.
- The employer attorney must stay focused on the events of the claim, and communicate regularly with the insured. They must support the mission of the corporation to save money.
- Generally more open to solution than plaintiff attorneys. However, some are more focused on the letter of the law than the spirit of the law, in protecting their clients.
- Protector of the company and assets.
- Usually good. Working with a good team is key. If anyone in that team is "off" it screws up the whole system.
- Dean Wermer summed it up to John Belushi: Fat, drunk and stupid (and Lazy) is no way to go through life!

C) From Consultants' Perspective

- Usually only there when appeals occur. If the claim had been adjudicated appropriately, you would have very few appeals.
- Whom I call defense counsel protects the legal rights of the employer.
- Used as the legal "expert" in combating the Plaintiff attorney's quest for maximum Industrial Injury award.
- Assist in keeping claim cost down & getting full/final resolution.

D) From Athletic Trainers' Perspective

- Make sure the company doesn't get screwed, but give the plaintiff what they deserve. Hold the plaintiff accountable. Make sure the company doesn't lose out because the plaintiff attorney was crazy greedy.
- The company watch dog - making sure the employer is not taken advantage of.
- Individual looking over the interest of the company.

E) From Occupational Medicine Specialists' Perspective

- Cases are best not allowed to reach the point of needing legal council. But the attorney can be very helpful when brought in, particularly in reality testing for the employer and clarifying possible outcomes.
- Just helps the employee achieve greater benefits in disability, making the employees mind set that he is more disabled.

F) From Exercise Physiologists' Perspective

- Employer attorney is concerned about two things—case cost and looking good to their client (employer). Necessary representation when plaintiff attorney is involved.
- A necessary evil, most of the time, otherwise, when they advocate for their clients in good faith, they are needed professionals.

G) From Insurance Professionals' Perspective

- Useless and very frequently an obstacle to conclusion and rarely in the best interest of the employer.
- To ensure patient is not taking advantage of workers' comp benefits.
- Employer attorneys are very important because they are the insured's voice in a litigated claim.
- Does not always appear to have sense of urgency in resolving matters.
- Police Officer...they are only there because of Plaintiff counsel. An extreme waste of money, talent and time.

H) From an Employer's Perspective

- Another shark in a suit.

I) From Advocates' Perspective

- I have worked cases in which employer's attorneys do their ethically and morally. I have worked others in which the opposing attorney can only be described as evil. Some will do anything to win, including withholding medical records from their IMEs. The ethical employer attorney hires IME physicians who actually practice medicine, treating patients on a daily basis. Unethical—an entire industry of experts-for-hire have grown up around workers' compensation law. Many treating physician's openly call those providers "insurance whores."
- I view the legal profession as a required nuisance within the workers' compensation system and should be involved as little as possible rather than the first call by the employer.

Role of the Judge in Workers' Compensation Cases

A. From Case Managers' Perspective

- Resolve conflict between worker comp carrier and applicant attorney.
- The judge needs to remain impartial and should have no connection to the company employing the patient.
- Jaded, occasionally miss the forest for the trees. Judges are put in an invidious position which can so easily be avoided if injured workers', employers and adjusters take the time to deal more honestly and promptly with each other.
- Moderator, providing fair judgment. Though I do feel the company is put on the defensive, but as a judge explained to me...workers' comp was to protect the worker and that is their focus.
- It doesn't mean anything to me.

B) From Consultants' Perspective

- Very few understand the system.
- The judge resolves legal disputes that may arise in a claim.
- Should be to dole out a fair injury award based on Factual evidence and medical diagnosis/treatment. Unfortunately given the **volume** of cases that are assigned to them, shortcuts in expediting resolution often occurs.....whereby a fair hearing of factual evidence and medical diagnosis/treatment does not occur.
- Generally does not view all details they should. Usually claimant friendly.

C) From Athletic Trainers' Perspective

- Fair, competent, upholds the law as well as fairness to the patient.
- Huge! Listens to both sides, weigh in on what's right or wrong. Hold both parties accountable to be honest and to do what's right to resolve the case in a **timely** fashion.
- The fair unbiased decision maker in terms of legal issues

D) From an Adjuster's Perspective

- They should be an impartial adjudicator of disputes and should apply existing law, not make new law. Too often, this does not happen.

E) From Occupational Medicine Specialists' Perspective

- In my experience, generally fair and objective. When an occasional bias is evident, it tends to support the employee.
- Judges need to understand medicine, evidence based guidelines, issues of impairment. Most judges have too many cases, too little training and interest.
- Should adjudicate as quickly as possible to avoid delays in the process of how disabled the employee "really is."

F) From Exercise Physiologists' Perspective

- Hard position—needs to be arbitrary, look at the facts, and make tough decisions that most likely nobody will be entirely happy about.
- A necessary evil, most of the time. If they are impartial triers of facts, we need them.

G) From Insurance Professionals' Perspective

- They have lost their sense of impartiality. Too chummy with plaintiffs counsel in way too many cases.

- Final arbiter, final obstacle, sometimes exasperating.
- Resolving benefit disputes.
- Judges can be an unpredictable key in the final settlement of claims. There are good ones and there are bad ones. Getting the right judge on a case can be the difference between a reasonable settlement and a crazy settlement.
- In Illinois the judge is an arbitrator who is looking out mostly for the injured or alleged injured party.

H) From Advocates' Perspective

- In most states, disputed cases are heard before an administrative agency. The experience and education of the decision maker(s)—and how they are selected for the position -- plays an important role. Their job is to make decisions based on substantial evidence; insuring due process is afforded to the parties. Their job is complicated because many injured workers' are not represented by attorneys, have little or no experience with the law, and simply do not understand the process. In those cases, the decision maker must be a teacher and guide -- all the while making sure no favoritism takes place. Talk about a nightmarish, impossible job!!!
- Detestable. If a workplace injury requires a hearing at any level of the legal process then the process has gone astray for all the people involved.

Role of the Arbitrator in Workers' Compensation Cases

A). From Case Managers' perspective

- Inexpensive way to come to resolve conflict between parties.
- Arbitrators can use their experience to work with the adjusters to learn the best way in which to approach the patient and then work with the patient in a respectful manner.
- Having been one, I viewed my role as trying to get the parties sort themselves out, before I did it for them...it was somewhat like a mother role - "if you can't sort it out, I will and no one will be happy!" I do not have a legal background. This confounded the attorneys when I was an arbitrator. They were looking for a fight. I was looking for a solution. Fortunately, most of the cases I was involved with were resolved by agreement rather than binding decision.
- A listener and deciding factor in the interest of the injured worker.
- As a bleeding heart democrat who gives in to these losers who don't need things done.
- The root word for Arbitrator is Arbitrary in Illinois. They do not write their own decisions but simply adopt the brief submitted by whichever attorney they side with. They have to do their job, but rehab people. Should never lose sight of providing for a positive rehabilitation outcome win or lose "at the commission."

B) From Consultants' Perspective

- Should be to dole out a fair injury award based on Factual evidence and medical diagnosis/treatment. Unfortunately given the VOLUME of cases that are assigned to them, shortcuts in expediting resolution often occurs.....whereby a fair hearing of factual evidence and medical diagnosis/treatment does not occur.
- Generally does not view all details they should. Usually claimant friendly.

C) From Athletic Trainers' Perspective

- Fair, competent, upholds the law as well as fairness to the patient.
- Draw out the obvious that become not so obvious when you're wrapped up in a situation. Be objective.
- The referee in terms of the legal issues.

D) From Insurance Professionals' Perspective

- Useless.

- Resolving benefit disputes.
- Arbitrators are like judges, it depends on who you get.

E) From an Employer Attorney's Perspective

- A good arbitrator will look at the evidence presented in an honest, unbiased way and make a determination from there. At times an arbitrator can be extremely helpful in helping the parties resolve difficult situations.

F) From an Advocate's Perspective

- Basically the same as a judge—insuring information flows openly and smoothly, that both parties fully understand the process.

Role of the Physical Therapist in Workers' Compensation Cases

A) From their own Perspective

- PTs are a valued resource to the patient to promote good outcomes. They should not be biased in their care of the patient and should become familiar with the patient's goals. They need to provide a customized treatment program to achieve the desired PDL in addition to reaching the pt. goals at a difficult time in their lives.
- Important to document subjective and objective findings.

B) From Case Managers' Perspective

- Provide treatment as prescribed by MD, obtain authorization before commencing treatment, be aware of treatment guidelines per ODG. Report clearly and promptly, report noncompliance ASAP.
- The physical therapist is important from the initial treatment, which is critical for the patient to resume usual and customary activities. The physical therapist is a source of great teaching for the patient to avoid future injury.
- The physical therapist must avoid marketing devices such as H Wave and placing the patient in a precarious position of being taken for a ride with unethical companies who would take advantage of the patient and the employer.
- Physios are great for getting the "real story" re: what a worker is feeling as well as how he/she is recovering. Injured workers' talk much more to physios than Drs. Physios can sometimes be overly worker-focused. The ones who treat *ad nauseum* perpetuate the "victim" mentality. This seems to be a much rarer occurrence these days, than in the 80's 90's, with insurers and regulators strongly focused on clinical guidelines and peer reviews on prolonged treatment.
- Encourage/facilitate the injured worker to return as close to pre-injury state as possible. Also plays a major role in education.
- Instrumental in getting the case done properly. That's why I use ATI so often. I am 97% happy with ATI.
- Therapy works!

C) From Athletic Trainers' Perspective

- Decrease pain, improve ROM, and increase strength.
- Help the client get better. Allow them to see what the goals of the future are and how the client will get there. Push them. Hold them accountable for time, effort, and attendance. It sure seems like we are their "first line" as far as explaining how the system works. Work with the client, their Nurse Case Manager, MDs, Attorney, etc. to get the person where they need to be...working again.
- A major key in the final outcome for the patient—make or break.
- They start the rehabilitation process of the patient and help direct the correct course of treatment plan with MD approval, increase pain tolerance, range of motion, basic strengthening, alignment.

D) From an Adjuster's Perspective

- Assist in rehabilitation by doing aggressive modalities and teaching the injured worker home exercises.

E) From Occupational Medicine Specialists' Perspective

- No different than in any case, usually helpful to support patient's recovery. Some PTs go beyond my concept of their role and suggest additional (often expensive and sometimes unnecessary) interventions that patients' latch onto, making it difficult to deny and still maintain a positive relationship.
- Limited role; emphasize self-care, home exercise program, education and active modalities. Very little role for passive modalities.
- Very important, helps the employee alleviate pain, work with ease and helps find appropriate work skills or work area changes to help the employee return to work.

F) From Exercise Physiologists' Perspective

- Necessary for orthopedic injuries. PTs essentially guide the injured worker through the acute phase of their injury and back to function.
- Should be a problem solver who is unafraid of any other medical professional (including, maybe, their boss, the physician). Should be unafraid to advocate for treatment—or advocate for discharge. Should rely a lot less on theoretically-based clinical tests, most of which rely on the patient's response to interpret.

G) From Insurance Professionals' Perspective

- Sometimes good sometimes not so good. A good P.T. like a good adjustor can be worth their weight in gold.
- Very important, as most patients will see therapist more frequently than any other health care professional.
- Physical therapists are very important. Their work helps to get the claimant back to his before-injury state. The faster that happens, the easier the claim.
- Respect the physical therapist - they again need to work with the treating Dr for best outcome
- The party who helps the injured party recover faster through their treatment.
- Can be extremely effective if they work in the field at the employee's worksite.

Role of the Physical Therapist in Workers' Compensation Cases (from an Employer Attorney's Perspective)

- This is huge. A physical therapist will be the one person who spends the most time with the injured employee. Therefore, the therapist needs to be well qualified and dedicated to his work. If not, you will run into a lot of problems.

H) From Consultants' Perspective

- Can be a real help. They know about dealing with curative rather than palliative care.
- The PT provides psychological recovery assistance to the injured worker.
- To challenge workers' and force their bodies to conditioning levels that will ultimately assist in injury recovery process.
- Assist in recovery - important.

I) From Advocates' Perspective

- The physical therapist is an important medical professional—no less significant or necessary than antibiotics in a bacterial infection. She or he is a healer, teacher, cheering section, advocate, facilitator... words fail me. Then, I have been a patient, with serious physical injuries—more than once or twice. If a good patient-therapist relationship is not established, the treatment may fail and permanent disability increases. If a good doctor-therapist relationship does not exist, communication fails—again, treatment fails, healing is delayed, permanent disability increases.

- All medical people need to set themselves to understand that the injured worker is the only reason that they are involved. The best possible outcome for the injured worker is what needs to be the focal point.

Role of the Athletic Trainer in Workers' Compensation Cases

A) From their own perspective

- Complete: Early Symptom Intervention; Acute Injury Management; Rehab; Return to Work; Wellness.
- Total case management from the injury evaluation to physician referral to patient care following surgery/injury to performance testing to return to full duty. Monitors return for a month to assure employee is doing well, and if not—supplements activities.
- Provide functional strengthening exercises to allow patient to return to previous level of functioning.
- Help the client get better. Allow them to see what the goals of the future are and how the client will get there. Push them. Hold them accountable for time, effort, attendance. It sure
- seems like we are their "first line" as far as explaining how the system works. Work with the client, their NCM, MDs, Atty, etc to get the person where they need to be...working again.
- Depends on their part played in the rehab. Ultimately, I would say it is the same as the physical therapist.
- Helps finish the rehabilitation needs of the patient by providing a more aggressive treatment with work conditioning / work hardening. Increases the strength, endurance, tolerance to activities.
- Are the specialists to deal with activity/athletic injuries.

B) From Case Managers' Perspective

- Work conditioning and FCE only.
- No role for athletic trainer in the workers' comp case.
- Exercise Physiologists can be great if the worker sees themselves as responsible for recovery. Otherwise, Exercise Physiologists tend to be viewed as young whippersnappers who are biding their time until they realize that workers' comp is a tough gig and move on to more rewarding avenues in personal training/corporate health.
- Critical in the "push" of work conditioning outcome.
- When push comes to shove, and the blue collar guy needs to have a reliable guide as to what he will be able to do at work, the AT is invaluable. A good one that is!

C) From a Consultant's Perspective

- To challenge workers' and force their bodies to conditioning levels that will ultimately assist in injury recovery process.

D) From an Adjuster's Perspective

- No role. Injured workers' are not athletes.

E) From an Occupational Medicine Specialist's Perspective

- Important in getting the unfit worker back to maximum fitness in his attempt to return to work.

F) From Exercise Physiologists' Perspective

- Athletic Trainers can serve a great role in advanced workers' comp cases by providing Work Conditioning/Hardening services and Functional Capacity Evaluations. WC/WH programs enable injured workers' to get strong enough to return to manual occupations, while FCEs are necessary oftentimes for WC case closure. Very underrated asset to difficult workers' comp cases.

- Should be a problem solver who is unafraid of any other medical professional (including, maybe, their boss, the physician). Should be unafraid to advocate for treatment—or advocate for discharge. Should rely a lot less on theoretically-based clinical tests, most of which rely on the patient's response to interpret. They are in a turf war with the PTs but the ATs tend to be more oriented to function.

G) From an Insurance Professional's Perspective

- Not a fan.
- Not applicable normally.
- Can be extremely effective if they work in the field at the employee's worksite.

H) From an Employer Attorney's Perspective

- His role is very important as well. A trainer can help the patient not only recover from the work injury, but also how to improve his life in general from a physical standpoint.

I) From Advocates' Perspective

- Same as a physical therapist -- many trainers are physical therapists.
- All medical people need to set themselves to understand that the injured worker is the only reason that they are involved. The best possible outcome for the injured worker is what needs to be the focal point.

Role of the Psychologist/Psychiatrist in Workers' Compensation Cases

A) From Case Managers' Perspective

- Appropriate in select cases of PTSD, head injury.
- Most are too "patient" oriented and do not deal well with their responsibility to be objective.
- Occasionally a psychologist or psychiatrist is useful to ascertain the mental health of the patient. Good observation of the patient's patterns of behavior or need for professional support after a traumatic loss of a body part is critical before prescribing psychological care.
- Generally disconnected to the WC process. Psychology/Psychiatry just doesn't fit within workers' comp benefit timelines. They are often the bane of other stakeholders' existence (except the worker they are treating) because they take a much more holistic view of influence, diagnosis and treatment. They do not (cannot?) limit themselves to '**just**' the work-related issues.
- Specialist in his field that can cut through the underlying mental status that can be hindering recovery.
- Typically bleeding heart democrats who address issues unrelated to work injury.
- Psychology is another unavoidable aspect of work comp claims, but like voc rehab, the provider is usually a fruitcake who couldn't counsel a cat to try and catch a mouse.

B) From Athletic Trainers' Perspective

- Needed once in a blue moon....don't have a lot of interaction but when I do I am glad they are there.
- Helpful sometimes when the patient is down for a long period of time with serious injury/illness. Must be part of the entire treatment team and support the team and patient.
- Some people can't handle it and get "down." Help them back up by listening, acknowledging the issues but don't overstep on the workers' comp side that may not be their area.
- An important component to have available when needed.

C) From an Adjuster's Perspective

- Ask a shrink if you need treatment and they will say yes. No one is normal in their view.

D) From Occupational Medicine Specialists' Perspective

- Not particularly helpful in managing routine claims. Usually reluctant to communicate and collaborate. Seldom provide helpful documents or notes. Generally not willing to be involved in any of the conflicts that characterize a case, e.g. causality, workplace relationships, role of outside relationships, etc. Can help guide case management by providing IME or fitness for duty evaluation in particular circumstances.
- Extremely important. Many people have fears or become depressed and need this type of intervention. Where I am seeing no results is in people who do not want to RTW and use this as the crutch when everything else fails. The person is cured, is ready to RTW, but that lingering fear or depression just keeps me out, it seems to be advantageous to a few.

E) From Exercise Physiologists' Perspective

- Due to the face time involved with PT and WC/WH, PTs and ATCs become the psychologist/psychiatrist. ;-) There are oftentimes many underlying issues with workers' comp injuries that a psychologist/psychiatrist could assist with for sure.
- Personally, I think that Robyn Dawes did a pretty good job of answering this question many years ago. Depression in the comp patient that is situational is resolved with the situation goes away. All other depression is related to bad potty training and a world of pre-morbid factors outside the control of the employer.

F) From Insurance Professionals' Perspective

- Wish they didn't exist.
- In more complex case, very beneficial. However, they can be over utilized.
- In most cases would not see involvement.
- Usually not applicable.

G) From an Employer Attorney's Perspective

- In my opinion, all injured employees should have a consultation with an experienced, well qualified psychologist/psychiatrist. Why? Many employees are angry, afraid, and dealing with many emotions that will have a profound effect on how the person recovers. The law should provide for consultations for everyone.

H) From Consultants' Perspective

- If you get to this point, it says to me you have lost control of the claims adjudication.
- The psychologist helps the injured worker identify and resolve cognitive and affective barriers to recovery and return to work.
- To help diagnose subjective injury complaints to hopefully determine which could be bio-mechanics and which are psychosomatic.

I) From Advocates' Perspective

- Emotional support for the injured worker and their family is an integral part of treatment. The relationship between chronic pain and depression is well-documented. Mental health providers must be keenly aware that workers' compensation is HIPAA exempt. This situation can severely hamper therapy. While the mental health provider must have unlimited access to very personal information, they must also fully understand that everything placed in the clinical record is not private. Everything can, and will be used against the injured worker in a strongly contested case.
- All medical people need to set themselves to understand that the injured worker is the only reason that they are involved. The best possible outcome for the injured worker is what needs to be the focal point.

Role of the Chiropractor in Workers' Compensation Cases

A) From Case Managers' Perspective

- After 6 sessions if the injured worker is not better, consider sports medicine approaches because it is active as opposed to passive in chiropractic.
- Better a physiatrist.
- For some patients the chiropractor is the correct individual to guide a portion of the care rendered. Chiropractors must have clear guidelines to allow for a cap on the number of visits to prevent lengthy periods of care and unreasonable expectations on the part of the patient and employer.
- Mixed views. Some workers' swear by them. Most insurers, Drs and Physios look askance at them. Acceptance of chiro treatment has improved generally in the 25 years I've been in the workers' comp sphere. Possibly improved in the same way that physio treatment has improved, with clearer clinical guidelines and peer review.
- I'm a believer in chiropractic medicine and especially in some of the chronic cases of back pain, neck pain. Again, with the aging workforce, surgery is not always the option, but the worker needs to learn how to manage his symptoms.
- The chiropractor should **never** have a role in any work comp case!
- No scientific support but what the hell they work--sometimes!

B) From Athletic Trainers' Perspective

- What role? They don't have one.
- Generally not helpful.

C) From an Adjuster's Perspective

- While there are some decent ones, too often they are just like the shrinks. Never met a person that didn't need treatment now and into the future.

D) From Occupational Medicine Specialists' Perspective

- Similar to any clinical role for chiropractic. In the proper situation can be very helpful to facilitate recovery. Subject to the same temptation to over treat.
- Limited to those treating injuries where chiropractic has been shown to work: certain low back pain.
- Same as PT.

E) From Exercise Physiologists' Perspective

- Depends. If the injury is simple and treatment duration is short, Chiros can be helpful. However, for difficult cases and big injuries, I haven't seen them be effective.
- Similar to the PT, however chiros tend to like having "patients for life."

F) Insurance Professionals' Perspective)

- The biggest cheats in the system.
- More often than not they are ineffective and only add cost to the claim without improvement.
- Not sure.
- I have never felt very comfortable about chiropractors getting involved in workers' comp claims. I've seen too many instances where it seems they were taking advantage of a situation in order to continue receiving compensation.
- Depending upon the amount of treatment and what guidelines are used to refer outside of their practice

- If necessary to help improve injuries to backs.
- Voodoo

G) From an Employer Attorney's Perspective

- Unfortunately, many chiropractors who treat injured employees just abuse the system and end up hurting the patient more than assisting in their quick recovery.

H) From a Consultant's Perspective

- More than worthless.
- In **rare** situation provide limited therapy on subjective complaint matters. It is troubling to see the number of Chiropractors who fail to acknowledge their limits of injury treatments. They often continue to treat well beyond what is deemed as being reasonable.

I) From Advocates' Perspective

- For many years chiropractic was considered to be medically useless "snake oil." Research has proven otherwise -- in limited applications. Back pain is one area in which this treatment modality has been recognized as appropriate. The U.S. Military now recognizes and employs chiropractic care in their medical facilities. As in any other medical professional, provider quality is an issue.
- All medical people need to set themselves to understand that the injured worker is the only reason that they are involved. The best possible outcome for the injured worker is what needs to be the focal point.

FRAUD AND ABUSE

Subjects were asked to estimate the rate/level of fraud in workers' compensation and to ponder the source(s). As one could imagine, the results were very interesting.

Case Managers' Estimates:

- 5% of reported work injuries occurred outside of work
- Extremely high and from all sources equally.
- From my own work as case manager, fraud possibly occurs in about 9 percent of cases. This can be fueled by word of mouth dissatisfied injured workers', social networks, and company groups who discuss the worst of workers' compensation. Most patients were on the level.
- Workers' - 2% Employers - 15% - e.g., misrepresenting operations to qualify for lower rating (less physically demanding) industry classification, which means lower premiums - Practitioners - 10% - e.g., billing long consults when only a short consult occurred.
- I've always thought it was the employee, but as mod rates become issues with obtaining work contracts and the rising cost of workers' comp costs, it's probably spread pretty even.
- Depending what you consider fraud. Total bullshit from the beginning? 25%. Total bullshit with original injury and they're better and malinger 70%. "Fraud" is too strong of a word. It exists when an attorney tries to influence a negative rehabilitation outcome for money (See Walter Mathieu, aka Whiplash Willy in "The Fortune Cookie"), but what often looks like fraud is just a sad set of factors that are all too common and leads to years of unnecessary disability and frustration: from misdiagnosis, to insurance delays and incompetency, to social factors of patient, to employer apathy or in short, the "system."

Athletic Trainers' Estimates:

- 12%, internal benchmarks and experience.
- Fraud - from patients, I would say 10-15%; Physicians willing to perform surgery at the drop of a hat: 50-60%; Chiropractors who see the patients 3-5 times per week for care: 75%

- Unclear for me.
- That depends on how you define fraud. If you define fraud by malingering then I'd say it could be as high as 50-60%. If you mean fraud by totally injury free and faking it, 15%. Sources - experience, my employer, Nurse Case managers, and attorneys.
- 5-10%

An Adjuster's Perspective:

- Fraud comes from several sources. Injured workers' fake or exaggerate their injuries and complaints. Employer's under-report payroll to keep premiums low. Carriers and TPAs intentionally understate reserves so their financial strength looks better than it actually is.

Physical Therapists' Estimates:

- Possibly 5-10% at the patient level.
- 30% other therapists' experience

Occupational Medicine Specialists' Estimates:

- I have no data, but experience suggests it is significant in this state where WC provides greater secondary gains than other insurers. This is reinforced by the fact that some conservative legal changes some years ago resulted in a significant decrease in workers' comp cases.
- Employer 10%, Injured worker 5%, Broker/agent 5%, Physicians 10%, Insurance carrier (adjuster)1%.
- About 25%. Mostly employees who are having poor performance and are looking for a way out.

Exercise Physiologists' Estimates:

- 1-10% fraud rate. Based on my 10 years experience in an outpatient rehabilitation center.
- 5% outright fraud. 30-40% soft fraud (i.e., the person has adjusted to being off work and has subconsciously decided to keep it that way.)

Insurance Professionals' Estimates:

- The amount of intentional fraud is likely very low. What seems to be high is "unintentional" fraud. By this, I think of examples of employees whose subjective complaints do not match the objective findings. Oftentimes, they have whined to themselves so much that they now actually believe that things are as bad as they say....but the objective findings do not support those complaints. Employees who would rather be off work completely rather than work modified duty are a form of fraud. Drug seeking behavior is a form of fraud.
- There is some element of fraud in 40% of all cases. Either the injury is totally fraudulent or exaggerated to extremes that result in higher costs than should be appropriate.
- 5% actual fraud.- 15% abuse such as extended lost time and over utilization, whether med's, chiro or P.T.
- 5% outright fraud. 15% malingering.
- I don't think that it is as bad as most people think. However, the few bad apples have definitely made most employers very cynical about their claims.
- Less than 10% and this is from my own experience being an adjuster.
- I think it is quite prevalent in the form of exaggerated injuries or the prolonging of treatment to delay going back to work. It is a subjective opinion based on what I see day to day.
- 100 in every legal situation. It is simply not needed. When an attorney is involved in WC it's illegal in my mind because they are taking money out of injured workers' pockets they would have already received.

Consultants' Estimates:

- 20%. Most of this comes from people who have prior injuries disguising their injuries as work comp.
- I define fraud as behavior which a typical workers' comp or civil course judge would deem fraud and would render decisions influenced by this finding. This is a relatively tight and appropriate definition, but not as tight as requiring that the behavior be prosecuted. About 1% to 5% of claimants commit fraud. About 1% of medical providers commit fraud. About 5% to 10% of employers commit fraud with respect to premium setting.
- I think this is tied directly to U.S. Social economical conditions. When unemployment is high and jobs are scarce, I think the % can be as high as 25-30%. In good economical times the number is probably closer to 10-15%. The Primary source is from injured workers' themselves submitted fraudulent claims.

Advocates' Estimates:

- Actually, research has proven that the majority of workers' compensation fraud is perpetrated by employers. Injured workers' account for less than 1% workers' compensation fraud. Those figures were established based upon the actual dollar value, as well as, actual number of occurrences. The real problem is the individual beliefs of Administrative Law Judges, medical professionals, lawyers and insurance adjusters. The media plays a significant role in the development of bias against injured workers'. News has become entertainment—surveillance photos of the exposed cheater makes an attention-grabbing story. A story which is frequently shown on national television.
- Less than 1% by injured workers' and over 10% by the professional strangers who required a high number of injured workers' to be circulated within the workers' compensations system/process. So the amount of white collar fraud would be the
- over-servicing of the injured worker, or the writing of reports that lead to further reports being required instead of telling the full truth. Even the overuse of medication to keep the injured workers' from being fully aware of all that is going on. Independent Medical Examiners who write reports based on the case managers questions rather than the attending medical reports. Independent Medical Examiners who fail to view x-rays or read MRI reports but still write a report that indicates that there is no evidence of injury. Independent Medical Examiners who charge the system for an hour but spend less than 10 minutes actually with the injured worker. This is all fraud that costs the workers' compensation system a great deal of money with no outcome for the injured worker.

Next the authors asked a variation on the Fraud and Abuse theme, i.e; respondents were queried to **estimate out of an average 100 cases, what number are malingering?**

Case Managers seem to have the widest variation, followed by Physical Therapists (albeit only n=2), and perhaps not surprisingly, Advocates (again, n=2) estimate the least amount.

Case Managers	ATCs	Adjuster	PTs	Occ Med	Exercise Physiologists	Insurers	PA	Employer Atty	Consultants	Advocates
0–1%	1-2 %	5%	<5%	<1%	5% outright fraud. 30-40% soft fraud (i.e., the person has adjusted to being off work and has subconsciously decided to keep it that way.)	~ 0.5%	10%	30-40%.	5%	<1%
1% start out malingering, 9% move to malingering	5 – 10 %		30%	1%	20 – 40%	10-15%			5–20%	2%
9%	9%			15%		15%			20%	

15%	10%	15%
20%	15%	15%
25%	15-20%	20%
35%		25%
96%		>25%

For the final section of the survey, the authors wanted to tap into some of the most "personal" experiences and opinions of the respondents. To do this, subjects were asked about what they considered to be the hardest part of their job as well as what is the most satisfying part of their job in working with workers' comp cases? They were queried what they would do to improve the current workers' compensation system and/or describe what they would consider to be an ideal model from their perspectives. Finally, the survey concluded with a request to describe an interesting or challenging case or two (maintaining patient confidentiality) that the subjects felt was representative of their work with workers' compensation cases or the system, and as a result some interesting stories were found.

Case Managers considered the following to be hardest part of their job in working with workers' comp cases:

- Establishing rapport with injured worker.
- The employee that is enjoying being disabled and does not want to RTW.
- Taking the brunt of the calls which adjusters will not take, but then the discussions with the patients are enhanced when the nurse can step in and cool someone who is upset at the adjuster, so it's also enjoyable. Working with the managers who push the injured workers' to heal faster than their bodies allow.. Seeing companies avoid training individuals, and seeing companies save money by not repairing modern conveniences that can keep workers' from being hurt (e.g. using manual jacks).
- Managing the expectations of all stakeholders - mainly employers, workers', insurers.
- Companies that just don't get it. No matter what the injury, they are not responsible, and the person is faking or hurt somewhere else, and doesn't follow the restrictions that the physician has outlined. The outcome is never what it could have been because the injured worker is already at a disadvantage.
- When the patient continues to have subjective complaints & there is absolutely no diagnostic indication that it is accurate and the treatment goes on & on & on & on.
- When I enter a hostile situation and I have to prove that if I do my job correctly injured worker, physician, attorney and insurance company will all benefit.
- Missing opportunities to be successful with the IW due to factors outside of my control. For example, an employer who misses an opportunity for a return to work or for training to a vexatious petitioner attorney denying his client a positive outcome for specious reasons.

An Adjuster considered the following to be hardest part of his/her job in working with workers' comp cases:

- Plaintiff attorneys who prefer to keep the injured worker disabled so they make more money from a settlement and judges who view workers' compensation as a social welfare program.

Insurers considered the following to be hardest part of their job in working with workers' comp cases:

- Employees who are unmotivated to return to work. Prescription medication addictions. State workers' compensation legal systems that perpetuate disability mentalities for their citizens.
- Pushing all parties to resolve open claims in a fair and equitable manner.
- Getting all of the players to be efficient and to remove the lag time between actions and inactions.
- Patient compliance.
- Keeping everyone involved calm and making sure that the claim file is being handled in the correct manner.
- Volume of cases.

- Dealing with malingering situations.
- Understanding that the injured worker is oftentimes taken advantage of by many people.

An Employer's Attorney considered the following to be hardest part of his/her job in working with workers' comp cases:

- Meeting my client's expectations while making sure that I do everything by the book. Sometimes you have to remind the client of how the workers' compensation system works and what you can't and can do.

An Employer considered the following to be hardest part of his/her job in working with workers' comp cases:

- Seeing the system sustained at the expense of the injured.

Consultants considered the following to be the hardest part of their job in working with workers' comp cases:

- Getting the adjuster to do what he/she needs to do to move the case to resolution. Way too much delay. Part of it being that most adjusters handle too heavy of a workload. So they only pay attention to the squeaky wheel.
- Passivity and ignorance of claims staffs, and the lack of high level medical intelligence in the insurer community.
- Sometimes it is to convince Clients/employers that they should consider accepting a matter as being a work injury.

Athletic Trainers' considered the following to be hardest part of their job in working with workers' comp cases:

- Working with the "frequent filers" that throw land mines in their treatment path.
- There are few patients that have been caught malingering which drain my energy. I'm often irritated by these people because I feel I could be helping someone who needs my care. There are few who act entitled and don't act responsible. In a sense, these people are nudges.
- Explaining release from care & return to work duties.
- Getting employees in to see physicians following a traumatic injury within 48 hours.
- Keeping patients compliant.
- Day in day out dealing with someone that is always down in the dumps, always in a bad mood, doesn't seem like they want to get better, doesn't work at getting better and on top of it takes all that out on you.
- The delays in authorizing care and the arbitrary limits placed on length of care.
- To convince the public, health care providers and workers' comp administrators that athletic trainers are well trained individuals to deal with workers' comp patients.
- Working to get approval for extended authorization because many people believe every case is the same as per guidelines. Or working with a patient that is known to be a malinger and have to keep them because of keep getting referred back to WC/WH or therapy.

Physical Therapists considered the following to be hardest part of their job in working with workers' comp cases:

- Dealing with unhappy patients who are not cooperative with treatment.
- Malingerers.

Occupational Medicine Specialists considered the following to be hardest part of their job in working with workers' comp cases:

- Trying to develop a supportive relationship with a resentful, suspicious employee.

- Having physicians follow evidence based guidelines.
- Those who refuse to get well when everything else says the contrary.

Exercise Physiologists considered the following to be hardest part of their job in working with workers' comp cases:

- Getting all parties to understand that we are there to help a person (injured worker) get back to work. They are not a claim or a diagnosis. They are people with real problems, who actually need to get back to work for themselves and their family. Whether they want to or not.....
- Dealing with adjusters who simply do not know very much about the medical side of the equation.

A Physician's Assistant considered the following to be hardest part of his/her job in working with workers' comp cases:

- Paperwork.

Advocates considered the following to be hardest part of their job in working with workers' comp cases:

- Remaining emotionally detached. Some of what I see turns the stomach.
- The hardest part can be rebuilding the self dignity and respect for self of injured workers'. The workers' compensation process can be destructive for injured workers', they are told that they are broken, they are told that they have limitations, they are told that they are having a tax payers holiday, they are told that they are costing the system a lot of money, they are told that no one believes them, they are told as many negatives things as possible in order to be controlled by the system/process. Sometimes I have no choice but to accept that my only way forward is for me to walk away from the injured worker as they have no desire to actually improve. But all that pales into nothing when I attend the funeral of an injured worker who has taken his/her own life. To stand and speak to try to find words that offer support and hope for all who have been left behind to try to resolve the confusion is almost unbearable. Suicide is a reality within the workers' compensation systems but it is rarely spoken about. For mine suicide is proof that the whole system needs to be re-focused and taken back to the original intent of betterment for injured workers'. I can never give a tipping point for most suicides; there is normally a multiple of issues that become too much for the injured worker to cope with. Suicide is a silent thief of a valuable life and it needs to be addressed in the open rather than spoken about in hushed tones behind closed doors.

Next, the authors asked the converse, "What is the most satisfying part of your job in working with workers' comp cases?" Here is what was learned:

Case Managers' considered the following to be most satisfying part of their job in working with workers' comp cases:

- Returning an injured worker to his previous condition, life work and play.
- Seeing the employee's life get back to normal.
- Working with the injured workers', explaining medical terminology, forging a communications bond with the patient and also with the doctors' offices so that reports can be made available.
- Resolving misunderstandings about the RTW process / potential.
- Good outcomes in the eyes of everyone involved with the claim.
- Catastrophic cases because the family is usually very appreciative & typically, the worse the injury, the better the patient.
- When I with my expertise as a nurse help the physician and patients, the patients. get well, move on, return to their previous life/work.
- Being a part of a successful team where an injured employee is dealt with from day one in a competent, empathetic and successful manner. They maintain their employment status and the companies build morale and consistency in their approach to this system.

An Adjuster considered the following to be most satisfying part of his/her job in working with workers' comp cases:

- Getting the best possible outcome for a seriously injured worker.

Insurers considered the following to be most satisfying part of their job in working with workers' comp cases:

- Very rarely, you do have a claim for an employee who is grateful for the benefits, is a hard worker and wants to return to their employment and who simply wants to get better with the least invasive treatment available.
- When fraudulent claims are identified, and the perpetuators are prosecuted.
- There isn't any. It's time consuming, frustrating, and costly and job threatening.
- Assisting injured worker get back to work, and normalcy.
- When everything runs smoothly, the claimant is taken care of and is able to return to work quickly and the claim closes at minimal cost to the insured.
- Returning the employee as much as possible to pre-injury status.
- Having the employee back to work swiftly and both the employee and employer feeling they were treated fairly.
- Working with great people and great employers.

An Employer's Attorney considered the following to be most satisfying part of his/her job in working with workers' comp cases:

- Accomplishing what I told my client I would do. Earning your client's trust is the most satisfying part of any job. That and getting a "zero award" at trial.

Consultants considered the following to be most satisfying part of their job in working with workers' comp cases:

- Watching employers catch on about how to manage a work comp claim. My clients are excited that they may have a bit of control over what happens.
- The delivery of very expert medical care, which requires a well designed provider network, composed of clinicians who make very few medical errors and understand the predicaments as noted above.
- Seeing a claim that is viewed as being fraudulent successfully denied by the Arbitrator/Commission.

Athletic Trainers considered the following to be most satisfying part of their job in working with workers' comp cases:

- Helping the people that are really hurt get better; busting the frauds and fakers.
- Seeing a motivated workers' comp patient return to full duty is most satisfying.
- Seeing a smile on their face when they leave satisfied with their care.
- When the system works in a timely fashion.
- Making a difference in the lives of patients.
- The person that comes in wondering what will happen to them and you get to explain it to them, watch them work, watch them progress, hear them say things like "thank you, I could never do that before" and they leave with their confidence and their life back...maybe to their old job, may be not.
- Having the pt. reach a high level of function and seeing how happy they are on returning to "normal" life.
- Getting the individual that is really motivated to get back to work and is grateful of the accomplishments you help achieve throughout the process.

Physical Therapists considered the following to be most satisfying part of their job in working with workers' comp cases:

- Seeing a patient return to their previous employment in a relatively rapid time.
- People get back to work at the appropriate level.

Occupational Medicine Specialists considered the following to be most satisfying part of their job in working with workers' comp cases:

- Successful recovery of employee with return to work with positive outlook.
- Decreasing disability by providing education.
- Seeing very ill persons get well and productive.

Exercise Physiologists considered the following to be most satisfying part of their job in working with workers' comp cases:

- Getting good outcomes and hearing satisfied patients and customers (MDs, Adjuster, NCM, attorney, etc.).
- Demonstrating that a person who has been suspected of being unmotivated is falsely accused---and has been proven to have a true functional deficit. When I can bring in both axes of information (medical and behavioral) and affect a turnaround in how a case is handled, I am extremely satisfied.

A Physician's Assistant considered the following to be most satisfying part of his/her job in working with workers' comp cases:

- Return injured individuals back to work.

Advocates considered the following to be most satisfying part of their job in working with workers' comp cases:

- Helping an individual regain self-respect. Lessening the fear that they, or their family, will not be hungry and homeless.
- The most satisfying is when an injured worker is able to stand on his/her own again, returns to work and is back fully in charge of his/her own life. The most satisfying outcome I have ever had was when an injured worker was placed with a small courier business for a 6 week work hardening program then was employed by the courier company, then went out to buy the company. I know that doesn't happen very often, but it shows what is possible if the support required by the injured worker is in place.

It was the opinion of the authors that this sample of respondents, being professionals with varied perspectives in workers' comp, could provide informative perspectives as to how they would improve the workers' compensation system or describe what they considered as an ideal model. Here is what was learned:

Case Managers conceptualized an improved workers' comp system as:

- To eliminate attorneys (which raise cost of claim), force employers to provide mod duty, control medical providers including physical therapist by advising them of the ODG and only pay for treatment that is within the guidelines.
- To increase the level of personal responsibility and the penalties for not being personally responsible.
- Have a company would spend a month training full time employees, and two weeks training part timers. Employees would invest in repairing broken equipment, thus preventing injuries and long future medical charges. A nurse for every patient. A way to have each patient meet face to face with someone in order to have a perspective about what is happening and avoid the use of *sub rosa* to assess the patients.
- Have proven disability management techniques acknowledged by the Illinois Legislature and enacted into law. This would include early intervention strategies, return to work time frames, light duty, and

other employer centered responsibilities. For their efforts, employers could receive tax incentives for enacting them to offset their additional costs.

An Adjuster conceptualized an improved workers' comp system as:

- Having medical charges the same as group health. Strict controls on narcotics, and no off-label pharmacy. Indemnity benefits that encourage workers' to rehabilitate. Indemnity should be a hand up, not a hand out.

Insurers conceptualized an improved workers' comp system as:

- The legal system is pro-employee when it comes to awarding benefits, which it should be. But it should also be pro-employee in terms of helping the employee to focus on remaining a productive, gainfully employed citizen. Instead, I see a focus by the courts on benefits, disability, SSDI, perm total, etc. There doesn't seem to be any "tough love" with employees in regards to job searches, transferrable skills, or a productive future as a taxpayer.
- Model the State of Indiana system.
- Remove attorney involvement. Remove appointed judges. Mandate treatment directives. Mandate modified duty of all employers. Mandate MPN usage in all states. There is no ideal model but California, Florida, Illinois, Pennsylvania, and New York ARE NOT the models to use!
- Too much variance in laws/statutes from state to state. Would like to see a more uniform and consistent approach.
- The current process in IL is a very slow process - both parties should be able to move claims forward - there should be timeframe in which to accept compensability and then no starting/stopping benefits based on the insurance carrier's doctor's opinion. This only slows the process from treatment, to settlement.
- Implementing a collective bargaining system or a system to eliminate the need for attorney involvement.
- Keep attorneys out completely. 100% Employer Medical Direction (like Indiana).

An Employer's Attorney conceptualized an improved workers' comp system as:

- We need to make sure that we know who is responsible for paying any outstanding bills. The way the system currently works is problematic. Also, it may be a good idea to offer injured employees in general psych consults, even to those with injuries that are not as traumatic.

An Employer conceptualized an improved workers' comp system as:

- It's a Sisyphean task - the system is self sustaining and has discarded all viable stakeholders that could have made a difference.

Consultants conceptualized an improved workers' comp system as:

- Have a system where we choose the appropriate physician. Allowing claimants to doctor shop is stupid.
- Have a system that takes into account pre-existing conditions. Right now, you have to fight to get any information even though work comp is excluded from HIPAA.
- Have a time limit for pysch issues just like long term disability.
- Significant improvement in insurer practices with regard to working with quality medical providers; fast and attentive response from employers post injury; much faster resolution of legal disputes.
- Add more Arbitrators and Judges to move cases along quicker.

Athletic Trainers conceptualized an improved workers' comp system as:

- Boosting the economy over all so my client's business does better. Other than that our system could benefit from less paper work that our client requires simply as "CYA" paperwork.

- Everyone should be under surveillance, but have the chance to defend their actions. Pictures don't tell the whole story. Run it just like work - whatever sick time you have you have, whatever PTO time you have you have, whatever you get paid for you would get paid for in the same way. And make it universal. Many people live/work in diff. states and that just messes with their RTW when you have all the issues that cross state boarders. Unify it. Have a WC counselor assigned to every case. That person will sit down and tell someone "this is how it will go, this is what will/wont happen, this is what you will/wont do and this is what you will be held accountable for."
- Have Physical therapists and/or MD decided plan of care of rather then a Nurse.

Occupational Medicine Specialists conceptualized an improved workers' comp system as:

- As noted above, no fault health care, where there would be no need to establish causality, and eliminate the tension and double standard that issue creates. All citizens would receive optimum treatment for their injuries or ailments. Supported by monies from a central government source, rather than a for-profit insurer, while employers might be expected to contribute additionally in some manner to cover unique costs of their employees, but generally all would benefit equally. In a country as affluent as ours, there should be no place for inadequate care, especially for productive employees.
- A no fault system where the objective is to get people back to being functional, even if they have a loss of some function. Where an arbiter sits with the employee and the employer and gets the best of both worlds so that the employee and the employer are satisfied as to the end result, searching for the appropriate and adequate means of RTW.

Exercise Physiologists conceptualized an improved workers' comp system as:

- An ideal model would include more face time with the patients, more physical rehabilitation than pharmaceutical drugs, less denied payments and attorney involvement on both sides, less marketing dollars spent by insurance companies, an agreed upon reimbursement rate for providers that allows providers to keep the lights on and make a good living and give quality treatments to injured persons. That's the big picture. Who needs details?
- Free market for the providers. Better systematic review of outcomes by the carriers---a review that goes far beyond "price of service." Better assessment of the relevant behavior (here again, at that seminal moment in a case, the FCE). I hate to beat this to death, but the FCE has been a missed opportunity since their inception, simply because to quantify function, you must quantify behavior **objectively**. Otherwise the outcome is dependent on the relative skills of the attorneys, the mood and understanding of the judge/arbitrator and possibly the whims of a jury.

A Physician's Assistant conceptualized an improved workers' comp system as:

- Eliminate it and require employers to contribute more to personal health insurance - which all employees would then have. Employee would use own insurance for treatment - work would be responsible for holding position for return and for paid leave during disability - all with limits.

Advocates conceptualized an improved workers' comp system as:

- I would like to see nationalized medical and disability benefits. The majority of the expense in disputed cases arises from the industry that feeds on the litigation. Too many uneducated, blue-collar workers' simply give up.
- This is a "dangerous" question to ask me. I would remove so many things, such as the investigations of claims before they are accepted, I would remove Independent Medical Examinations for the first 12 months of the claim just accept that the treating medical team actually do know what is best for the injured worker. I would have a many support systems in place not just for the injured worker but for the family of the injured worker as well. I would ensure that the case managers understand that they are dealing with a person not a claim number. Every claim file would have a photo of the injured worker so as there is a reminder to everyone that there is a need for dignity and respect.

The authors conclude with a sampling of case studies provided by the respondents. They are organized by profession:

Case Managers' Case Studies:

- A young, very dedicated full time patient had a big spine surgery. Back problems had ensued from the overworked conditions and the company's saving money by using manual labor versus conveniences to prevent injury. The patient had physical therapy which we extended until the patient was able to function on land based exercises. When it came to the attention of the adjuster that the patient's physical therapist was adjacent to a commercial gym and the patient could have some supervision for appropriate exercises, I advocated for the approval of the gym membership prescribed by the spine surgeon, although the adjuster went into the Cost benefit mode and refused. I explained that the initial investment would be useful to keep the patient on the job, and eventually the patient got the 3 month membership. On other cases I also illustrated to the adjuster and managers that the patient's initial care would eventually allow the patient to be more productive for the company and that not providing the exercise training would cost them much more in the end.
- I implemented vocational rehabilitation on a 50 year old mechanic when he was 10 days post op-rotator cuff repair. After 10 months of rehab and post-op care, he had a Associates Degree and 3 semesters of Spanish. With his other skills, he was a great job placement candidate when he reached MMI. The costs of an Associates Degree was about $5K. The client was motivated and maintained motivation throughout; his attorney was supportive to the rehab plan, etc.

An Employer's Attorney's Case Study:

- The most challenging cases I have had, have always been those in which the treating doctor wants to treat forever and the patient believes in this doctor. I once had a lady who had about 5 surgeries to her elbow, arm and hand and probably 3 of them were not needed. But this doctor kept telling her that her next surgery was going to "heal all of her pain" and she believed him. It wasn't until we convinced her to switch doctors and see a well respected arm surgeon that we got things to turn around. But it was amazing to me to see the power that this doctor had over her.

A Consultant's Case Study:

- A worker sprained his back. Weighs 400 lbs. After being off 1 1/2 years, now alleging psych even though the employer knows the family history and previous psych and back issues. Challenging to get the info about past injuries and getting an IME that takes into account prior psych issues. This guy is using the system to keep him from ever going back to work.

Athletic Trainers' Case Studies:

- If they were interesting or challenging they wouldn't be representative of the case load now would they (smile)?
- Getting the TPA adjuster to understand the importance of timely physician intervention.
- Not so good - The patient had multiple injuries while on his job. He had previously hurt his arm, but had documented proof he had equal strength and AROM prior to getting hurt with that arm (so his previous injury shouldn't matter, right?). This guy tried WC/WH and did not, but his UE injuries limited him. He kept getting MD & IME appt. rescheduled by the insurance company all the while he apparently has severe damage and needs surgery. He has been in limbo with that for over a year now.
- I had a patient that came for WC/WH that was approved for 4 weeks but as soon as the script was finished, all other visits were to be denied even though it was medically necessary for the individual to continue due to the requirements of the job. Even with filing an appeal through the insurance company only one additional visit was authorized. This is due to a utilization review of documents being misread.

Occupational Medicine Specialists' Case Studies:

- A middle-aged mill worker presented with a complaint of sciatica he attributed to routine work activities a month earlier. He denied any specific incident but filed a WC claim based on bending over at work. In the interim he had already sought care from his PCP and a chiropractor, with whom he continued to treat. Apparently, when he realized the cost of his co-pays with his indemnity policy, he opted to defer to the employer's WC policy. As physician for the employer I confirmed the clinical diagnosis and requested records from the treating providers. A very thorough History note from the chiropractor carefully documented the absence of any injury, insult or work activity on his presentation last month! I shared that discrepancy with the employer's Human Resources manager who confronted the employee with the doctor's report, and the employee opted to withdraw the WC claim rather than challenge it's veracity. The employee continued to report to me regularly as requested, completed his course of manipulation with complete recovery, and willingly returned to full duty, from the restricted status I had imposed.

- The employee indicates that he fell on a table and hurt his back. Notifies on a Monday after a long weekend. No physical findings of loss of function or muscle tone, just pain. Patient works at a nonphysical job, that requires standing and sitting. Never returned to work, at the last alleging severe depression due to his physical loss and pain.

An Exercise Physiologist's Case Study:

- Patient came in for an FCE stating that her MD (ortho) did not want her to return to work based on the level of injury to her knee. She had been at her employer for 7 years, was a single mother, and wanted to RTW. Patient was completely functional during testing, so I had her perform additional tasks above and beyond the FCE -- wrote a strong RTW letter, called all parties and made a RTW recommendation -- and the patient went back to work. The Orthopedic MD was very upset about this outcome, but went along with it due to my recommendation and pressures from the other parties. In this case, the patient wanted to RTW and we should not stand in the way of her employment—especially with few transferrable skills. At least, she could go give it a try.
- Second case -- while performing WC/WH on a patient, the NCM called at the 3 week mark and told me that the client will RTW after 4 weeks (1 additional week). It was my recommendation that he would need another 2-4 weeks to progress to the HEAVY PDL required of his job. NCM did not agree and said she would not authorize. I wrote a progress note for the 4 week MD appointment and obtained a prescription for the remaining 2-4 weeks. NCM was very upset and denied treatment. We treated anyway, based on the prescription from the MD. We obtained a HEAVY PDL functional outcome and a RTW at the 8 week mark. In the end, the patient RTW and is a productive again in society.

Advocates' Case Studies:

- One case in particular stands out in my mind. The case was referred by a doctor's wife who volunteered in a soup kitchen. The injured worker and her two children were living in their care. She had learning disabilities that made it impossible for her to read and write. She was barely able to walk due to a work-related back injury. She obtained government disability and medical benefits, for herself and her children -- and ultimately a workers' compensation settlement that provide a significant special needs trust.
- A difficult case for me is the one that I am involved with at present, the injured worker was working as a career and an enrolled nurse. Her injury was caused when an elderly patient fell on her breaking her neck and shattering her shoulder blade. There have been many surgeries and now the lady has had her neck repaired and her shoulder blade rebuilt. There is limited movement in her neck and limited movement in her shoulder. However the biggest tragedy in all of this is the lady is going blind due to a non-compensable illness. The claims agent has shown no compassion at all, refusing to have home help in place that is the same person every time so as the injured worker can be reassured that everything will remain in place in her own home. The claims agent has stated that the blindness is of no concern to them, the requirement is for home help and nothing more. The only option we have had is to negotiate a redemption for the injured worker who will never be able to return to work in her chosen field. Because of the workplace injury will now be excluded from any form of retraining to return her to work as a result of her blindness, not the compensable injury.

The authors would again like to thank all of those who took the significant time required to complete this survey, and they hope to provide an annual update henceforth.

CHAPTER 8

Getting Justice: The Unintended Consequences of the Dispute Resolution System

Robert M. Aurbach

Uncommon Approach, Inc.; E-mail: Bob@uncommonapproach.com

Abstract: The adversarial process of dispute resolution in workers' compensation claims that occurs in most American jurisdictions creates significant costs and delays for all parties. These proceedings also have significant unintentional consequences with respect to the long-term outcomes of many injured people. Delay in case resolution, and circumstances that require the workers to repeatedly focus on their disability, tend through the mechanism of neuroplasticity, to habituate the association between physical symptoms, emotional responses and the events focusing the workers on their condition. This combination of symptoms, emotions and thoughts helps to explain why the probability of returning to full productive life drops as the length of time away from work increases. The actions of attorneys in the dispute resolution system are particularly pernicious contributors to this phenomenon. There is a discussion of some mechanisms for adjusting dispute resolution to improve outcomes.

INTRODUCTION

Two workers suffer the exact same injury. One recovers from the physical injuries as expected, undergoes physical therapy to regain function, returns to the pre-injury job and is awarded a nominal award for permanent impairment. He resumes his life with minimal disruption and long-term effect.

The second worker undergoes a normal course of recovery from the initial presenting injury, but has lingering pain that does not have any clear medical etiology. He undergoes a long series of treatments by an increasing small army of doctors to find and treat the cause. He attempts physical therapy, but is guarded and resistant, fearing re-injury. His case goes into protracted litigation, with the employer questioning the legitimacy of the currently reported symptoms and the worker pressing, through his attorney, for the largest possible award. The worker becomes despondent about his future and the impact on his degenerating family life. He becomes addicted to pain medications. Eventually he "wins" an award of permanent total disability, of which the attorney gets a sizable percentage, and finds that it is insufficient to restore or maintain the lifestyle he had prior to injury. He has no hope of returning to productive life, and seeks support from the Social Security disability system for continued maintenance.

In examining this phenomenon, it is important to avoid confusing the outward manifestations of a complex mechanism with its causes. Much has been written about the predictive value of psychosocial factors in understanding the difference between these two workers (Fulton-Kehoe *et al* 2008). As an explanation it is instructive, but insufficient. Psychosocial factors may contribute to the result, directly or indirectly, or they may be co-morbid with the failure to recover as expected, but they do not cause it. Developments in the understanding of how the human mind works and reshapes its internal networks to adapt to stimuli give added depth to the understanding of why some claimants thrive and return to life, and why others spiral into disability and emotional dysfunction. The way that we treat people and the expectations that we create in the course of processing their claims through the dispute resolution system can have significant impact on their ultimate outcome. Many of those that we teach to act like victims learn so well that they never stop. This process, sometimes referred to as iatrogenic disability, system-made disability, or needless disability, has been well documented in medicine. There is strong indication that a similar phenomenon is created by the adversarial nature of dispute resolution in workers' compensation claims.

IATROGENIC DISABILITY AND NEUROPLASTICITY

I have asked over 5000 persons in audiences across the United States and Australia the following question: " Suppose I gave you a blank check. You could write it for any amount up to, say, $50 million dollars. How many of you would accept a life altering injury in exchange for that check?" To date, not one person has volunteered to accept the trade.

Chris E. Stout, Matt Kruger and Jeffrey Rogers, (Eds)

When our system for resolving disputes forgets that that no one voluntarily chooses to live a altered by disability in exchange for a monetary payout, the system abandons the desires, as well as the best interests, of the injured.

Iatrogenic disability is that disability that is caused by the system in which the disabling event is treated or adjudicated. When a physician administers a treatment that is contrary to that indicated by best practices as informed by the best available empirical evidence and the result of the treatment leaves the patient in worse condition than they were prior to the doctor's visit, any resulting disability is iatrogenic (Aronoff & Feldman 2007; Brigham 2003; Mitchell 2000).

Although the use of the term in medicine is fairly common1 the concept of injury caused by the treatment provided for a particular presenting condition can be profitably applied to other areas in the workers' compensation world. It is of particular importance to consider the relatively understudied impact of litigation and the involvement of attorneys on the long-term outcomes of those presenting disputes for resolution by our workers' compensation systems.

To understand iatrogenic disability, it is important to understand the mechanism by which the mind incorporates experience into the literal structure of the brain. The mechanism relies on the ability of the brain to alter the organization of its neural networks based upon experience, a phenomenon known as brain plasticity or neuroplasticity (Duffau 2006; Kolb & Wishaw 1998; Doidge 2007; Strang 1985). Brain plasticity continues throughout life, and is the mechanism for all kinds of adaptive behavior. Repetitive experience creates connections between parts of the brain, facilitating responses in the presence of certain stimuli. It is variously associated with repair by the brain of certain kinds of organic damage, such as stroke, habit and addiction formation, creation of muscle memory in athletes and enhanced playing ability in musicians. Famously, Dr. Doidge coined the phrase most often used to describe the phenomenon; "Neurons that fire together, wire together."

The significance of this new understanding of brain function is that it explains a lot about the formation of the link between ideas, emotions and physical sensations. When a person feels pain and a doctor tells them that he or she has a permanent condition, the feeling of pain becomes associated, over time, with the diagnosis, the emotional response to the diagnosis and factors associated with the diagnosis[2]. This is particularly true when the injured person has to validate and/or defend, over and over, their non-working status by disclosing their diagnosis to others, defending their status in court, and brooding over their status during the period any dispute resolution process is pending. With this repetition of the association, the synapses adapt to make the connection between sensation and diagnosis more automatic. The diagnosis also associated becomes with various emotions: helplessness, fear, injustice and all of the other components of what we commonly refer to as the role of a victim., or "learned helplessness" At that point, an experience of pain, reminder of diagnosis, or the situation invoking the victim's role each trigger the other experiences, and the creation of a disabling outcome is complete. The injured person has adopted to the role of the victim. As repetitions of this cycle continue to build while the claim for benefits awaits resolution, the worker sinks deeper into the role of the victim, the neural network of associations becomes stronger and with it the role becomes harder to break. It is no wonder that the literature is rich with studies showing that when a worker is off from work for a period of time the probability of their eventual return to work decreases. Most of these studies suggest that if a worker has not returned to work in 12 - 24 weeks, the probability of their eventual return is cut in half (Benyahya *et al* 2004;Bouter *et al* 2006; Bruns & Disorbrio 2009; Hay *et al* 2008; Jin *et al* 1995; Johoda 1982; Kinicki *et al* 2005; Main *et al* 2007; Martikainen& Valkonen 1998; Mathers & Schofield 1998; McGill 1968; Meyers & Sander 1986; Nachemson 1983; Stewart 2001; Strang 1985).

Psychosocial factors likely have a role in this process. Some people feel despair when additional stressors (like the rigors of recovery and dispute resolution) are added to their life, where others are able to shrug off the additional load. The degree to which someone is resistant to an emotional reaction to additional stressors is likely influenced by the nature and cumulative impact of the other stressors in their life. Collectively, we call these other stressors "psychosocial factors" and note that a high level of those kinds of stimuli correlates with the acquisition of the complex of physical sensation, emotion and ideas that we call "learned victimization", or "learned helplessness".

Once we understand that the way the human brain processes information is adaptive and facilitates connections that

---

[1]The National Library of Medicine, National Institute of Health research database Pub Med lists 216 records on a search of the term in late April, 2010.

[2]In this context, the phrase, "maximum medical improvement" has the ominous ring of a life sentence to many workers.

render connections between sensations thoughts and emotions habitual, the connection between delay and repetition of behaviors modeling disability during the dispute resolution process and poor outcomes for some of those utilizing the process becomes understandable. Time focusing the attention of the injured worker on the diagnosis, circumstances of injury, current physical sensations and prognosis all tend to focus the injured party on his or her disability, and render it habitual. Repetition of behaviors associated with the disability also cause habituation, through exactly the same mechanism. Therefore, when avoidance of iatrogenic disability is the goal, time in the disadvantaged state and repetitions of the disabled behavior patterns are the enemy. Unfortunately, the processes used in the U.S. to resolve disputes over workers' compensation claims generally do not incorporate this understanding, and therefore rationally must be considered a potential source of iatrogenic disability.

DISPUTE RESOLUTION IN WORKERS' COMPENSATION

Dispute resolution in Worker' Compensation in the United States is almost always a bewildering and counter-intuitive process for the injured worker. He or she is confronted by a claims adjuster who is often taxed by their case loading beyond the reasonable ability to respond to the worker with the same urgency as the worker attributes to their issues. The services of the treating physician may be questioned, and treatment delayed. The physician may not be the injured worker's choice of health care providers. Neither situation in health care is likely to be consistent with the common experience of the worker with respect to the care received in other contexts. The terminology utilized in the process is unfamiliar to inexperienced claimants, and some terminology (i.e. "maximum medical improvement") is used in ways that have industry specific meanings.

If there is a dispute, the mechanism(s) for resolution of the dispute may be unfamiliar, and the rigors of presentation of a case for formal dispute resolution require an understanding of the rules of evidence and procedure in effect in that tribunal, an understanding of the specific facts that must be proven to prevail and the ability to present the case, examine necessary witnesses, solicit supporting documentation and successfully argue their position.

While the worker is recovering from their injuries, they are subjected to lawyer advertising and the advice of friends, both tending to create fear of attempting to handle the requirements of the system without help and concurrently creating an expectation concerning the monetary rewards that are expected at the end of the process. During the pendency of the dispute the worker may feel cut off from their support systems present at work, and their identity as a productive person and family bread winner. He or she may feel alienation from his or her employer, friends and family. The worker may, with the reduction of income suffered during time off from work, experience financial pressures, especially if their claim has been denied. These stressors, separately or in combination, may push the worker into seeking the aid of an attorney to assist in the collection of their claim.

Dispute resolution processes vary considerably from jurisdiction to jurisdiction. Some systems utilize some form of alternative dispute resolution mechanism. Models range from true meditation (e. g. the Navajo Nation[3]) to mandatory non-binding arbitration (e.g. New Mexico[4]) to voluntary arbitration (e.g. Mississippi; Quarles, L 2006). Whether or not there is a mechanism for alternative dispute resolution available, the majority of jurisdictions have a captive first level formal dispute resolution mechanism. These include internal administrative law judges[5] and internal boards or commissions.[6] In all U.S. jurisdictions there is eventual access to the civil court system, at least for access to the appellate process.

THE ROLE OF ATTORNEYS IN WORKERS' COMPENSATION CASES

Plaintiff's Attorneys

There are two distinct varieties of plaintiff's lawyers, operating under different economic models and therefore subject to differing influences upon their motivations. The private plaintiff's lawyer is generally compensated by the plaintiff, most often out of the proceeds of the recovery from the case. The private attorney works for the claimant,

[3]15 NNC 1010
[4]Section 52-5-5 NMSA 1978
[5]For example, in California and New Mexico
[6]For example, in Arizona and Arkansas

and owes ethical allegiance to him or her alone.

The public attorney is paid a salary by an entity for which he or she works, and provides services to the plaintiff without expectation of compensation from the plaintiff. The public plaintiff's attorney still owes ethical allegiance to the claimant, but also is subject to certain controls, formal and informal, within their employing entity. Regardless of the role and source of compensation, the role of the plaintiff's lawyer is to win the case before him. The lawsuit is, to the plaintiff's attorney, a classic "zero sum" game where one party wins and the other loses.

Cases are accepted on a variety of criteria. The majority of plaintiff's attorneys are paid only upon obtaining a positive outcome for the injured party. Therefore the plaintiff's attorney will often make an economic decision concerning the viability of the case, both in terms of it's probability of success and in terms of the economic potential for fee generation under the applicable standards controlling attorney remuneration. This can make it hard for worker with a case in which there is a small dollar value in controversy to get representation, even if the issue is of great significance to the worker. This is particularly true in cases where only medical benefits are in dispute. One exception occurs when the case presents a possibility of creating precedent applicable to other cases. The notoriety and opportunity for future business attendant the creation of favorable precedent may provide sufficient motivation for the attorney to accept a case for which a substantial profit is unlikely.

Private plaintiff attorneys are often partially motivated by management of the caseload assigned to them. They may be tempted to utilize tactics to maximize the probability of a settlement of the case. Settlements are desirable, despite generally resulting is some reduction in compensation in the individual matter, because they allow the attorney to undertake representation of a larger number of clients over any period of time. The trade then becomes resolution of more claims at a reduced level of compensation versus maximization of the return on a particular case. The settlement strategy also reduces the probability that a given case will go entirely uncompensated. Tactics utilized include the bringing of questionable claims, accompanied by a willingness to settle them at less than the cost of the defense of the claim, and the bringing of claims for excessive items and amounts of claimed benefits (particularly indemnity benefits) so that the claim will contain items that can be compromised to obtain a settlement. Ethical constraints (which are generally quite loose if the attorney can argue that he or she is seeking an "extension of the law") personal responsibility, and the oversight of administrative and civil courts act are factors limiting such behavior.

Public attorneys may also be motivated to settle cases due to the need to manage their caseload. They may be rewarded for processing more cases in a given period of time, or may be motivated simply by avoiding the sensation of being overwhelmed by their assigned cases, but there is no direct economic motivation to maximize the award for the worker. Public attorneys are often seen as of inferior quality, but that impression ignores the fact that such practitioners are among the most experienced members of the bar in their particular specialty, and that they usually do not have the distractions of the economics of law practice to cloud their judgment or divert their attention.

Defense Attorneys

The defense attorney most often is a member of a law firm that contracts with the payer to handle those claims that require services that are beyond the role of claims adjuster. Attorneys may be statutorily required for the representation of corporations. In such a model, the purchaser of the services is the either the claims adjuster on the case or someone in authority to make such decisions in the payer organization, and the attorney will very likely be mindful of the need to please the hiring entity to obtain further work.

If not a member of a law firm, the defense attorney may be an employee of either an insurance company or an employer that was authorized to assume its own risk of on the job injury. In such cases the attorney may have significant direct control over the positions taken on particular cases and the general style of case handling within that environment.

The defense attorney often faces situations where the possibility of "winning" the case reducing the employer's liability to zero is remote. In such cases, the creation of conditions where a settlement of the case at less than the maximum possible liability is considered a victory. A variety of strategies are utilized for that purpose including delay of the case (to create economic pressure to settle), forcing the claimant to prove their case even when its merits are apparent (in hopes that the other side will make a mistake that can be exploited) or using "scorched earth" tactics

- contesting every possible issue to the maximum extent - to raise the cost of prosecution of the case to the level where a settlement at a compromised level of liability becomes attractive. Countervailing pressures exist to hold down the use of these tactics. They include ethical constraints, personal beliefs, and the desire of the entity paying for defense services to strike a balance between aggressive defense and the cost of the defense in attorney fees and litigation related expenses.

THE ROLE OF ATTORNEYS IN THE CREATION OF DISABILITY

The impact that attorneys have, under the system of compensation of attorneys and resolution of disputes currently prevalent in the United States, in the creation of systemically induced disability is sufficiently unique, that it deserves its own term. For purposes of this Chapter, it will be referred to as "attorneyogenic" disability.[7]

Attorneys, as might be expected, are highly resistant to the notion that their activities might cause disability. To be sure, most attorneys have no idea that they are harming their clients, and would be concerned if they considered the implications of their practice. Some are sufficiently aware to avoid such harms.

THE ROLE OF ATTORNEY FEES IN CREATING DISABILITY

In the United States, most attorneys who accept workers' compensation and/or personal injury lawsuits do so on a contingent fee basis. That is, the attorney representing the injured person does not get paid for their services unless they are successful in obtaining a judgment for the injured party, and they take a percentage of that judgment as their fee. The percentages vary with local practices, but often run between 25% and 33% of the ultimate award for personal injury cases, depending on a variety of factors, including the extent of court proceedings in the case. In workers' compensation the practice of being paid on a contingent fee basis is often controlled by statute, and/or is subject to governmental approval of attorney fees.[8] However, in either case the principle remains the same – the attorney gets paid more, the larger the size of the award received by the injured party. Since the injured party gets a larger award, based upon measures of damages such as loss of wages, expectations of future lost wages, degree of permanent physical impairment, pain and suffering (in personal injury, but not workers' compensation) and medical bill, it is literally true that the attorney gets paid more, the more disabled the injured party is found to be. Thus, the rational economic interest of the attorney representing the injured party is to present him or her to the world as disabled, helpless and without prospects of future improvement, so as to maximize the award.[9]

The impacts of such a system can be both overt and subtle. A worker who has returned to work cannot make a convincing case that they are too disabled to work, and deserving of a higher award on that basis. Workers report, not infrequently, that they were advised by their attorney not to return to work when they felt ready to do so, for fear of compromising the award that they would get at the end of the case.[10] Significant impact also occurs when the attorney publicly refers to the injured party as someone who is no longer able to work, seeks an award based upon the expectation that they will be dependent on others indefinitely, or coaches the client on how to appear at hearings, doctor visits and other occasions where the degree of their disability will be judged. As we have seen above, the modeling of a particular behavior can create associations that make neural connections between the behavior and a whole complex of

---

[7]The term was coined by a physician, whose name was unfortunately not recorded, at the 2009 American Occupational Health Conference of the American College of Occupational and Environmental Medicine. It also appears in a chapter entitled "The Legal System and Behavioral Health" in Warren, P., The Handbook of Behavioral Health Disability: Innovations in Prevention and Management, Springer Publishing, pending publication.

[8]Attorney fees must be approved by the court or administrative body in 37 states, according to "Workers' Compensation Laws, 2d edition – a Joint Publication of IAIABC and WCRI", June 2009

[9] This action, adverse to the long-term best interests of the client, might be considered a conflict of interest. Interestingly, the Rules of Professional Conduct suggest otherwise. Contingent fees in civil cases (except domestic relations) are specifically approved. See, Model Rules of Professional Conduct, Rule 1.5 (C.), American Bar Association, 2004. Conduct adverse to the client's interests is not considered in the general rule on conflict of Interests. Model Rules, *supra.*, 1.7. The issue could be raised under the following language: "Unless otherwise required by these rules, a lawyer shall not represent a client if the representation of that client may be materially limited by….the lawyer's own interests" *supra,* 1.7 (B.), however the rules also provide an exception to the rule prohibiting acquisition of a proprietary interest in a claim for contracting for a contingent fee. *Supra*, rule 1.7 (j.) (2)

[10]The evidence for such events is only anecdotal, but many experienced workers' compensation claims adjusters relate such stories. Personally, I have heard more than a dozen workers relay similar tales, in the capacity of investigator of allegations of fraud, and as an investigator of allegations of attorney misconduct.

beliefs and emotional responses. In common parlance we speak of "self-fulfilling prophecy" or the "Pygmalion effect" rather than speak in terms of the creation of neural pathways, but the outcome is the same regardless of the level of detail invested in the description of the mechanism – the injured party who is treated as if they are disabled, or counseled to act disabled, often becomes the story that is told to the outside world. Thus, some attorneyogenic disability arises as a result of the plaintiff's attorney seeking a larger award, and consequently, a larger fee.

Far from being seen as an inherent conflict of interest, the plaintiff's bar defends the practice on several grounds. First, it is asserted that the use of contingent fees is necessary so that economically challenged individuals can afford to pursue their claims without risking their own resources, already taxed by the loss of work and medical bills attendant the injury. This supposition is only valid in an environment where each party pays their own attorney fees. The system of each party paying their own attorneys fees (sometimes modified by workers' compensation statutes[11]) is called the "American system" of attorney compensation. It is contrasted with the "English system" (Kritzer 1992) in which the losing party pays the costs for representation assessed for both parties. The American system is defended on the ground that other systems suppress meritorious claims from being brought due to the risk of the economic burden of loss. The same system is subject to the criticism that it allows frivolous lawsuits, "strike suits" (litigation brought with the hopes of a settlement for less than the cost of defense) and "professional plaintiffs" litigation (the practice of a small number of very litigious people to make some or all of their living by maintaining multiple lawsuits, against multiple parties, in the hope of sufficient income for economic viability). The majority of the world follows some variant of the "English" system.

Second, the plaintiff's bar asserts that the contingent fee arrangement is necessary to afford access to representation. They argue that, since the plaintiff is always at risk of non-recovery and therefore the attorney representing plaintiffs is always at risk of non-payment, the percentage of fee generating cases has to carry the risk of loss and the burden of economic viability of the entire caseload. Put another way, the winning cases have to finance the losing cases. This argument would be more persuasive if the attorneys representing the injured were required to accept the cases presented to them. The opposite is the case. Attorneys often will not accept cases that they feel have a poor chance of failure in the courts, and even routinely refuse to accept meritorious cases when the potential for fee generation is insufficient. For instance, it is common for a worker that has no claim for wage replacement or indemnity benefits, but who has a dispute about some issue concerning medical care (medical-only claims) to have difficulty finding an attorney that will accept their case. This is because the fee generation potential with regard to a medical services that might result in an award of a few thousand dollars is less attractive than a case involving wages replacement benefits in the tens, or hundreds of thousands of dollars, while consuming equal amounts of the attorney's time and energy.

Finally, the contingent fee system is defended on the grounds that it motivates the attorney to do the very best for the injured party. This argument does not survive much scrutiny. Other professions, including some that are involved in the treatment of injured men and women, seem to survive the test of motivation without making their fees contingent on outcome. Physicians, and related health professionals are often paid on according to schedules for the procedures that they perform, regardless of outcome. This is usually justified on the ground that the physician is not entirely in control of the outcome, which is subject to multiple independent intervening variables. Interestingly, the argument that physicians will put forth better efforts if they are paid contingent on the outcome of their treatment is not considered appropriate.[12] Moreover, like doctors, ethical principles concerning the practice of law already require the attorney to use their best efforts on behalf of their clients.

Defense attorneys are not immune to the lure of additional fees in the practice of workers' compensation. Although there is a growing trend for defense attorneys to be compensated on a flat rate per case basis, the majority of defense practice is done on an hourly fee basis. The creation of additional work results in higher fees, and the practice of an attorney "churning" the case to generate additional billable hours is a well-known hazard with which claims personnel are quite familiar. The difficulty with such practices, as will be discussed below, is the creation of additional delay in the resolution of the case and additional circumstances in which the injured party must model

[11]For example, in many cases the employer and claimant statutorily split liability for the claimant's attorney fees. See e.g. Section 52-5- New Mexico Statutes, Annotated., 1978.

[12]A recent "hot topic" for discussion of in workers' compensation has been the possibility of "pay for performance" for health care professionals. Interestingly, this debate is not based upon an assertion that the doctors will be more motivated to heal the injured worker if their fee structure depends on outcome, but rather on the notion that such a scheme would motivate health care professionals to utilize empirically proven techniques in preference to less effective or more experimental medical procedures.

disabled behavior. As we have seen this additional time and repetition of the associations between the injury and the emotional and intellectual attitude of disability make it more entrenched and harder to overcome.

OTHER FACTORS CREATING "ATTORNEYOGENIC" DISABILITY DELAY

Delay in the resolution of any disputes in the case causes harm. It creates more time in which to habituate the behaviors that model disability. It creates time where the injured worker may obsess upon their condition, the people who have wronged them and the unfairness of the system in failing to compensate them. The obsessive behavior varies among individuals, but where present, it results in repeated association between the injury, the emotional loading of the concern that gave rise to the obsessive behavior, and the worker's status as someone unable to resume their accustomed role in their life. Through the mechanisms discussed above, the worker's neural network adjusts, allowing those associations to become habitually linked, and very difficult to break.

Delay also causes direct hardship, where the worker has medical treatment or benefits necessary for the maintenance of their lifestyle held up by court disputes. These hardships are stressors that increase the tension experienced by the worker and with it the physical symptoms experienced (Copeland 2009; Gatchel, *et al* 2010; Kritzer 1992; Okifuji & Turk 2002). As the delay stretches on, the delay, the resultant stressor, and the increased perception of physical symptoms may habituate themselves, causing a complex association of thoughts feelings and emotions that has become part of the neural makeup of the worker. They may truly experience the negative results of delay, even though those results were never intended.

Delay may come from a variety of sources. It can be a tactic utilized by the defense to put economic pressure to settle on the injured worker (also known as "starving the worker out"). Delay can occur because the attorneys, in an attempt to maximize their own incomes (or in the case of public plaintiff attorneys, because the resources devoted to the function are outstripped by the demand) simply have too much on their respective plates to give each case attention at the first instance when the case is subject to the next step in resolution. It is common to see attorneys have schedules too full to allow quick scheduling of hearings, and the practice of attorneys seeking continuances of matters set for hearing is a continuing problem in judicial administration (Goerdt 2000). Similarly, the crush of a large caseload often stretches available adjudicatory resources, resulting in delays in resolution caused by the inability to obtain a hearing date from the relevant adjudicatory body. Decisions from the courts can be delayed, after hearing, for the same reason. Delay is also caused by the need to coordinate the care, examinations, and reports from multiple physicians, therapists, rehabilitation specialists and other professionals. Regardless of the source of the delay, it all has deleterious effect upon the party seeking to resume their pre-injury life.

ENCOURAGEMENT OF BEHAVIORS FOR THE PURPOSE OF ENHANCEMENT OF THE CASE

The degree to which attorneys functioning within the dispute resolution system to directly or indirectly encourage their clients to model disabled behavior is not well documented. By it's nature, the phenomenon is difficult to study quantitatively, because the perceived economic interest in the pending dispute resolution, and eventual award of benefits, could be compromised by disclosure of tactics that are perceived as being questionable. There is, however, significant anecdotal evidence to suggest that lawyers on both sides either intentionally or inadvertently encourage the injured worker to act in a disabled manner over a longer period of time than is necessitated by their physical condition and repeated in multiple demonstrations of disability. This time in the "disabled" state and repetition of behavior tends to habituate the development of associations between physical sensations, emotional reactions and behavior.

Experienced health care providers and claims management personnel are familiar with the not-infrequent assertion that a worker's attorney told the worker that, "going back to work will damage your case". It is, of course, unknown what percentage of those cases represent actual advise from the workers' attorney and what represent an attempt by the worker to justify their avoidance of return to work, a mis-communication between worker and attorney, or the mis-attribution by the worker of advice obtained from some third party. Nor is it likely to be possible to quantify such behaviors, since an admission by the attorney may be considered a breach of the Rules of Professional Conduct[13] governing the ethical constraints of attorneys. Nonetheless, the persistence and frequency of such reports suggests that the phenomenon is real. Assuming *arguendo* that such reports are sometimes legitimate and accurate,

[13]Model Rules of Professional Conduct, Rule 3.3 a 1 and 3 and b. American Bar Association, 2004.

the holding of a worker out of work for longer than is necessary has clearly been shown to have a detrimental impact on their ability to eventually return to work at all.

Nor are the attorneys representing injured workers the sole source of such deleterious effects. When an attorney engaged in the defense of a claim questions the legitimacy or severity of the disability or its causes, the likely outcome is to force the worker to model the disabled behavior more often and for longer periods of time, with outcomes that are predictable in light of our understanding of neural plasticity and the formation of the "disabled persona"[14]. This effect can be magnified in an atmosphere where there is an expectation that an investigator will be watching the claimant in an attempt to catch them acting in a manner inconsistent with disability.

PROFESSIONAL ENABLING

Even where the motivation of the attorney representing the injured worker is entirely the pursuit of the workers' enlightened best interests, the role of attorney, by its nature, tends to exacerbate the possibility that an injured person will develop habituated disability behaviors. "Enabling" is a term applied, often in the context of alcoholism, or other issues involving family dysfunction, to describe actions by another, which tend to separate or protect someone from the consequences of their actions. An alcoholic's enabler might work an extra job to keep familial finances under control, make excuses for absence from work, create inaccurate explanations for family and friends for the alcoholics behavior and even deceive themselves intro thinking that everything is normal, or at least an appropriate response to stressors in the environment. The enabler acts from a desire to maintain the appearance of normalcy and stability rather than from any motivation inimical to the best interests of the alcoholic. Unfortunately, the actions of the enabler often allow the behavior to develop to the extent that the addiction is much harder to address and the chances for a positive resolution are diminished (Wegscheider-Cruse 1989).

Professionals can also take the role of an enabler. A lawyer acts as a professional enabler when seeking to shield the client from the consequences of his or her actions. The most obvious example of this is the role of a criminal defense attorney. Such attorneys conceive their role to be to "get the client off" the charges, or at least to minimize the punishment for the offense, if liability for the criminal act cannot be successfully avoided. Parallel roles often occur in the context of employment law, marital and familial situations, and economic dealings.

The role of enabler in workers' compensation involves the promise of outside intervention to spare the worker the consequences of taking responsibility for their recovery and return to normalcy. The television lawyer advertisements proclaim that "you may be entitled to a large cash award", or similar phrasing. The frequently used terms, "award", "settlement" and "compensation" all imply that the status of the worker has changed. The term "entitled" is often used to describe the relationship between the change in status and the "award". The message is that the worker is owed something by the world –they should not focus on their own resources and choices but should rely upon the world providing compensation for the wrong that has been done to them. This focuses the injured party on the outside world as the source of their problems and the lawyer as their salvation. This belief system, while a very good advertising practice, focuses the injured worker on their helplessness and, by repetition of the message, creates dependency. Unfortunately, when the case is over, the attorney will move on to the next case, pulling the support from the worker, who now has to confront abandonment issues as well as their acquired disabled persona. Unfortunately for the worker, the cash settlement is never sufficient to make them whole as compared to the wage earning potential they have as a working person (Barth *et al* 1998; Biddle *et al* 2001a; Biddle *et al* 2001b; Reville 2001).

CHARGES OF SYMPTOM MAGNIFICATION AND MALINGERING

The terms "symptom magnification" and "malingering" are often used, incorrectly, as being synonymous, but both give rise to dynamics that encourage the worker to model disabled behavior longer and more frequently, with predictable, if somewhat ironic, results.

---

[14]"Disabled persona" is a useful term for the personality organization of a person who, by reason of the habituation of associations between their injury, their experience of physical symptoms, and emotions such as depression, anger, helplessness and hopelessness begins to see themselves as a victim of their circumstances, unable to take control of their situation.

"Symptom magnification" in the legal context is the tendency for a person to focus on physical symptoms that exceeds "normal" expectations. "Normal" however, is in the eye of the beholder. Most people have had the experience of getting a bruise or cut and not remembering how they got it. Many people have experienced themselves, or someone else, overreacting to a relatively minor injury or condition. "Normal" reaction lies somewhere along the continuum between these two responses. The person who focuses on their perception of physical symptoms also tends to focus upon the anticipation of future experiences of the physical symptom and fear associated with those anticipated future events. The complex of physical symptoms, emotional responses, and worries about the future becomes habituated through the mechanism of neural plasticity, and symptom magnification is established.

In this context, the defense attorney, often at the suggestion of a health care provider, investigator or employer, may seek to establish that the worker is magnifying their symptoms in an attempt to gain a larger award. By doing so, the worker may perceive an attack on his or her credibility. The natural tendency of someone under such a perceived attack is to defend himself or herself, often by modeling the disabled behavior that they are accused of magnifying, to demonstrate to the world that the symptom is real. Moreover, the accusation will likely cause delays in the resolution of the case, and an increased probability (whether perceived or real) that the worker's actions and activities will be scrutinized by an investigator. Thus, the charge of malingering ironically causes the worker to focus more and longer upon the very symptoms he or she is accused of magnifying, causing either an entrenchment of the behavior, if it exists, or in some cases the creation of the magnifying behavior. It becomes a classic case of self-fulfilling prophesy (Tauber 1997).

"Malingering" is a much more serious charge, and generally a more value- loaded accusation under the law. "Malingering" is the conscious creation, extension or magnification of symptoms or limitations in the anticipation of "secondary gain" (Aronoff *et al* 2007; Canyock *et al* 2002; Conroy & Kwartner 2006; Reid 2000). Secondary gain is, in turn a neutral term to which a value loading has become associated, and implies the seeking of an external reward for a particular behavior (Gatchel & Shultz 2005). Secondary gain can range from increased attention and sympathy from loved ones through permission to avoid disagreeable tasks, to behavior aimed at maximizing the economic payout from a particular incident. Where the worker is consciously seeking secondary economic gain that they are not otherwise entitled to, the malingering becomes a species of fraud.

Like symptom magnification, the ability to demonstrate the requisite mental state is critical to proof of the allegation. Similarly to symptom magnification, the proof of the charge is necessarily indirect, and the allegation itself causes the worker to feel threatened and attempt to defend him self or herself. Often this defensive behavior contributes to the habituation of it, and the resentment of the treatment at the hands of the employer's agent may lead to a sense of justification for intentional creation, maintenance or extension of symptoms for economic recompense. Ironically, in such cases the behavior of defense counsel may actually create the problem it was designed to eliminate or defend against.

The ethical plaintiff's attorney will not encourage malingering or symptom magnification. Aside from ethical considerations, all claimant advocates quickly come to understand that people who are overly focused upon their symptoms tend to be difficult and demanding clients. However, the actions of the plaintiff's advocate are not necessarily benign. The attorney is more highly compensated, the more disabled the worker is shown to be. People who are focused on their symptoms tend to present them as more severe to evaluating physicians and tend to be more credible in defense of those symptoms as witnesses. It is difficult to counsel a client on how to present themselves as a witness without inadvertently communicating the message that the more convincing the worker is about their condition, the better the outcome of the case.

CHANGE OF LOCUS OF CONTROL

The legal process is one where the claimant is almost always subject to a loss of sense of control. Control is lost to the lawyers and judges running the process of dispute resolution, a health system that casts the patient in to the role of passive recipient and claims examiners who may control the means to obtain the basic needs of day to day living. The transfer of control over the necessities of daily living has been shown to be a good predictor for increased disability. In this context it is usually referred to as a change in the perceived locus of control (Lefcourt 1982). This is a systemic variant of "medicalization" of a claim, involving the larger actions of the entire medico-legal system in the process The resulting encouragement of an identity as a disabled person, internalization of limitations consistent with that role and change of perceptions so that experience in the world is interpreted to reinforce those limitations has been sometimes called "learned helplessness (Gatchel & Turk 2002; Gatchel 2004; Maier *et al* 1993)"The legal system has shown no conscious awareness of the impact of this phenomenon on the plaintiff's long term well being, although there is a tendency for the plaintiff's advocate to assert that the diagnosis, once established, is a permanent condition. Unfortunately, the legal process itself may help fulfill this prophecy.

ABANDONMENT

In general, the legal system stops when the claim is resolved. There is no follow up to see if the litigants have resolved their issues and moved on with their lives. The advocate for the claimant has no systemic motivation to assist him or her after the claim is completed, depriving the claimant of what may have been their only support system during the pendency of the litigation. Planning for functional adaptation and treatment after the dispute is resolved is often lacking. Once the projected future costs of functional recovery are reduced to a monetary figure and an award is made, the claimant is most frequently left to their own devices with regard to actually obtaining services.

CATASTROPHIC THINKING

In the process of presenting the best possible case for a large award of damages, the natural tendency is for attorneys to project the worst possible case into the future, for the purpose of creating motivation for the award of maximized future damages. When an individual projects the worst case scenario into the future, behavioral health experts are likely to refer to the phenomenon as "catastrophic thinking" and take therapeutic steps to assist the person in recasting their thinking into more useful directions. When the same behavior takes place in the courtroom, it is considered good advocacy, and the lawyers involved seem unconcerned that the claimant may internalize the characterization, engage in his or her own catastrophic thinking about their condition and prospects and habituate the disabled behavior that was being projected (Horwitz & Wakefield 2007; Barsky & Borus 1995). Indeed, conversations with plaintiff attorneys about their clients are usually scattered with reference to lives that have been irretrievably shattered, with no hope of meaningful restoration and only a large award as solace. If the worker's guide to this mysterious process has given up hope for his client's recovery, the claimant's opinion is likely to follow.

MULTIPLE MEDICAL EVALUATIONS AND TREATMENT PROTOCOLS

A very significant occasion for development of needless disability comes at the hands of the medical profession, when it is invoked by the legal profession in the process of dispute resolution. In this sense, the drive to maximize awards for disability engenders contact with the medical profession that is sometimes problematic, and the circumstances for the creation of needless disability can be legitimately be said to arise from the legal context.

In the course of a dispute, if one side has a doctor providing an opinion concerning a critical issue, odds are that the other side will want its own medical expert to give a contrary opinion. The potential for this feature of dispute resolution to act as a cost driver is exacerbated by the fact that some U.S. jurisdictions allow, when each side has a contrary medical opinion, the engagement of a "neutral" third medical provider to create a tie breaking opinion.[15] Diagnostic testing is multiplied, additional delay for examinations and opinion generation is encountered and the worker is subjected to repeated deliveries of the message that they are subject to the control of others in the process of dispute resolution. Moreover, the message is often confounded by the variance between professionals.

Differing opinions amongst doctors as to the diagnosis, medical causation, and level of permanent impairment lead to the sense that no one knows what they are doing, or that the medical professionals are not objective and interested in the worker's best interests.

Perhaps more serious is the repeated message that the worker is a diagnosis, rather than a functional human being. It is not uncommon to hear workers refer to themselves by their diagnosis rather than in more personal terms. The negative effects of this phenomenon should be clear, given out understanding of neural plasticity and the

[15]See, for instance, http://www.lni.wa.gov/ClaimsIns/Providers/Treatment/IME/About/default.asp, describing the procedure under WAC 296-23-302-392 for an IME to be requested by an insurer. See, also Section 52-1-51, NMSA 1978 for an example of the procedure in effect for the parties to request a "tie-breaker" IME.

"medicalization (Harvard Magazine 2009; Conrad 2007)" of patients. The focus on the connection between injury at work and disability, the worker's personal identification with a diagnosis, and the process of multiple evaluations of impairment repeatedly sends the message of disability, limitation, and inability to resume a normal life to the worker. Like the classic case of the child, told by a teacher that he or she is stupid, conforming to the message in their performance at school (Tauber 1997) it is not surprising when the worker acquires a disabled lifestyle and develops what is for them a genuine inability to return to productivity and normalcy.

This unfortunate cycle is partly perpetuated by the fact that the payment system for medical services is based, for the most part on diagnosis as a condition precedent for payment.

Medical practice guidelines and impairment ratings are almost universally diagnosis based, and most payers for medical services in the workers' compensation and personal injury arenas are organized to recognize the provision of services only in the context of a diagnosis. This has led to the description and naming of a number of "diagnoses of exclusion", that are the diagnostic label put on people who exhibit what appear to be genuine complaints, but for which there are no objective signs or symptoms (Conrad 2007). The placement of these labels on the injured worker creates an opportunity to refer to the various complaints with greater facility, leading to repetition of a consistent message and creation of links between that message and other factors in the life of the worker. Thus, the worker who can refer to the cluster of complaints they are experiencing with the easily uttered phrase, such as "chronic pain syndrome" will be more likely to reinforce their identity with the diagnosis.

Moreover, these "diagnoses of exclusion", by naming the cluster of complaints, tend to give a air of objective reality to them. In a process of modern shamanism, the naming leads to a chain of faulty reasoning: "If it's got a name, then it's got to be something real. If it's something that medical science regards as real, then it's something that I have to look to an outside professional to treat. If I'm not getting better with treatment, then I must be disabled." Unfortunately, since the original diagnosis was based on the exclusion of all diagnoses for which the etiology and treatment were well understood, the probability of a poor outcome is significant.

THE IMPACT OF CURRENT DISPUTE RESOLUTION PRACTICES -THREE STUDIES

While it is clear from the above that the impact of our dispute resolution mechanisms for workers' compensation in the United States can and does inadvertently create significant additional disability, the costs associated with such disabilities are essentially impossible to isolate. The myriad of confounding factors, including the entire array of psychosocial factors impinging on each individual, and the significant differences among attorneys with respect to the extent that they engage in practices that facilitate the formation of "attorneyogenic "disability, present factors for which it is impossible to control with accuracy, given the current state of data collection in the field. But these are not the only costs of attorney involvement in the dispute resolution system. The payments made in benefits and payments made to third parties for services to the worker are more accessible for study. While the state of the art with regard to research in this area still is problematic, the results of the few studies that are available are suggestive.

The discussion of the impact of attorney presence in workers' compensation is often confounded by a mis-perception about what the issue is that is under discussion. For purposes of this chapter, I am unconcerned about the amount of money directly paid to plaintiffs or defense counsels in exchange for their services. The costs vary somewhat from state to state, but seldom is the total of defense and plaintiff's costs in excess of 10% of total loss costs. For purposes of this analysis, I will consider that sum to be a necessary expenditure, notwithstanding that it may be reduced by implementation of some of the suggestions enumerated at the end of this chapter. Rather, the impact of attorney involvement discussed here is the *indirect* effect of attorney involvement. The focus is on the additional costs caused by the creation of needless disability, the multiplication of costs in the resolution of disputes, the multiplication of medical/legal costs and the costs of diagnostic treatment, multiple examinations and re-examinations and other factors that are co-incident with attorneys representing clients.

THE DIFFICULTY IN STUDYING THE INDIRECT COSTS OF ATTORNEY INVOLVEMENT

The difficulty in studying the costs of attorney involvement is based in the difficulty in establishing comparable populations for study. An examination of the differences in total expenditures between populations of workers represented by an attorney and populations that resolve their disputes without representation is well within the capability of many workers' compensation research entities. The difficulty with such comparisons is that they often do not tell us very much. Attorneys for workers will counter that the workers who come to them tend to be the most severely injured, and that differences in benefits paid out between represented and unrepresented cohorts are due to them successfully obtaining results for the workers that they could not obtain on their own. Accordingly, severity – a measure of how injured the populations to be compared are, and outcomes – a measure of how successful the representation of the worker was, must be controlled if definitive statements about the cost of attorney involvement in our dispute resolution systems are to have credibility.

The best model for study would be a case of a jurisdiction that changed the involvement of attorneys directly or indirectly by statute under circumstances where it had collected compatible data sets concerning system costs and outcomes over periods before and after the change of sufficient size to allow the length of the "tail" on workers' compensation claims (the period of payout of benefits) to be largely completed. Ideally, this change would be the sole change in an otherwise stable period of statutory history, to minimize the confounding factors on behavior generated by other changes in the law, leaving only inflation and changes in the demographics in employment over time as factors for which the data had to be normalized. This situation has not existed at any time in the United States, and by the nature of legislative reform, is unlikely to ever exist. Any motivating factor of sufficient magnitude to result in significant changes in the interaction of lawyers with a segment of the legal system is highly unlikely to be the only component of the efforts undertaken to resolve the situation. Moreover, data collection efforts have only relatively recently become sufficiently sophisticated to allow such research.

Such a model would work because the size of the samples before and after the change in the law would be sufficient that the severity of accidents could be reasonably presumed to be constant, and the variations of outcomes could be measured by the overall awards of benefits and normalized across the data. The closest example that comes to mind is that of the state of Western Australia, which, in November of 2005, reauthorized the use of attorneys in workers' compensation cases, under a fee schedule for their services, after a period of statutory prohibition from representation of workers before the dispute resolution scheme. Unfortunately, serious challenges with the data collected, together with confounding changes in other portions of the law make a study of that case infeasible at this time.

In the absence of large populations that can be presumed not to contain significant variations in severity over time, a proxy metric for severity must be found for such studies to be more than suggestive.

THE DELAWARE RATING BUREAU RESEARCH

In 2005 the Governor of Delaware enlisted the author and significant internal resources in the State to assist in an effort to reform the workers' compensation law in that state. Delaware utilizes a captive insurance premium rating bureau (shared with Pennsylvania) for the purpose of advising the Insurance Commissioner in the setting of insurance premiums for workers' compensation in the state. The rating bureau was highly cooperative during the reform process. One interesting piece of data obtained from the rating bureau was suggestive, but not definitive. The rating bureau analyzed the most recent two complete premium years available at the time and compared the total medical costs paid and total indemnity benefits paid for both represented and unrepresented workers for those two years. The results for medical expenditures were eye-opening, but consistent with the notion that the more serious cases tend to be the ones with attorney representation. For each year, the medical expenditures for represented workers were about 11 times higher than that the expenditures for unrepresented workers.[16]

When the indemnity benefits were examined a similar pattern appeared, but at a much greater magnitude of difference. Represented workers received approximately 30 times the indemnity benefits of unrepresented workers. This seemed to be something other than the effects of differences between the groups in the severity of the injuries. The cohorts examined for medical and indemnity costs were the same, and logic (and the results of the Swedlow study, discussed below) would suggest that any differences in severity of claims between represented and unrepresented claimants should be reflected, if not equally, then in some understandable relationship. No such

[16]Unpublished report from the Delaware Compensation Rating Bureau, May 2006, prepared as a part of workers' compensation law reform in that state.

relationship has been found to describe the fact that there is a nearly 300% differential between the observed differences in medical payments and indemnity payments, except that the mechanism for compensation of attorneys was based largely on the size of the indemnity payments the worker received. No follow on research concerning this phenomenon has been published. While the results of this study were suggestive of a significant phenomenon, there was no control for severity or outcomes. Ultimately, the statutory reforms adopted did not lend themselves to further study of this

THE SWEDLOW STUDY IN CALIFORNIA

In October of 2003, a study was published in the CWCI Research Notes (Swedlow 2003) that measures the level of attorney involvement in more than 1.7 million claims in California from 1993 through 2000, average legal and benefit costs of those claims and information concerning the timing of attorney involvement and the method of claim resolution. The study, other than looking at significantly more claims than the 2005 Delaware study, also was able to access considerably more detail about the claims resolution process and exposed significant issues about the timing of attorney engagement in the case and the kind of cases that attorneys were likely to accept. Like the Delaware study, the normalization of the data with regard to injury severity in comparisons between cases in which there was representation and those in which there was not representation was not attempted.

The study found that attorneys were involved in 14% of claims during the period but that the distribution of attorney involvement in claims was seriously affected by the nature of the claim. Only 2.7 % of medical only claims had attorney involvement as compared to 90.5% of death claims and 81.2% of permanent disability claims where vocational rehabilitation was involved. Permanent disability claims amount to almost 80% of all expenditures in the system.

The study found that attorney involvement was highest in cumulative injury claims (over 84% of all permanent injury claims) and was highest in multiple body part and back cases when looking at the body part affected. Attention was given to the permanent disability cases, where attorney involvement was highest, to see if there was any pattern in the distribution of attorney involvement. Attorney involvement ranged from nearly 70 % for those cases with the lowest permanent disability ranges to 96.4% for cases of 100% physical impairment.

Interestingly, the study showed an inverse relationship between employer size and attorney involvement rate for all but the smallest employers. The researchers theorized that larger employers have more resources to devote to allaying the fears and anxieties of injured workers, more opportunity to facilitate return to work, and better safety and benefit plans. Each of these factors was seen as one that potentially affects the incidence of litigation, although the study calls for more analysis of these factors.

The study calculated and analyzed the "frictional costs" associated with claims – the sum of attorney fees and litigation related expenses. The study found that defense costs were higher than plaintiff costs, but it noted that defense attorneys were involved in some case types (i.e. medical-only claims) where the claimants were seldom represented. Not surprisingly, litigation costs are higher in case categories showing higher attorney involvement. Claims with a high permanent disability rating had much higher litigation costs than other claims.

The study looked at the total expenditures on benefits for represented versus unrepresented claimants, and found results similar to those reported in Delaware. Average benefit payout for all closed claims that had an attorney involved was 23 times the average paid benefits for claims in which the claimant was unrepresented. The percentage was lower when looking only at indemnity claims, and lower still in permanent disability claims, reflecting the higher level of attorney involvement in those claims. Interestingly, the California study did not replicate the differential in impact on medical versus indemnity losses found in the Delaware study, and showed a higher multiple for medical benefits when an attorney involved than when an attorney was not present.

Finally17, the study analyzed the method of claims resolution by attorney involvement. Settlement of claims accounted 63.8% of cases where an attorney was involved. About 12% of cases resulted in a dismissal or zero judgment. The rest of the cases had a stipulated award (8.1%) findings and an award after hearing (8.8%) or some other resolution.

[17]The also study analyzed various other factors, such as region, industry and cost by claim type, not germane to this discussion.

THE BERNACKI STUDY IN LOUISIANA

Dr Edward Bernacki and Xuguang Tao published a study in the September 2008 issue of the Journal of Occupational and Environmental Medicine (Brenacki & Tao 2008) that attempts to utilize a proxy for injury severity to normalize the data as between cases involving attorney representation and those not involving attorneys. As background for the study, the authors cite to 11 studies showing increased costs when attorneys are involved (seven of which also show an association between attorney involvement and increased lost time from work). The study examined attorney involvement at four different levels of lost time, theorizing that claims with higher lost time values were more likely to attract attorney involvement. The cost distribution within each lost time category was then examined to determine if the cost distribution was proportionally consistent with the frequency distribution. If not, then the differences in cost would appear to be related to the involvement of the attorney. "Lost time" was also used as a proxy for injury severity when looking at: claim duration, differences in indemnity and medical costs of claims, and the time of initial involvement by an attorney.

The study confirmed findings in previous studies that attorney involvement is associated with longer periods of lost work. When they controlled for lost time as a proxy for injury severity, total costs and claims handling costs were higher in claims where the worker was represented. Of particular interest was the finding that medical costs in cases involving attorneys were higher, when controlled for time away from work. The study went on to find that early attorney involvement was a significant predictor of higher claims costs and longer claim duration, especially in those claims in the lower categories of injury severity. The study suggests that the mechanism by which attorneys influence costs may be the lengthening of the time the claim is open.

WHAT THE ATTORNEYS SAY

It should come as no surprise that attorneys who represent injured workers are aghast at the suggestion that their involvement in the dispute resolution system has detrimental aspects for the workers they represent and the overall costs of the system. They assert mightily that their involvement is, if not an inherently good thing, a necessary concomitant of a system that pits economic powerhouses such as insurance companies and large self-insured workers against individual workers. Accordingly, the trial bar is likely to assert that their clients are the least likely to be able to protect themselves, especially after they have been injured. They will assert that insurance companies are soulless entities that take advantage of the inability and lack of sophistication of injured workers to collect premium and then make obscene profits by failing to pay out on claims.

Plaintiff attorneys will go on to assert that the whole system of workers' compensation has already resulted in the worker giving up his or her just right to appropriate compensation, including the real losses occasioned by pain and suffering loss of future earnings and the capacity to enjoy life in the future. They assert that the employer/insurer has already escaped these damages, that are inherent parts of the common law system of personal injury compensation, and that as a result they should have the greatest award possible.

Finally, representatives of injured workers will assert that the results of serious injury are lifelong, but their interaction with the workers' compensation system and their interaction with the attorney in the role of helper through that system are relatively brief. They may assert that the worker therefore must get what they can out of the system before it is done with them and has moved on to newer cases.

Defense lawyers will also defend their involvement in the dispute resolution system. They assert that testing the truth of claims is necessary because there will always be people who try to take advantage of the system and become unjustly enriched at the expense of others who follow the rules. There is a perceived incidence of "fraudulent" behavior, which apparently ranges from claiming for exacerbation of pre-existing injury at work, through symptom magnification of the consequences of legitimate injuries, to inventing of non-existent injuries and claiming workers' compensation benefits for non-work accidents. Defense counsel believe that the concerns of employers that they are being victimized by the assertion of claims that are not justified need to be addressed and that they act as a deterrent to such assertions.

In a similar vein, defense counsel assert on behalf of employers that employers have a legitimate interest in getting the fruits of their efforts to do the right thing in the workplace.

Workers' compensation is designed as a "no-fault" remedy, in that the worker need not show the existence of a duty and breach of that duty by the employer and the employer does not have a defense based upon the negligence of the worker in the occurrence of the injury. Nonetheless, there is a tendency for employers to resent the costs of accidents which they tried to prevent through provision of safety education and equipment, and to blame the victim when such accidents occur through no fault of their own. Since the employer has done the right thing by way of attempting to avoid the accident that gives rise to the injury, the thought is that they really ought not to have to pay.

There is also a perception that attorneys representing injured workers, and the doctors that are often chosen by them (where the law permits such choices) to examine and treat injured workers, are actively conspiring to mutually support each other for the purpose of maximizing the profitability of their own businesses. Defense attorneys may assert that if they don't "hold the line" on expenses, the cost of insurance for workers' compensation will increase to the point that it impacts the ability of business to operate profitably, and therefore compromise the ability of businesses to hire and adequately compensate a workforce. In the alternative they would assert that the cost of workers' compensation insurance is passed on to the ultimate consumer in the form of higher prices, and that there role is necessary to protect the economy.

All of these assertions are both partially correct and, at the same time, misleading. Injured people are often bewildered by the counterintuitive system that we use for resolution of disputes. Arcane rules of evidence and procedure act as traps for the unwary. The process is stressful and time consuming and the injured worker is among the least likely to be able to withstand the rigors of the process. The insurance company (or self insurer) isn't as malevolent as portrayed, but the economics of claims adjusting keep the caseloads too high for the adjuster to seem responsive or engaged in the recovery of the worker, regardless of their personal proclivities. However, the perception that insurance companies make their profits through underwriting is erroneous: most insurers profit from the investment of premium before it is needed for payments and hope to break even on the balance between claims costs and premiums.

The assertion that awards should be as high as possible because of the failure of the system to pay for pain and suffering and other forms of tort damages misconceives the nature of the remedy. Workers' compensation is not designed to provide a replacement of the income lost as a result of injury. Theoretically, to do so would be to provide an economic incentive for staying at home from work. Practically, no state has come close to full wage replacement (Reville 2001; Biddle *et al* 2001b; Biddle *et al* 2001a; Barth *et al* 1998). Trying to make the system look more and more tort-like has had a negative effect on overall benefit structures insofar as the response of many legislatures has been to restrict access to benefits by setting statutory qualification criteria higher.

The contact with the workers' compensation system for most workers is relatively brief, but the mistake in the assertion that a worker must get what they can while the claim is active presupposes that the object of the worker in the system is the same as that of the attorney. The attorney wants to get paid and move on to the next case. The worker wants, generally, to get on with his or her life, and to return to normalcy, rather than a life of disability. The worker may need some continued support to do so, and if that is the case, then a system that leaves him or her without assistance once the benefit check is delivered does not fit the bill.

The perception that claimants are bad people who generally try to game the system is not supported by the research.[18] However, that perception leads to the significant delay in the resolution of claims, and other activities that actually make workers less likely to return to work. In this respect, the defense attorneys are as guilty of perpetuating mythology that supports their income making opportunities as are the claimant's attorneys. The relatively few cases of intentional fraud are likely to be caught by monitoring cases and selectively investigating, and the wholesale use of tactics that also exacerbate the severity of the claim does not serve the employer or insurer.

In a social insurance scheme, such as workers' compensation, the concept of fault has no more place than it does in general health insurance. In both cases the worker will sometimes conduct themselves in ways that are inconsistent with

---

[18]Claimants are not the only parties to the system that commit fraud. Employers commit various forms of premium fraud by underreporting and misclassifying their employees. It has been suggested by the Coalition Against Insurance Fraud that employer fraud may be more significant than worker fraud.

their best health outcomes. In either case the behavior is not always completely shaped by the employer's best efforts at prevention or proactive intervention. The difference is that there is an inappropriate stigma attached to the workers' compensation claimant that is not attached to the person who merely becomes ill or injured outside of work.

Finally, the assertion that the worker's side has their own specialized representatives and health care provider is true. And it is true that the defense has it's own specialists in both law and medicine. The fact that alliances form is not inappropriate in a system where the dispute is handled like a zero sum game, where my win is your loss, and vice versa. If both sides are doing the same thing, then the suggestion that one side or the other unilaterally "disarm" is contrary to reasonable expectations.

BLOOD IN THE WATER – THE SYSTEM IS WHAT NEEDS TO CHANGE

Workers' compensation is conceived of as a mechanism for insuring that injured workers are not thrown on the scrap heap of life, but are given the proper opportunity to heal and return to productivity and self-reliance.[19] This discussion should not be read as an attempt to blame the attorneys engaged in the industry for the deleterious outcomes discussed with regard to the workers' compensation system. While the empirical research supporting the extent to which attorneys drive indirect costs of their involvement in the system, including the creation of "attorneyogenic disability", is not (and for the reasons discussed above, may not ever be) available some might conclude that the proper response is to blame the attorneys for what's wrong with the system and lament that if they were driven out of the system everything would be fine.

When there is blood in the water and sharks go into a feeding frenzy, we do not think that regulating the sharks for their bad behavior is likely to be an effective response and we do not morally judge the sharks for obeying the instincts that have led to their survival. Similarly, when attorneys look at a dispute and try to push it into a model of dispute resolution that existed for hundreds of years prior to the development of workers' compensation at the beginning of the 20th century,[20] we should not morally judge them nor look for direct regulation of their activities to be wholly effective. Litigation as a system of dispute resolution was born in the conditions prevalent in 13th Century England. It may not be well suited to complex dispute resolution with regard to matters that were not conceived of until more than 725 years had passed. The current system of dispute resolution is weighted down with the mythology, expectations and the collective weight of hundreds of years of development in the resolution of different disputes in the seductively similar, but entirely different, environment than that presented by a no-fault social insurance program. Whether or not the current model of legal dispute resolution is still functional in other contexts, there is good reason to question its coherence with the intention of modern workers' compensation schemes. Dispute resolution in workers' compensation damages some of the lives it is intended to help heal (Lippel 1999; Guthrie & Monterosso 2009).

To understand why we are stuck in this dysfunctional pattern, it is necessary to understand something of the structure of legal education and the politics of the legal world. When a person goes to law school in the United States, they are taught to "think like a lawyer". The phrase is really shorthand for a two-pronged socialization process. In the first instance law students quickly learn that the purpose of the law is not the seeking of justice, but rather the resolution of disputes. It is not nearly as important to derive a just decision, as it is to derive a final decision upon which precedent can be based, allowing for predictability in the future.

The validity of this observation is quickly appreciated with a minimum amount of reflection about the creation of law via judicial decision. In the first instance, the evidence the decision is based upon can, and often is, restricted in accordance with other policy priorities. Accordingly, we may see issues arise in workers' compensation litigation involving the admissibility of probative evidence, based upon considerations of how the evidence was collected, or whether regulations concerning activities such as communications with health care providers or the conduct of investigations and surveillance were followed. Moreover, the case will be presented by a particular set of advocates that may or may not have an interest in pursuing a particular issue to the fullest extent in that particular case.

---

[19] A listing of treatises on the history of workers' compensation is presented on the IAIABC website at http://www.iaiabc.org/i4a/pages/index.cfm?pageid=3299

[20] The first U.S. system to withstand constitutional challenge was adopted by the State of Wisconsin in 1911.

Nonetheless, when the case is decided, and precedent concerning the issue is established, subsequent parties are bound by the precedent without regard to the skill or motivation of the original litigants. Thus, the law is properly seen as a mechanism for the resolution of disputes and the creation of precedent that lends predictability to the future, with little regard for what we would call individual justice.

Second, law students are taught to dissociate from their personal feelings concerning the justness of a particular position and to be able to argue either side of any legal question. This results in several phenomena that can be problematic. First, it allows a lawyer to take a position, which they might find, in another context, morally repugnant. Much of the consternation experienced by the lay public with regard to the actions of lawyers is traceable to this aspect of their training. Second, it enables a lawyer to take a position that might seem absurd when viewed by the public from a perspective of common sense and common cultural values, and press for an "extension of the law" - an expansion of an existing legal principle into a new context where it its application was never intended - when first conceived. This allows lawyers to press for extension of a precedent that might have made sense in one context or under one set of facts, into an entirely new area of application. This phenomenon gives rise to the creation of new legal rights or obligations that sometimes test the bounds of societal values, as when liability is found for failure to warn about a cup of hot coffee actually being hot.

Finally, it is necessary to remember that the alleged defenders of the public from the dangers of legal decision-making run amok – the judges – were themselves likely practitioners in the same context as the lawyers that they now attempt to control. Judicial selection procedures are often influenced by the politics of a particular jurisdiction, such that the judiciary disproportionately represents the views of the local political majority. Moreover, with the exception of those judges appointed for life, the pressure to maintain one's position often subtly influences judicial decisions. The judge has friendships amongst the trial bar, influencing their decisions in some cases. If for purposes of reporting judicial performance to the public, a judge is going to be evaluated by the local bar the judge is likely to be mindful of actions that would likely result in dissent from that quarter. But most of all, the judge is inculcated with a particular view of what's right, based upon his or her experience. As the old adage goes, "If the only tool in your toolbox is a hammer, every problem looks like it can be solved with a nail."

With sharks, we let the blood dissipate in the environment before venturing back into the water (or go in protected by cages). With our current system of dispute resolution, the system must be allowed to change to better suit the current environment. Attorneys will still have a role, but in the majority of cases that role can be more supportive of rational outcomes than the current system. That should not be surprising. The perceptions offered to justify the actions of the attorneys on both sides are born of thinking that starts with the assumption that our system of dispute resolution is immutable and necessarily pits the employer/insurer against the worker in a winner take all contest. If the desirable end result is seen as resolution where the interests of both sides is advanced, then the promise of workers' compensation – "quick and efficient delivery of medical and indemnity benefits to injured and disabled workers at a reasonable cost to employers"[21] can be fulfilled.

WHERE DO WE GO FROM HERE

Some Examples of Different Approaches to Dispute Resolution

The Navajo Nation is the largest Tribal Sovereign in the United States, with reserved lands in an area covering parts of Arizona, New Mexico and Utah. As a tribal sovereign, they have the right to adopt a mechanism for dealing with injuries to their workers in whatever manner they wish, subject to certain minimal standards imposed by virtue of their status as a "gaming "tribe subject to compacts pertaining to Indian gaming with the states in which they have gambling operations. The Navajo Nation has had its own workers' compensation program since 1978 and pattern it generally off state law in the states in which they are present, but with an increasing percentage of unique provisions designed to be consistent with their cultural and demographic uniqueness.

With respect to dispute resolution, the Nation has a unique program that incorporates a cultural value encouraging people to work out their differences. Formal dispute resolution is invoked only after the worker goes through a multi-layer alternative dispute resolution process. The process involves multiple opportunities for the Workers'

[21]Section 52-5-1 "Purpose, New Mexico Workers' Compensation Administration Act" New Mexico Statutes Annotated, 1978.

Compensation Program and worker to come to agreement. The first layer, based on cultural tradition and values,[22] ensures that the claimant and the claims "analyst" (the same role as a claims adjuster) will talk directly (and usually face to face) about any concerns before the matter goes further. This step is not codified, but is nonetheless consistently utilized with a high rate of success. There is an additional codified informal dispute resolution step required before the matter can go on to formal hearing. This step requires a discussion between the claimant and both the program supervisor and the department supervisor with responsibility over the program.[23] Matters brought to this level ensure that personal issues between the claims analyst and the claimant do not affect the outcome of the claim. The case goes to a formal dispute resolution hearing only if there is still an active dispute after these informal discussions. Legal representation is prohibited for both sides at the informal resolution levels, and discouraged indirectly at the formal hearing level. The claims "analysts" do not use an outside lawyer to represent them, but rather use a tribal court advocate, employed by the Nation, who specifically is charged with the preservation of traditional values and protection of the worker in the representation of the Program. The Program does not pay any portion of the attorney fees of claimants.

The outcomes experienced by the workers' compensation Program are quite unusual. The alternative dispute resolution process undertaken makes the parties feel as though they are heard, and provided them with a combination of a "day in court", an opportunity to present their side of the dispute clearly, and an opportunity for the claims staff to inform them more fully of their rights and obligations under the law. As a result, the formal dispute resolution mechanism is very rarely used. The final legal appeal in the system is to the Navajo Nation Supreme Court. In the 12 years since the program adopted its present dispute resolution practices, there been only one case submitted to the Supreme Court, and it was resolved and withdrawn before the matter was decided. Since, under Navajo traditional law[24] the claimant has a right to file a claim solely on the grounds that he or she felt the workers' compensation settlement was unfair or inadequate, the virtual absence of litigation appears to reflect worker satisfaction with the system, and not overreaching by the Workers' Compensation Program. It should be noted that there is a strong emphasis placed on informing claimants of their rights and assisting them in getting all that is due to them, so these results also do not reflect lack of claimant knowledge.

Similarly, the State of New Mexico has had mandatory "mediation" - actually a non-binding arbitration – as part of its law since 1991[25]. Historically, the percentage of cases resolved before getting to the formal dispute resolution process has been over 90%, with the resolution rate at "mediation" maintaining at about 70% (New Mexico Workers' Compensation Administration 2008). By statute, this result is obtained within 60days of lodging the dispute with the agency (although the average in 2008 was just over 61 days), where only 11 percent of claims submitted for formal proceedings were completed within 270 days of filing.26 These results strongly suggest that alternative dispute resolution procedures can be highly effective in achieving resolution of claims in a timely and efficient manner.

Some jurisdictions have experimented with different methods of compensating attorneys for their services. The state of Western Australia (2007) in Australia has implemented fee schedules for attorney services that are based upon the work done, rather than the results obtained. The pay system is highly analogous to the fee schedules often utilized for medical personnel. It has been suggested that the utilization of such a schedule will impact adversely on the motivation of the attorney to maximize the benefits obtained by the worker. It is not usually suggested that doctors expend less efforts in healing patients because they are paid by the procedure. Indeed, the concern with regard to doctors has been over-utilization of medical services, rather than flagging interest. Although changes in the pattern of utilization of the court system in Western Australia have not been documented, it remains a subject of which regulators have awareness and vigilance.

A similar mechanism is utilized in the state-run insurance scheme for personal injury arising from traffic accidents in Victoria, Australia. The Transport Accident Commission utilizes a flat rate fee schedule for achievement of specified levels of case processing by attorneys (TAC Road Safety 2010). The results appear to be encouraging.

[22] The concept of *Ke'* a Navajo word without an English translation that denotes kinship or clan identification is the basis for this level of interaction.

[23] 15 Navajo Nation Code Section 1010

[24] The concept of *nayeleh* captures the idea, but again has no direct English translation.

[25] Section 52-5-5, NMSA 1978

[26] Ibid, page 13.

Attorneys are motivated to achieve the various stages in case progress as efficiently as possible, and appear to be assessing the relative payoff of the next level of involvement before undertaking that stage in representation. The clear message of these initiatives is that claimants and employers can get representation of their interests under models of compensation that do not include perverse incentives such as paying higher fees for higher disability.

In the State of California the phenomenon of "carve-outs" has been given statutory imprimatur.[27] Carve-outs are captive programs replacing he state workers' compensation program with a negotiated agreement concerning the rights and benefits for workers' compensation that is part of a collective bargaining agreement. These programs have become popular, where the eligibility criteria can be met, largely because they contain provisions concerning dispute resolution that substitute informal dispute resolution procedures on a very quick time table for court proceedings to resolve disputes, and because they specifically allow for the utilization of lay advocates (usually union based) to represent injured workers. It is said that the costs of such programs is markedly lower, the return to work rates higher and the worker satisfaction greater than with the conventional system.[28] While obviously applicable only in circumstances of collective bargaining, the popularity of the carve out programs with both employers and worker representatives indicates that satisfaction with alternative mechanisms for the resolution of disputes is significant.

Some other steps to take that could make a difference in reducing disability caused by the current system of dispute resolution.

As promising as these attempts at making the system work better in terms of preventing system – caused disability, there are likely several additional steps that could be taken to good effect that would also be effective if properly implemented. Some of these opportunities have seen limited implementation, and others are merely examples of possibilities yet to be put into practice.

LEGAL PRACTICE GUIDELINES

The advent of evidence-based medical practice guidelines has arguably been the greatest advance in recent memory in improving the quality of care in workers' compensation (Glass 2004). The addition of a computerized interface (Ford & Stanhope 2006) with the medical practice guidelines of the American College of Occupational and Environmental Medicine (ACOEM) that allows non-medically trained claims personnel to utilize the ACOEM Guides as a tool for evaluating the reasonableness and necessity of proposed medical care has also made the development of these tools a powerful mechanism for controlling the costs of the provision of health care to injured workers.

The utilization of evidence based guidelines for the practice of law in workers' compensation also has appeal. Like medical practice guidelines, legal guidelines could improve the quality of care given to injured workers and prevent some needless disability by instructing less experienced counsel and claims adjusters concerning the expected course of progress of legal matters. Is a claim for permanent impairment for a simple fracture of the non-dominant radius usually asserted? What evidence is necessary for the assertion of a claim of retaliatory discharge? Research into the effective practices of law could also inform injured workers of the efficacy of asserted claims, setting more accurate expectations and could be utilized in conjunction with legal services fees schedule for the control of any observed tendency of lawyers to make up for lost income by multiplying the pleadings, hearings and other scheduled components of a fee schedule.

The obvious issue with the implementation of such an idea is the lack of empirical research in the field. Hundreds of papers are published yearly on the efficacy of various medical procedures, but virtually no research is conducted with regard to the efficacy of various techniques in legal practice. Such research is not more difficult, in principle than that addressing medical practice, but there is no current source of funding nor pool of researchers to facilitate such explorations.

[27]California Labor Code Section 3201.5

[28] Compare the results reported by the Division of Workers Compensation in its 2008 annual report of alternative dispute and carve out programs (http://www.dir.ca.gov/dwc/Carveout/CarveOutReport2007.pdf) with the report of the National Academy of Social Insurance of it's research on claims costs for the same year, in Reno, V & Sengupta, I 2010, 'Drop in California's Workers' Compensation Spending Slows Growth in National Spending in 2007', *IAIABC Journal*, Vol. 47, No. 1.

Issue Trending Research

The regulatory process is one that has been described as a dance of opposing forces. The regulator imposes an attempt to control a perceived problem within the workers' compensation system. The regulated parties, having no wish to relinquish the income generated by such activity often respond by developing a "work-around" strategy that renders the regulation ineffective. The regulator, after a time lag necessary for the recognition of the work-around, promulgates a control strategy for the work around, and the cycle restarts, with the regulator always just a bit behind in his or her response. The "dance" continues indefinitely as long as the regulator fails to recognize the larger trends that give rise to the underlying behavior sought to be controlled.

It is clear that attorneys on both sides of the bar discuss not only strategy pertaining to individual cases but also long term trends in the "development of the law" amongst themselves and at continuing education conferences. They promote new approaches to the maximization of awards, identify what they perceive as vulnerabilities in the law and recruit cases and litigators to press for desired results. These efforts will be disclosed, over time, in the mixture of cases coming to decision and going on to appeal. Examination of the issues being brought for hearing may be the only way of getting information about these developing trends before they are entrenched.

Moreover, the surveying of case decisions with regard to the issues raised in them is an underutilized mechanism for identifying dysfunction within the system. A persistent emphasis on litigation over medical causality, for instance, may disclose some structural deficit that can be addressed by statute or regulation. Accordingly, such `analysis could result in changes regarding the standard of proof, the qualification of opinions concerning the subject or other issues that may give rise to practical mechanisms for the streamlining of adjudication.

Requirement for "Good Faith" in Claims Handling

There has been a well recognized common law cause of action for bad faith practice in the handling of claims by insurers. These lawsuits have not been particularly effective in the deterrence of sharp practices by payers, for several reasons. First, the remedy requires independent litigation and may be too remote in probability of success and time to resolution to be of much interest to individual workers who have been mistreated. Second, without the collection of complaints by a centralized authority, patterns of behavior that cannot be discerned in one case can be disclosed and dealt with. But most of all, the problem with bad faith causes of action is that they only control the most extreme examples of abuse, and therefore do not address the perception that payers are likely to abuse workers who do not have the protection of a lawyer to ensure fair treatment.

The necessity of a requirement that the payer act in good faith in claims handling has been asserted in several jurisdictions, without notable success. The usual reason given is that the judiciary is not eager to create a cause of action that is so subject to frivolous assertion and consequential overloading of the courts with cases that are likely to be unique on there facts. There is also a concern that a remedy for failure to act in good faith would be either too low to create an economic incentive for change by the payer or high enough to create a concern about unjust enrichment of individual claimants (and their attorneys). These concerns are legitimate if the model foe resolution of the issue is litigation by individual workers. Nonetheless, there is substantial appeal in addressing the common fear, often expressed in lawyer advertisements, that the insurer will take advantage of an individual who attempts to perfect a claim without legal representation.

All the concerns about the difficulties inherent in bad faith litigation and inherent in a litigation approach to enforcement of a good faith requirement are addressable if the enforcement of the requirement is vested in an administrative agency rather than in individual enforcement through litigation.[29] An administrative remedy for fact in good faith in claims handling would allow the accumulation of cases beyond the means of any individual lawyer or litigant. It would allow the administrative authority the opportunity to identify problematic practices and assist the payer in taking corrective action, obtain restitution for the affected workers and prevent workers from having their return to normalcy delayed by prolonged individual or class action litigation. Most of all, such a remedy can be controlled, such that a "feeding frenzy" is not created and expectations of additional awards or the fees based upon them are not encouraged.

---

[29]Guthrie, R and Aurbach, R. "Preventing Harm to the Harmed by Changing the Battleground", under review by the International Journal of Social Security and Workers Compensation.

Public Support for Advocacy Assistance in Qualifying Cases

The need for advocates in a dispute resolution system is directly related to the level of formality and the presence of arcane rules of evidence and procedure in the system. It has been noted widely that the law has its own language, and rules. Words are often used in unique ways that are different from the way we use the same word in a normal context.[30] Applicable rules of evidence or procedure are sometimes counter-intuitive or obscure. These features of traditional legal systems tend to limit full access to all but the initiated (or those with exceptional personal resources) forcing the retention of lawyers to navigate the intricacies of the system. The maintenance of those institutions in their present form may, in fact, be designed exactly for that purpose.

Notwithstanding the concerns expressed above pertaining to the impact of attorneys and the current dispute resolution system in workers' compensation, elimination of the role of advocate entirely simply is not an outcome that is practical. Some issues will be too complex or technical for the injured worker to present for decision, regardless of the structure of the system used for dispute resolution. Some workers will have challenges with language or will be unsuited by temperament or behavioral health concerns to present their own position, regardless of the level of formality of the proceedings. Some workers will be unable to undertake presentation of their own issues at the time advocacy is necessary simply because their injuries are insufficiently healed to allow that level of participation. There doubtless are other categories of cases in which the presence of an advocate would be essential for the fair presentation of the worker's position in any advocacy setting.

Where the dispute resolution systems in place look more like a traditional model of court-like, win-lose contests, the need for advocacy is even greater. As noted above, the current mechanism for the compensation of lawyers in workers' compensation cases discourages the representation of workers with small cases, particularly ones in which only medical benefits are in issue. So too are other small dollar value claims that may make an important difference in the life of a worker. Claims for vocational rehabilitation services, and workers' compensation system remedies for retaliatory discharge, are examples of such claims.

Recognizing that there will always be the need for advocacy in special circumstances, regardless of the dispute resolution system, does not leave us inevitably joined at the hip to the current model of representation by private attorneys. Some states[31] provide a public advocacy function as part of their systems. In such systems, a claimant may apply for the services of a public advocate to assist them through the presentation of their case. Other systems that utilize an ombudsman role to assist in the avoidance of unnecessary disputes[32] may also allow the ombudsman to assist the worker in the preparation of their case up to the point of the beginning of the informal dispute resolution proceedings, and may provide materials to the injured worker that will assist in the presentation of their case.

Another possible mechanism for supporting advocacy where it is needed is the provision of subsidies for traditional legal representation. Qualifying small cases that would not generate a sufficient fee to attract the interest of a lawyer on their own could be eligible for supplemental funds from the state paid directly to the attorney providing representation. This system, which has been proposed, but not adopted, in legislation, would not discourage litigation in the traditional model, but would address the access issues inherent in the present mechanisms for paying attorneys.

Retooling the Way we Look at Industrial Injury and Disease

As noted above, virtually no one wants to exchange his or her current quality of life for a life-changing injury, regardless of the monetary award accompanying that injury. That having been said, the question still remains whether the person who is already injured will have the same attitude. The expectation in the United States, and elsewhere[33] is that, once injured, the orientation of workers is to get as big a payout as possible as the primary response to the injury. The facts differ from the perception. The vast majority of workers who are injured at work

---

[30]For instance, the “foundation” for the admissibility of a piece of evidence is an entirely different concept than the “foundation” of a building.

[31]15 states are listed in “Workers’ Compensation Laws, 2d Edition – A Joint Publication of IAIABC and WCRI” as having either ombudspeople or public advocates for workers. Nevada is a clear example of a state with a well developed public advocacy program. See Ballantyne, D. Workers’ Compensation In Nevada: Administrative Inventory, Workers’ Compensation Research Institute, WC-06-15, 2006.

[32]Ibid, Workers’ Compensation Laws, 2d Edition, *supra.*, Table 15.

[33]This question was posed in a discussion of the prevention of needless disability to the senior staff of Comcare, the Australian federal program for public sector employees workers’ compensation program.

return to a productive life (Melhorne 2004). People who look to workers' compensation benefits as a replacement for the wages that they were earning prior to injury are invariably dismayed to find that such benefits are not adequate for that purpose(Barth *et al* 1998; Biddle *et al* 2001a; Biddle *et al* 2001b; Reville 2001). Indeed, it may be rationally argued that workers' compensation was never designed to replace income, but rather to provide support and subsistence until the desired outcome of return to productive life could be achieved. Moreover, all United States systems have limitations on the length of time for which benefits are payable, except for the most profoundly injured. Transition of workers from workers' compensation benefits to the Social Security Disability system is a fact of life that has attracted significant critical comment (Burton 2007).

The idea that people who are injured at work should be "compensated" is a created societal expectation, and one of relatively recent vintage. Lawyer advertising ("You may be *entitled* to a *large* cash *award,"* emphasis added) and "viral advertising" (Joe got a big settlement for his injury...) have contributed to an environment already infused with the concept that anyone who suffers any adverse experience is a "victim" who "has the right" to be "compensated" for the wrong that has been done to them.[34] True progress in avoidance of needless disability requires attention to this cultural phenomenon, at least in the workers' compensation context.

There are several examples of significant initiatives for the accomplishment of this wider societal goal. In Australia, where the emphasis on empowering injured workers to return to work is arguably stronger than in the United States, there are several employer-based initiatives of note. Australia Post, the Australian counterpart to the U.S. Postal Service, has an award winning, albeit controversial, program of very early intervention and return to work for all but the most severely injured employees. RiskCover, a major third party claims manager in Western Australia runs a program known as "Injured, But Still Part of the Team" that is designed to maintain engagement between the worker and the workplace and counter the tendency for time away from work to create psychological distance that interferes with return to employment. More broadly, Dr. Mary Wyatt and Robert Hughes, of Victoria, Australia have created and maintained a subscription website providing a broad range of resources pertaining to returning injured workers to work, known as "Return to Work Matters"[35]

In the United States, the most significant initiative to help reverse the preconceptions that have been fostered concerning the outcomes of the workers' compensation system is the "60 Summits Project". 60 Summits is a grassroots initiative to create local mobilization of resources to prevent needless disability and promote return to work. The name refers to the desire to spread the message through the convening of "summits" in every state and the 10 Canadian provinces (Christian 2009). The initiative is based on the "Guidelines for the Prevention of Workplace Disability" issued by the American College of Occupational and Environmental Medicine (ACOEM 2006) and has resulted in 20 summits in 14 jurisdictions as of this writing.

Another initiative that appears to be responsive to the current perception that dispute resolution in workers' compensation has led to a breakdown in the system is under consideration in California. In that state employers and workers are mandated to participate in an employer based short-term disability insurance program. The state has also considered the adoption of a mandatory employer based 24-hour coverage health care plan. If the health care program is adopted, the initiative suggests that workers' compensation, as we presently know it, should be deconstructed to cover only long-term disability. The primary impetus for such a move would be the avoidance of litigation of most issues. The reasoning goes that, if most injuries resolve relatively quickly, and do not result in long term disability, then efficiencies can be obtained by combining the systems for work and non-work health care and short term disability and disputes that are often litigated earlier in the claim than would be necessary under the proposed system could be deferred until the long term disability threshold, eliminating the cost and unnecessary disability created by avoidable litigation.

This initiative raises the entire question of whether workers' compensation as a separate system of social insurance, should be better integrated with our other social insurance programs. Workers' compensation was the first social insurance program adopted in the United States, and many programs have been developed subsequently that are, in some instances, poorly coordinated with workers' compensation. The poor quality of coordination is understandable,

---

[34] The sources of this mythology are the subject of a different, and much lengthier, discussion.

[35] http://www.rtwmatters.org/

given that workers' compensation is a state based system, and that many of the other societal safety net programs are either federally based or federally mandated, with the policymakers in Washington either unaware or unconcerned about the impact on the state-based systems. Arguably the well-documented tendency for medical costs in workers' compensation to be higher than those in general health (Mealy 2010) would create sufficient incentive to consider integration. The ability of other disability and medical insurance programs to resolve disputes efficiently and without resort to tort-like litigation in the vast majority of cases may present an even more compelling argument.

More broadly, it is necessary to reassert the proper aims of workers compensation and spread the message as broadly as possible to employers, doctors and insurers as well as to workers. Perhaps the message that needs to be communicated is that the proper goal of any workers' compensation system should be "return to life"[36] for those who have experienced workplace injury or illness, rather than maximization of awards for the injured and profits for those who feed off the system.

REFERENCES

ACOEM Stay at Work and Return to Work Process Improvement Committee 2006, *Preventing Needless Workplace Disability by Helping People Stay Employed*, viewed 14 July 2010 http://www.acoem.org/guidelines.aspx?id=566.

Aronoff, G, Dorto, A, Genovese, E, Klimek, E, Maitz, E, Mandel, S, Staats, T 2007, 'Evaluating Malingering in Contested Injury or Illness', *Pain Practice*, vol. 7 no. 2, pp. 178-204.

Aronoff, G & Feldman, J 2007, 'Preventing Iatrogenic Disability from Chronic Pain, *Current Pain and Headache Reports*, Vol. 3, No. 1 pp 67-77.

Barsky, AJ & Borus, JF 1995, 'Somatization and medicalization in the era of managed care', *Journal of The American Medical Association,* vol. 274, no. 24, pp. 1931-1934.

Barth, PS, Peterson, MA, Reville, RT, Stern, RK 1998, *Compensation Permanent Workplace Injuries: A Study of the California System*, RAND Corporation, Santa Monica, CA.

Benyahya, R, Fayad, F, Fermanian, J, Lefevre-Colau, MM, Poiraudeau, S, Rannou, F, Revel, M, Revel, M, Wlodyka Demaille, S 2004, 'Chronicity, recurrence, and return to work in low back pain: common prognostic factors', *Ann Readapt Med Phys.* vol. 47, no. 4, pp. 179 –189.

Biddle, JE, Boden, II, Mardesich, C, Reville, RT 2001a, *An Evaluation of New Mexico Workers' Compensation Permanent Partial Disability and Return to Work*, RAND Corporation, Santa Monica, CA.

Biddle, J, Boden, L, Reville, R. 2001b, 'Permanent Partial Disability from Occupational Injuries: Earnings Losses and Replacement in Three States', in P Budetti, R Burkhauser, J Gregory, & HA Hunt (Eds), *Ensuring Health and Income Security for an Aging Workforce,* W.E. Upjohn Institute for Employment Research, Kalamazoo, MI, pp. 263-290.

Bouter, LM, Jellema P, Stalman, WA, Van der Horst HE, van der Windt, DA, Vlaeyen JW 2006 'Predictors of outcome in patients with (sub) acute low back pain differ across treatment groups', *Spine*, vol. 31, no. 15, pp. 1699 –1705.

Brenacki, E & Tao, X 2008, 'The relationship Between Attorney Involvement, Claim Duration and Workers' Compensation Costs', *Journal of Occupational and Environmental Medicine*, vol. 50, no. 9, pp. 1013-1018

Brigham, C 2003, 'Iatrogenic Disability: Avoiding Needless Illness Behavior and Disability – Focusing on Function', Presentation to Academy of Independent Medical Examiners of Hawaii, January 16, 2003.

Bruns, D & Disorbio, JM 2009, 'Assessment of Biopsychosocial Risk Factors for Medical Treatment: A Collaborative Approach', *Journal of Clinical Psychology in Medical Settings*, vol. 16, no. 2, pp. 127-147.

Burton, J 2007, 'The Mystery of Workers' Compensation Reform Solved', *IAIABC Journal*, Vol. 44, No. 2, pp.49-68.

Canyock, E Condit, D Mittenberg, W. Patton, C 2002, 'Base Rates of Malingering and Symptom Exaggeration', *Journal of Clinical and Experimental Neuropsychology*, vol. 24, no. 8, pp. 1094-1102.

Christian, J 2009, 'The 60 Summits Project: A Grass Roots Initiative to Prevent Needless Work Disability by Helping People Stay Employed – in the Real World', *IAIABC Journal*, Vol. 46, No. 2, pp. 113-152.

Copeland, M 2009, 'CBT for Pain Management', *IAIABC Journal*, vol. 46, no. 2, pp. 77-92

Conrad, P 2007, *The Medicalization of Society*, Johns Hopkins University Press, Baltimore, MD.

Conroy, MA & Kwartner, PP 2006, 'Malingering', *Applied Psychology in Criminal Justice*, vol. 2, no.3, pp. 29-51.

Doidge, N 2007, *The Brain that Changes Itself*, Penguin Books, New York, NY

Duffau, H 2006, 'Brain plasticity: From pathophysiological mechanisms to therapeutic applications', *Journal of Clinical Neuroscience*, Vol. 13, No. 9, pp. 885-897.

[36] I suggest that phrasing as a psychologically more appealing – and accurate – statement than the more frequently repeated "return to work".

Ford, J & Stanhope, M 2006, 'The Critical Role of Evidence-Based Decision Support Systems to Deliver the Intended Benefits of Treatment Guidelines in Workers' Compensation', *IAIABC Journal*, Vol. 43, No. 2, pp. 35-60.

Fulton-Kehoe, D, Franklin, G, Gluck, JV, Sheppard, L, Stover, B, Turner, J, Wickizer, TM, Wu, R 2008, 'Early Predictors of Chronic Work Disability', *Spine*, Vol. 33, No. 25, pp. 2809 – 2818.

Gatchel, R, 2004, 'Comorbidity of Chronic Pain and Mental Heaalth Disorders: The Biospychosocial Perspective', American Psychologist, vol. 59, no. 8, pp. 795-805.

Gatchel, R, Kishino, N, Minotti, D 2010, 'The Clinical Effectiveness of Early Intervention for Musculoskeletal Pain Disorders', *IAIABC Journal*, vol. 47, no. 1, pp. 23-56.

Gatchel, RJ & Schultz, IZ (Eds) 2005, *Handbook of Complex Occupational Disability Claims*, Springer Publishing, New York, NY.

Gatchel, R, & Turk, D (Eds) 2002, *Psychological Approaches to Pain Management: A Practitioner's Handbook (2d Ed)*, Guillford Press, New York, NY.

Glass, L 2004, 'ACOEM's Occupational Medicine Practice Guideleines', *IAIABC Journal*, Vol. 41, No. 2, pp. 149-167.

Goerdt, J, McMillan,J, Steelman,D 2000, '*Caseflow Management: The Heart of Court Management in the New Millennium*', National Center for State Courts, Williamsburg, VA.

The Government of Western Australia 2007, *New cost scale for the DRD*, viewed 14 July 2010 http://www.workcover.wa.gov.au/News/New+costs+scale+for+the+DRD.htm.

Guthrie, R & Monterosso, S 2009, 'Preventing Further Harm to the Harmed- Towards a Therapeutic Approach to Workers' Compensation', *Journal of the International Association of Industrial Accident Boards and Commissions*, vol. 46, no. 1, pp. 115-142.

Harvard Magazine 2009, 'On the Medicalization of our Culture', *Harvard Magazine,* 23 April, viewed 14 July 2010 http://harvardmagazine.com/breaking-news/medicalization-of-our-culture.

Hay, E, Jellema, P, Main, C, Van der Windt, D 2008, 'Psychosocial interventions for low back pain in primary care: Lessons learned from recent trials', *Spine*, vol. 33, no. 1, pp. 81 –89.

Horwitz, AV & Wakefield, JC 2007, *The Loss of Sadness: How Psychiatry Transformed Normal Sorrow into Depressive Disorder,* Oxford University Press, New York, NY

Jin, RL, Shah, CP, Svoboda, TJ 1995, 'The impact of unemployment on health: a review of the evidence', *Canadian Med Assoc J.* vol. 153, no. 5, pp. 529-540.

Johoda, M 1982, *Employment and Unemployment: A social and psychological approach*, Cambridge University Press, Cambridge.

Kinicki, AJ, McKee-Ryan, F, Song, Z, Wanberg, CR 2005, 'Psychological and Physical Well-Being During Unemployment: A Meta-Analytic Study', *Journal of Applied Psychology*, vol 90, no. 1, pp. 53-76.

Kolb, B. & Whishaw, I 1998, 'Brain Plasticity and Behavior', *Annual Review of Psychology*, Vol 49, pp. 43-64.

Kritzer, H 1992, 'The English rule', *ABA Journal,* vol. 78, pp. 54-58.

Lefcourt, H 1982, *Locus of Control: Current Trends in Theory and Research, 2nd Edition*, Lawrence Erlbaum Assoicates Publishers, Hillsdale, NJ.

Lippel, K 1999 'Therapeutic and Anti-Therapeutic Consequences of Workers' Compensation', *International Journal of Law and Psychiatry*, vol. 22,nos. 5-6, pp. 521-546.

Maier, S, Peterson, C, Seligman, M 1993, *Learned Helplessness: A Theory for the Age of Personal Control*, Oxford University Press, New York, NY.

Main CJ, Sullivan MJ, Watson PJ (eds) 2007, *Pain Management: Practical Applications of the Biopsychosocial Perspective in Clinical and Occupational Settings*, 2nd edn, Churchill Livingstone, Edinburgh, Scotland.

Martikainen, PT & Valkonen, T 1998, 'The effects of differential unemployment rate increases of occupation groups on changes in mortality', *American Journal of Public Health*, vol. 88, no. 12, pp. 1859-1861.

Mathers, CD & Schofield, DJ 1998, 'The health consequences of unemployment: the evidence', *Medical Journal of Australia*, vol. 168, pp. 178-182.

McGill, CM 1968, 'Industrial back problems: a control program', *Journal of Occupational and Environmental Medicine,* vol. 10, no. 4, pp. 174-178.

Mealy, D 2010, *State of the Line Report, slide 40*, viewed 14 July 2010 https://www.ncci.com/Documents/AIS-2010-SOL-Presentation.pdf

Melhorne, JM 2004, 'The Advantages of Early Return to Work', *IAIABC Journal*, Vol. 41, No. 1, pp. 128-147.

Meyers, J & Sander, R 1986, 'The relationship of disability to compensation status in railroad workers', *Spine*, vol. 11, no. 2, pp. 141-143.

Mitchell, K., 2000, The Dance of Invisible Impairments: Chronic Pain Syndrome and the Disability Insurer, American Pain

Society Bulletin, Vol. 10, No. 4, pp.1-8.

Nachemson, A 1983, 'Work for all – for those with LBP as well', *Clin Orth Related Research*, vol. 179, pp. 77-85.

New Mexico Workers' Compensation Administration *2008, 2008 Annual Report(pp. 12)*, State of New Mexico Workers' Compensation Administration, New Mexico, viewed 14 July 2010 http://www.workerscomp.state.nm.us/research/ar08/wca_annual2008.pdf.

Okifuji, A & Turk, D 2002, 'Psychological Factors in Chronic Pain: Evolution and Revolution', *Journal of Consulting and Clinical Psychology*, vol. 70, no 3, pp. 678-690.

Quarles, L 2006, 'Alternative Dispute Resolution on a Shoestring', *IAIABC Journal*, vol. 43, no. 2.

Reid, W.H., 2000 'Malingering', *Journal of Psychiatric Practice*, vol.6, no.4 pp 226 –228.

Reville, R 2001, 'The Impact of a Disabling Workplace Injury on Earnings and Labor Force Participation',in JC Haltiwanger, JI Lane, & JJM Theeuwes (eds), *The Creation and Analysis of Employer-Employee Matched Data,* Elsevier Science B.V., Amsterdam, pp. 147-172.

Stewart, JM 2001, 'The impact of health status on the duration of unemployment spells and the implications for studies of the impact of unemployment on health status', *Journal of Health Economics*, vol. 20, no. 5, 781-796.

Strang JP, 1985 'The Chronic Disability Syndrome, in GM Aronoff', (Ed), *Evaluation and Treatment of Chronic Pain*, Urban & Schwarzenberg, Baltimore, MD.

Swedlow, A 2003, *Attorney Involvement in California Workers' Compensation, 1993 – 2000, CWCI Research Notes*, California Workers' Compensation Institute, Oakland, CA, October.

TAC Road Safety 2010, *TAC Protocols - Legal costs effective from 1/1/2010*, viewed 14 July 2010 http://www.tacsafety.com.au/upload/Protocol%20legal%20costs.pdf.

Tauber, R 1997, *Self-Fulfilling Prophecy: A Practical Guide A Practical Guide o its Use in Education,* Praeger Publishers, Westport CT.

Wegscheider-Cruse, S 1989, *Another Chance: Hope and Health for the Alcoholic Family, Second Edition*, Science and Behavior Books, Inc, Palo Alto, CA.

CHAPTER 9

A Respondent's Perspective of the Workers' Compensation System

Martha Gely-Kruto

Attorney; E-mail: migely16@yahoo.com

Abstract: Many factors are going to determine the outcome of a workers' compensation case. There is a common misconception that in Illinois the system greatly favors the petitioner. Yes, the petitioner does have advantages, but in my opinion, whether you try or not the case in Illinois will have very little to do with the end result. How you approach the settlement or trial of a particular file, how good or bad your IME physician's report is and who the injured employee is, are more significant elements of whether you win or lose a case than the jurisdiction in which you practice law. The type of relationship you have with your clients, with the claim adjusters, with the Arbitrators and your opponents will also play a role in determining the outcome of a case. Also of importance is whether you need a report from an IME physician and why, who your doctor is and what kind of report he issues can make or break your case.

INTRODUCTION

In this chapter I will discuss the factors that, in my opinion, will impact a workers' compensation case from the respondent's standpoint. Obviously your relationship with your clients is one of the most significant aspects of any case. How you handle competing interests and expectations from multiple clients will not only determine how you resolve the case at hand, but also how future cases are taken care of and how much of a say you have in them.

Your relationship with your opponents and with the arbitrators will also impact how the case is resolved. Who the petitioner is will also have a profound effect in how quickly you can resolve the file. I have dealt with petitioners with devastating injuries who were committed to getting better and returning to their jobs and they accomplished both. On the other hand, I have also dealt with petitioners who suffered minor injuries, but refused to finish the medical treatment or return to work.

Like I previously stated, relationships with clients and with everybody else is extremely important. However, there is more to resolving a workers' compensation case than dealing with the parties you work with. A petitioner's average weekly wage or AWW, excessive medical treatment, and IME physicians, are also very relevant aspects of any comp case.

In the following subchapters, I will touch on all of the above while focusing on what the challenges are in dealing with multiple clients, what kind of obstacles we face before we can resolve a case and how I feel about IME physicians and the use of their reports.

RELATIONSHIPS WITH CLIENTS

Very often whenever I am handling a file, Petitioners' attorneys come to me because their clients need something. If I don't agree with what they need I am told "you don't understand, this client is going to be very mad at me." Petitioners' attorneys and sometimes arbitrators seem to forget that Respondent attorneys have clients as well and their interests are as important as those of the Petitioners.

Early in my career, I inherited a file that had been opened for a couple of years. There was very limited medical documentation available, but whenever the case was up for status or hearing it would be continued without any explanation. Needless to say my client was getting very frustrated.

I decided that the best approach to handle this particular file was to bring the client with me to the next hearing. As planned, I appeared before the Arbitrator and explained that my client was present and that before the case was automatically continued he would like to come and see him. As soon as my opponent came in, we met with the Arbitrator.

Chris E. Stout, Matt Kruger and Jeffrey Rogers, (Eds)

Was the case resolved at that time? No. Was it continued? Yes. However, several things changed. First of all, my client better understood how the process worked and that made my job a lot easier moving forward. More importantly, the Arbitrator explained to my opponent that unless he produced some medical records and also current information as to whether the Petitioner was still being treated or was at MMI[1], he would dismiss the case. Miraculously before the next hearing date I had all the information that I had been requesting for months and we were able to resolve the case shortly thereafter.

Relationships with clients can be tricky and challenging. It can be even trickier if you have more than one client involved and their interests are at odds. Take for example the relationship between a claims adjuster, an employer representative and the respondent's attorney. They all have the same goal in mind—to resolve the claim or case as quickly and as efficiently as possible. However, how each party goes about achieving that goal varies drastically depending on whom you talk to.

Claim adjusters have a very tough job to do. They handle every little detail of hundreds of claims simultaneously on a daily basis. Adjusters sometimes need to make serious decisions on the spot and most of the time whether they are right or not, no one is pleased with their decisions. Their job is insanely stressful at all times and they get very little sympathy or respect for the job they do.

Employers are also in a difficult position, even though most Petitioners' attorneys would like to disagree with me. An employer needs to run a business and make it profitable, while at the same time the company needs to take care of all employees—the ones who are injured and the ones who continue to work for them.

Employer representatives also are requested to make difficult decisions with very little time to think and sometimes with very little information. At times they need to try and find witnesses the day before a trial, even though the case had been set for trial for over three months. How would you feel if you were in that spot?

It is understandable then to see why employer representatives and claim adjusters can be at odds sometimes. Their objectives and expectations are different even though they share the same goal. This relationship becomes even more complicated if you have an employer who doesn't really understand how the workers' compensation system works or if you have an adjuster who believes that the attorney and the employer do not need to be in contact with one another.

It is very frustrating for me, as an attorney, to deal with adjusters who come from the old school of thought that believe that adjusters own a claim and the attorney is there just to take the case to trial. This line of thinking makes everyone's job extremely difficult and doesn't always lead to the best results. The earlier in the game that the attorney gets involved, the more protected the adjuster will be. Why? As much as the adjuster knows the claim, and they do know their claims, it is the attorney who knows and understands the law and how things work at the Commission.

I am the one who knows the Arbitrators. I know how much I can push a situation, when to sit back and wait, or when to take a case to trial immediately. I know my opponents. I know who has no clue of what the case is about and who is always ready and prepared to proceed. I am here to make the adjusters' jobs easier and it becomes very frustrating when I am not allowed to help out.

The other side of the coin is an employer who doesn't truly understand how the workers' compensation process works and has unrealistic expectations. More than once I have heard the "I don't like the guy" line. That's wonderful. I probably won't like the guy either, but that means absolutely *nothing* when it comes to determining whether an injury occurred and what our responsibilities are to the employee if any. We need to focus on what's important regardless of emotions. The "I don't like the guy defense" does not exist, so let's move on. Let's not waste time and money on something that is irrelevant.

As far as expectations go, it is tough at times to explain to a client that even though they are paying for everything they pretty much have no say on anything. Employers have to pay TTD benefits, medical bills, and many extras depending on the case, but it is the employee who chooses where to be treated and with whom. He can decline

[1] Medical Maximum Improvement.

having a nurse on the file and he pretty much only needs to show up for one IME[2] appointment to remain "complaint." That is a tough pill to swallow.

Communication between the parties, especially among multiple clients is key in making this process work to our advantage. Everyone needs to get involved from the very beginning and everyone's expectations need to be addressed at that time. The sooner we all agree in a strategy the more likely we are to succeed.

In my career, I have worked with some of the best, most dedicated claims adjusters in the business. They believe in what they are doing and truly want to do the right thing on every single file, for every single petitioner. We should show them a little bit more respect and consideration.

The same goes for employers. I have worked for some of the biggest companies around and I always walked away knowing that we did right for the injured worker. More than once I have seen companies go that extra mile to take care of the employee. They accommodate crazy restrictions, they create jobs to make sure that an employee makes it to his 25th year with the company, they pay an injured employee his full salary instead of TTD benefits while he recovers.

Somehow though, things like these are very rarely acknowledged or talked about, let's give credit where credit is due. Yes, we can all do a better job at what we do. But neither the employer nor the insurance company is the big bad wolf who is to be blamed for everything that goes wrong.

ARBITRATORS, OPPONENTS AND THE PETITIONER

Arbitrators who agree to pre-trial conferences can save you a lot time and expenses. You avoid having to go to trial just because you couldn't resolve let's say an issue of TTD[3] or a petitioner who believed he was entitled to a higher offer. Once the arbitrator makes her recommendation you can advise your client of where you stand and make an informed decision on how to proceed.

I also always appreciate an arbitrator who will talk to the petitioner or to my client depending on the circumstances. We may be able to avoid a trial if the petitioner understands what he really is entitled to or that if the case goes to trial he may receive an award of lesser value than the offer that I presented. If my client is the one with some concerns, it is sometimes easier to have the arbitrator talk to him. An arbitrator's assistance is priceless.

How you deal with your opponent is equally important. The Commission[4] is a small community where everyone knows everyone else. There are no secrets. Every so often who you are and how you conduct yourself will be the deciding factor between your opponent agreeing to a continuance to make sure that your witness can make it to the hearing or forcing the case to trial regardless of what your circumstances are.

You also have to consider what type of petitioner you are dealing with. You may get lucky and have someone who loves his employer and who will do everything within his power to get healthy and back to work in no time. He follows his attorney's advice and is compliant with the medical treatment. Then you have some petitioners who don't want to do anything, but who feel entitled to everything. Those are a real treat.

Most Petitioners fall within the middle of the spectrum though. They do want to get healthy, but may not be as committed to their medical treatment as they should. Or they may feel that they should be off work for a longer period of time than what is recommended. All of them have one thing in common—they want to be heard.

Once I had this case where as far as I was concerned there were no issues. However, the Petitioner continued to refuse to sign contracts and I was getting very annoyed. Finally, I received a call from my opponent stating that the Petitioner would not sign the contracts unless I agree to talk to him. A few days later we met at the Commission and he told me his story. We talked for maybe 15 minutes and then he signed contracts. He wanted to make sure that *I*,

---

[2] Independent Medical Examinations.

[3] Temporary Total Disability.

[4] Illinois Workers' Compensation Commission.

as the company's attorney, knew how he felt about his injury and the process. That's all it took. He didn't want an apology, he didn't want extra compensation, he was not mad at the company, but he needed to make sure we knew *his* version of what had happened. From that point forward I have always made myself available to talk to all petitioners, their moms, their spouses, the entire family as long as I can close my case.

For some people it may seem like a waste of time, but I have one goal in sight—to close out my case as quickly as possible and if talking to a few more people will help me resolve the case then why wouldn't I do it?

OBSTACLES WE FACE BEFORE REACHING A SETTLEMENT OR MOVING FORWARD WITH ARBITRATION

As a Respondent's attorney, my job isn't to deny anyone of his rights under the law. However, I will make sure that the injured employee doesn't feel like he just won the lottery either. Most Petitioners' attorneys will get all upset and tell me that their clients are good, decent people, who have been wronged by the employer and that I should be ashamed to think this way.

Some of these employees *are* hard working, dedicated employees who unfortunately got injured. I know that. But let's not kid ourselves. Some employees do take advantage of the system and some of them push the boundaries as much as possible. Some petitioners dislike their employers and want to use the opportunity to show the employer who really is boss. And finally, there are employees out there who look at an injury as a way to improve their retirement fund—jackpot!

Section 8 of the Workers' Compensation Act[5] provides an injured employee with very specific rights. The employer is ordered to pay for all medical bills regarding the injury under section 8(a). Section 8(b) provides for the payment of temporary total disability benefits or TTD benefits if the employee is unable to work due to his injury. Finally, once the employee reaches medical maximum improvement or MMI he is entitled to compensation for his permanent partial disability or PPD.

It should be a very simple process, but it isn't. You have Petitioners with unrealistic expectations, doctors and medical facilities who keep prescribing treatment to the point where it is unnecessary and unreasonable, and petitioners' attorneys who don't do a very good job at explaining the process to their clients. These are just a few of the obstacles that we have to deal with before the case is closed.

When trying to settle a case, one of the main problems that I face is the petitioner's average weekly wage or AWW. Whatever the petitioner was earning during the year prior to his injury is what will dictate how we calculate his PPD. I feel bad for someone who had a severe injury and whose compensation is low because of his wages. I get it. However, I didn't create the system, neither did my client so do not come to me asking for extra compensation. Besides, no one has ever offered to give me a credit or refund when dealing with a Petitioner whose AWW is at the maximum rate.

Another problem that we deal with is unrealistic expectations from the petitioner. People watch too much TV or listen to the wrong advice or both. I have had to try cases because of a petitioner's refusal to listen to anyone, including his own attorney and sometimes even the arbitrator. Then after the case is tried and the award is less than what was offered the petitioner blames everyone but himself.

A serious issue that is affecting everyone who deals with work comp cases is excessive medical treatment and the so-called-doctors who take advantage of people who are hurt and don't know what to do. As a respondent's attorney, sometimes you feel at a loss because there is not much that you can do to stop the situation. I can set up a million IME exams and it won't matter, I can meet with the petitioner and his attorney, I can bring the matter before the arbitrator and in the end if the petitioner wants to go ahead with an extra surgery or whatever he thinks he needs he goes for it.

Unfortunately, too many times the petitioner ends up in terrible shape and with lots of outstanding medical bills because he listened only to the doctor and ignored everyone else. In the meantime these medical facilities keep

[5] Illinois Workers' Compensation Act, 820 ILCS 305; Last amended 8/21/07; http://www.iwcc.il.gov/act.pdf

going forward in search of the next petitioner to make money off. It is shameful and somehow we need to find a way to put a stop to it.

INDEPENDENT MEDICAL EXAMINATIONS

Independent Medical Examinations or IME examinations[6] are a crucial part of a Respondent's case. Sometimes an IME report is all we have to defend our client. That being said, a bad IME report can also destroy your case. Don't assume that when I mean a bad IME report I mean a report that states that the employee was injured at work and requires further treatment. In fact, a bad report to me is one that lacks any kind of foundation whether factual, medical or sometimes both.

I once had a case in which our IME's report stated that "no accident occurred and therefore there was no work injury" etc. Most Respondent's attorneys would think that that is just what they needed. I did not. This particular employee was injured while assisting his supervisor move some lawn equipment. It was his supervisor who took him to the emergency room and contacted their human resources department to notify them of what had happened.

Now, my IME wants to tell me that no accident ever occurred. Really? Would you like to reconsider? That was a total waste of time and money for many reasons. First, if you do more than one IME your opponent will accuse you of "shopping" for a doctor and this negatively impacts your credibility and that of any doctor that follows your first IME.

Secondly, we lost our opportunity to truly determine what the best medical care would be for the employee and we have no control over it moving forward. A file that could have been closed in six months now can linger for a year or longer.

Yes, I can ask for another report from a different doctor. The problem is that the stigma of the first report will follow the case forever. Whenever a new doctor contradicts the treating physician my opponent will raise his arms up in the air and tell the Arbitrator about the first report and how the company that I represent is just trying to hurt the employee. This is not a good situation for the Respondent.

The best IME reports that I have received are those in which the doctor had the same or better qualifications than the treating physician. This doctor also had all the medical records and facts before he wrote the report. Finally, the doctor was fair, unbiased and took the time to listen to the employee. No, I am not advocating for the employee here. Think about it. If your doctor doesn't take the time to listen to what this person has to say how can he accurately determine what happened, how it happened and whether or not the injury could have happened as the employee tells it?

The examining physician needs to have all the MRI reports, all the physical therapy reports, etc. not just a handful. He will not be able to have a complete picture of the case without all the information. Why set up the exam in the first place if we are not going to give the doctor all the tools that he needs to write an efficient and accurate report?

We do not ever want to be in a situation where we need the doctor to write an addendum report to the original report because he received the information little by little. The doctor's credibility, for the most part, will diminish piece by piece for each extra addendum he was to write.

A problem that I often encounter is when adjusters or employers "marry" a particular IME physician. There are tons of doctors in Illinois! Why use the same one over and over again? The explanation seems to always be the same "I got a good report the first time." That's great, but now we are down to the 100th report and it's not looking too good. Now all we get are the cookie-cutter copies of the same report. Nothing changes except for the name of the petitioner.

How is that helpful? What really happens then is that both, petitioners' attorneys and arbitrators, "get to know" this doctor and the type of reports he writes. Whenever a report from such doctors comes in, the petitioner's attorney dances with joy and the arbitrator tells me "counsel, this doctor is not very reputable, so I am going to have to defer to the treating doctor." Why do we do this to ourselves? Why waste the money?

---

[6] Section 12 of the Illinois Workers' Compensation Act, 820 ILCS, 305

Let's not ruin a simple case with a bad IME. Before we set up the exam, we need to determine whether we truly need an IME or not. And no, we do not need IME exams on every single file. We also need to work with different doctors. Let's make sure that if we are setting up an IME because the treating physician is recommending back surgery that we set up the exam with an orthopedic surgeon, not just a doctor we like. Finally, let's save our best doctors for the very complicated cases.

On the other hand, we need to be fair to these physicians. Let's provide them with all the information that will help them formulate a good report. Make sure that he has all the medical records. Let's be clear and specific on the type of questions that we are formulating. We get one shot at getting this right, let's not blow it.

I strongly believe in the use of IME exams. A good report is like a diamond to me. However, for a report to be useful it needs to be done properly and by a well-qualified, prominent physician who knows what he is doing and who has all the necessary tools to give you what you need—an unbiased, accurate report that you can use to determine how to proceed with your case. Telling me what he thinks I want to hear is a complete waste of my time and I don't like it when people waste my time.

CONCLUSION

Regardless of whether respondents feel that the system favors the petitioner or not is truly irrelevant. This is the system that we have in Illinois and we need to do the best job we possibly can without looking for excuses. Yes, it is very frustrating to feel as if we have very little saying on how a case should proceed when it is the respondent who is footing the bill. I fully understand that. But the reality is, that the system is in place to make sure that people who suffered a legitimate work injury are taken care of. How do you argue against that?

More than fighting the system, I believe we need to take a stand against the many medical facilities that abuse the petitioner by continuing to prescribe medications they don't need and recommend procedures that are unnecessary. If somehow we can put an end to that, we will be able to control cost, we will be able to have petitioners return to work quickly and we will get the system to work in a more expeditious manner. Let's focus on what the real problem is and once we can resolve that issue everything else will fall into place.

CHAPTER 10

Performance Based Compensation: 'Just What The Doctor Ordered' For Workers' Compensation

Gregory Krohm

International Association of Industrial Accident Boards and Commissions

Abstract: Medical care delivery in workers' compensation suffers from a combination of poor incentives that promote overtreatment of injuries, particularly major surgical interventions, and shelters ineffective medical providers from quality and value based choices by purchasers. These malincentives include the lack of copayments by injured workers, the disconnection between the payer and the choice of service provider, and setting payments for services performed without regard to the effectiveness of the treatment. Finally, the selection of provider is very frequently made by the injured worker without any regard to the cost of service, and often little knowledge about the pattern of effectiveness and quality of care for that doctor. This paper focuses on the principles needed to govern a realignment of payment incentives and evidence on how well these principles have worked in the context of workers compensation medical treatment. An assessment is made of how current payment practices depart from ideal incentives for improving clinical behavior in the treatment of occupational injury.

INTRODUCTION

To frame the topic of this paper, let us briefly review the setting in the US, which is the focus of this paper: The US health care delivery system is a bad bargain. Granted, at its best, the supply of medical services and technology in the US defines world class. Yet, even its ardent defenders are hard pressed to refute the list of indictments against the US system of medical care:

- not only is the US the biggest per capita spender on health care in the world, the annual growth in per capita expenditure has been growing relatively rapidly over the past two decades (Kaiser, 2007).
- rapidly increasing prices and average expenditures per capita (much higher than average inflation) or the past 15 years
- no obvious return for the high expenditures, since health outcomes are mediocre overall when compared to other post-industrial nations
- there is substantial "waste" in the medical care delivery system, in the sense of spending that is not needed to produce a service with a given quality outcome (Gawande, 2009; Price Waterhouse Coopers, 2008)
- Access to doctors, especially primary care physicians, is restricted in some geographic areas and for some ethnic and impoverished populations.[1]
- inability to counter incentives created by indemnifying time off from work by motivating patients to return to work as soon as possible[2]
- legal friction costs when medical opinions clash with opinions of employers/payers about the management of a case
- in many jurisdictions, providers excessively wiling to call conditions work related because of relatively high fees payable
- iatrogenic injury from excessive surgery.[3]

[1]See Center for Study of Health System Change showing reduction in primary physicians per 100,000 population, website at: http://www.hschange.com/CONTENT/934/SP1.htm

[2]In a survey of neuro surgeons, the most frequent factors considered very important in the development of chronic neuropathic pain were psychosocial factors (64%), mechanism of injury (59%), workers' compensation or litigation (54%), and iatrogenic injury (48%).

[3]According to Hadden, "The conclusion is inescapable that iatrogenic and jurisgenic factors have a direct effect (in the cohort of cases analyzed) on the prolongation of medical care, and delay in returning to gainful employment, and, consequently, contributing to the high cost."

Chris E. Stout, Matt Kruger and Jeffrey Rogers, (Eds)

Workers' compensation systems throughout the world have struggled with medical cost containment. In the US, the problem is acute: medical claims cost has risen to 59% of insurance benefit payments, up from about 45% thirty years earlier.[4] The rate of escalation in medical cost per claim has substantially exceeded the rate of the CPI for medical services. Yet, indemnity cost per claim has consistently grown at a rate well below medical cost per claim.[5] Paying the bills for medical care is the biggest cost driver in workers' compensation today, and has been for over a decade.

From a humanitarian point of view, the greatest tragedy of the current workers compensation system is that it provides injured workers with irregular quality of care and an unacceptable risk of needless disability. Most workers receive orthodox care and are restored to their pre-injury functional condition and job with little problem. However, a few unfortunates fall into the hands of medical providers that cause unnecessary delay in proper treatment of the medical condition, expose the worker to invasive and unnecessary treatment, foster dependency on narcotics, and provoke needless delays in indemnity benefits through mishandling of medical reports to insurers or administrative agencies. In small fraction of claims, poor management or treatment of the injury by the physician results in a catastrophic new work disability far beyond what the original work accident would have created.

The thesis of this paper is that workers' compensation needs a massive shift toward more rational incentives for both medical providers and patients.[6] By incentives we mean the payments made to medical providers for the treatment of injured workers, or other administrative benefits associated with payments for services. "Treatment" here is broadly construed to include more than a typical procedure or service that might be billed by a standard Current Procedural Terminology (CPT) code. It could include all episodes of care related to a particular condition, including appropriate involvement in the return to work process. Designing incentives (and in some cases sanctions) to produce better outcomes for injured workers and lower system costs is the challenge which we wish to address here.

THE RIGHT INCENTIVES AS REMEDY FOR IMPROVEMENT IN MEDICAL CARE DELIVERY

Advocates for health care reform offer many --often conflicting-- remedies for the ailing health system. It would appear that the majority of health economists and actuaries consider deductibles and co-payments to be an essential part of a reformed system. They reason that consumers of health care, like consumers of all other goods and services, ought to have an incentive to shop for the most efficient and effective providers and treatments. Yet, critics of the insurance mechanism contend that insurers are forcing consumers into ever more costly and difficult self funding of care, which discourages prompt preventative care, the proper use of expensive pharmaceuticals, and other counterproductive behaviors designed to reduce out of pocket expense.

The Medicare drug deductible has drawn particular fire from the elderly, but drugs are a very high and rapidly expanding component of Medicare expenditure. Deductibles seem to be a system for controlling overutilization.

The benefits of a "single payer" system for payment versus competitive insurers are also hotly debated. These and other remedies boil down to a choice of economic incentives versus prescriptive rules/processes to control what care is demanded and supplied.

This paper focuses on incentives that might be applied to physicians. Physicians amount to about a third of the cost of medical care paid by workers' compensation.[7] In addition, physicians are the gatekeepers to other medical services, such as pharmaceuticals, hospitals, therapy centers, and durable medical equipment for patient use.

By extrapolation, similar issues and solutions arise in the practice of medicine by other medical practitioners, such as therapists and chiropractors. Likewise, direct incentives, albeit different structures, might be applied to hospitals.

---

[4] Based on approximately 30 states in which the National Council on Compensation Insurance provides rate making services. See Mealy, 2009

[5] Using the same state data cited above, NCCI found that indemnity cost per lost time claim increased at an average rate of 3.4%/year between 2002-2007, while medical cost increased by 6.7%/year over the same period. See Mealy, 2009.

[6] It is not within the scope of this presentation to address co-pays, deductibles and other incentives applied to workers' compensation claimants. This would be a radical and highly controversial move, though it would address the obvious need for patients to have some incentive to care about selecting highly dubious treatments or paying exceptionally high prices for services.

[7] According to the median value of the 14 WCRI Compscope states physicians were paid 35.4% of all payments for 2006/2007 Claims with More Than 7 Days of Lost Time.

PHYSICIAN PRACTICE SETTINGS AND TRENDS

Building better incentive systems requires understanding the organizational structures under in which physicians practice their profession and earn their incomes. By organizational structure we mean the form, size, and ownership and management of the organization in which the doctor practices medicine. The organizational structure and how it deals with the wide array of payers of medical services will have an enormous control over the degree to which workers' compensation payment mechanisms have any maneuvering room to provide good incentives.

Physicians are no less savvy about compensation and contingent ties to performance than any other profession. Like accountants, lawyers, and other professional service providers they understand monetary incentives as they affect their take home pay, risk of income variation. They understand the stress and conflict that some performance incentives creates relative to colleagues in the same practice group or partnership. Finally, like other professionals they are motivated by non-pecuniary factors, e.g., they derive personal satisfaction from professional autonomy in their decision making.

Notwithstanding the personal satisfaction and autonomy that an independent practice offers, economic stresses on the small independently owned medical practice are so great that this model appears to be steadily giving way to other forms of physician employment. Increasingly, medical professionals are part of groups, or networks, of providers.

The most recent look at ownership of medical practices was done in a 2005 survey by the Center for Studying Health System Changes (CSHSC). That survey finds that 51.8 percent of primary-care physicians owned their practices in 2005 (see Table **1**), compared with 54.3 percent in 1997. The greatest drop in practice ownership was greatest among medical specialists, which dropped to 47.3 percent from 58.1 percent. For surgical specialists, the percentage fell to 68.4 percent from 75.5 percent.

Table 1: Trends in "Independent" Medical Practices By Physician Type

Physician Type	1996-1997	2004-2005 *percent*	Relative Reduction
Primary-care physicians	54.3	51.8	4.6
Medical specialists	58.1	47.3	18.6
Surgical specialists	75.5	68.4	9.4

Source: *Data are from the Center for Studying Health System Change, August 2007.*

CSHSC data on size of practice is shown below (see Table **2**). The reduction in 1-2 doctor practices is the sharpest change, and the fastest growing practice size appearing in the 6-50 grouping.

Table 2: Doctors in Different Practice Group Sizes and Employment Settings

(Percentage changes shown from 1996-97 to 2004-05)

1-2 physicians, 40.7% to 32.5%, down 8.2%

3-5 physicians, 12.2% to 9.7%, down 3.5%

6-50 physicians, 15.9% to 21.8%, up 5.9%

Single specialty, 13.1% to 17.6%, up 4.5%

Multispecialty, 30.9% to 27.5%, down 3.4%

Source: *Data are from the Center for Studying Health System Change, August 2007.*

Bureau of Labor Statistics data supports the above CSHSC survey findings. Their annual survey data shows the proportion of self-employed physicians dropping from 30% in the year 2000 to 25.9% in 2007. The big discrepancy between the above two sources is based on very different survey methods. However, multiple sources attest to a clear trend away from small, independently owned medical practices, especially by non-surgeons (see also Jellinek and Isaacs, 2008).

In corporate or partnership practices, the individual physician agrees to adhere to a professional relationship with the organization via some contractual agreement. This might be a partnership agreement, employment contract or some other affiliation agreement. Communicating with doctors about their individual performance and individualizing incentives becomes complicated in a large practice setting. For the workers' compensation payer, individualizing payment incentives is aggravated by the fact that most medical practices the average doctor has few encounters with workers' compensation cases.

How are financial incentives or sanctions affecting the behavior of doctors? Jellinek and Isaacs (2008) research shows a high degree of self-reported feelings of autonomy and self direction in patient treatment by physicians. Surprisingly, the feeling of autonomy in the practice of medicine is higher among employee physicians than among owners of independent practices. If true, this suggests that large corporate organizations do not impose significant constraints on treatment practices, nor would it seem that incentive systems are binding or hampering the professional judgments of clinicians.

Greenfield (1998) asserts that, over the past twenty years less complex incentive structures have been build into physician compensation. Not many years ago employment contracts were complex and had a number of very different reward structures for a wide array of behaviors and accomplishments. Many of these goals had nothing to do with the practice of medicine per se. e.g., public service volunteering and increasing billings. Some of the goals were corrosive to the practice of good medicine, such as agreements to refer patients to a facility in which the provider had a financial self interest, or having a significant share of annual income come from net profits of practice owned diagnostic service centers.

Practice management software further constrains incentives. If the provider's software is inflexible or designed for other payment schemes, imposing a new reporting and payment system may be difficult. Workers' compensation is notoriously laden with special reports not required by general health plans.

One final trend that should be the most disturbing of all for workers' compensation stakeholders is the declining numbers of doctors specializing in occupational medicine. The number of board certified occupational medicine specialists has declined sharply since 1997 (LaDou, 2002). Likewise the membership of the American College of Occupational and Environmental Medicine has been in decline since the late 1990s. This should be of grave concern to insurers, employers, and labor advocates. Skilled practitioners in occupational medicine produce better outcomes in treating injured workers. They also have a familiarity with the workers' compensation system that is helpful for fostering good administration and good public policy.

For workers' compensation to insert a new compensation incentive into system it must deal with several changes in employment and compensation of physicians:

1. Fewer physicians will have the freedom or ease of accepting new compensation systems independent of their employing organization's management
2. Larger practices that are dominating the market will be increasingly more sophisticated in their administrative/payment operations, which have both pluses and minuses for dealing with the special demands of workers' compensation.
3. Specialists are increasingly being hired by hospitals and larger organizations and hence will not be negotiating their own incentive systems.
4. Payers need to exert influence in negotiations with the larger umbrella organizations that employ an increasing share of doctors but see workers' compensation as a tiny share of their revenues. Workers' compensation is only 2-3% of medical care cost in the US and hence most doctors' employers have scant incentive to modify their office systems and physician compensation procedures to respond to yet another standard of benefits, billing and reward system.

Given all the changes in practice settings, the challenge to workers' compensation is to devise a model that is:

1. reasonably compatible with the overarching billing and payment systems that govern general health care;

2. able to articulate a specific set of behavioral and performance goals for providers and the organizations that employ them
3. offers overall compensation packages that compete favorably with other payers in the market.

WHAT DEFINES GOOD TREATMENT?

A prerequisite to using incentives is having a good grasp of what goals you are trying to accomplish. What constitutes good outcomes in occupational medicine? Who decides whether a treatment path is good medicine?

At an abstract, conceptual level, the goals seem reasonably clear: care that improves functional status of the injured worker and enables rapid return to work both accomplished with a minimum of wasted medical or administrative resources. But what sort of medical delivery style gets us to this ideal? We need to consider more than the proper us of diagnostic and treatment options. Also important is the time spent with the injured worker uncovering all the issues that may potentially impede the ideal outcomes and counseling the patient on good treatment, therapeutic, and behavior that will advance the ideal outcomes.

Guidelines have become a touchstone for medical cost containment both in workers' compensation and general health care. Institute of Medicine (IOM) defines a guideline as "systematically developed statements to assist practitioner and patient decisions about appropriate health care for specific clinical circumstances."[8] They are used by clinicians to direct their decisions, and by claims adjusters to evaluate the reasonableness of treatment. Hence they are often at the core of incentive contracting arrangements.

For many important treatment issues, debate rages between groups of practitioners that consider best practices from their particular orientation in medicine. Various professional associations of doctors disagree on important issues. Some members of the public have shown a deep suspicions about guidelines, conjuring up images of "death panels" denying treatment for the terminally ill and attributing corporate greed as the basis for limiting diagnostic tests and therapies.

While not in the occupational medicine field, Dr. Jerome Groopman offers a rich example of the intractability of deciding on treatment guideline that will win public and government approval. In 2009, the Preventative Services Task Force sponsored by the federal Dept. of Health and Human Service touched off a controversy that eventually forced them to back peddle on what seemed to be a scientific consensus that routine mammograms are not required for woman between the ages of 40-49. Groopman comments as follows on the failed process:

The fault lines that erupted among medical providers were not uncommon in setting guidelines. Many informed woman found it patronizing that the Task Force was superimposing itself between a woman and her doctor. Does a woman need to be sheltered against anxiety, or have other decide what is best for her? Medical experts clashed: the American College of Physicians, composed of internists, agreed with the task force conclusions about mammography while the American Society of Clinical Oncology rejected the recommendation (Groopman, 2010).

Treatment guidelines have become increasingly popular with state regulators as a tool for controlling excessive utilization or unnecessarily expensive treatments. As of 2001, at least 20 states had enacted guideline, and many others have been studying the adoption of such guidelines. While there is broad agreement on some issues, the guidelines differ in scope and content. To illustrate the lack of consensus, the four most recent states to consider such guide for workers' compensation have all selected different approaches.[9]

In a study for the California Commission on Health, Safety and Workers' Compensation, the RAND Corporation identified five guidelines that are current, comprehensive, and reasonably applicable to workers' compensation (Nuckols *et al*, 2005):

1. AAOS—Clinical Guidelines by the American Academy of Orthopedic Surgeons

[8] See National Institute of Health at: http://www.nhlbi.nih.gov/guidelines/about.htm

[9] CA selected ACCOEM, TX selected ODG, WI adopted its own version of the MN guidelines, and MT is currently working on a hybrid of ODG and Colorado.

2. ACOEM—American College of Occupational and Environmental Medicine Occupational Medicine Practice Guidelines
3. Intracorp—Optimal Treatment Guidelines, part of Intracorp Clinical Guidelines Tool®
4. McKesson—McKesson/InterQual Care Management Criteria and Clinical Evidence Summaries
5. ODG—Official Disability Guidelines: Treatment in Workers' Comp, by Work-Loss Data Institute.

In addition to the above published guidelines, many insurers have their own internal guides to assist adjusters. Finally, clinical practice groups may have their own formal or informal guidelines for how they should approach problematic or complex injury situations.

These many guidelines sometimes overlap and are often roughly consistent on common injury types, e.g., low back sprain. However, it must be admitted that consensus breaks down on how to treat a great many diagnosis groups. This lack of consensus may be due to a lack of solid empirical evidence on treatment outcomes, or it may be do to the many complicating factors that make treatment predominantly case specific.

The reaction to clinicians to guidelines has been mixed. Doctors are rightly proud of their training and need to exercise professional judgment in their work. In general medicine the tough judgment calls stem from such needs as early diagnosis and end of life care. As discussed below, workers' compensation has its own peculiar set of issues over which sound judgment must be exercised to justify one treatment in favor of another. Another major difference between occupational injury and other injury is the need to promote and manage the return to work process. Occupational medicine can justify early use of diagnostic measures and aggressive treatment if it can reasonably be thought to facilitate the early return to work (this is the so called "sports model").

In a practical sense, guidelines are really only needed for a relatively small subset of the overall mix of workers' compensation claims. The vast majority of injury cases involve relatively straightforward medical treatment and present low costs to the system In many jurisdictions, two thirds of all injury claims or more are "medical only." Most of these are often handled by routine office visits and minimum diagnostic testing. To illustrate the relatively well focused and uncomplicated nature of most claims, the top four "nature of injury" descriptors in 2008 for the State of Washington workers' compensation cases are described in Table **3**.

The Washington injury data was used because of its detail and inclusion of all medical cost. Federal OSHA reported injuries have a different reporting system and do not include medical costs. The OSHA data also suggests that the majority of workplace injuries are—generally speaking-- relatively simple traumatic injuries. According to 2006 OSHA reports for the US, the leading specific classes of injury by percent of all reported are (see Table **3**): "Sprains/Strains" at 39.9%, "Cuts, Lacerations, and Punctures" at 9.7%, and "Bruises" at 8.6%.[10]

Table 3: Workers' Compensation Injury Claims in Washington 2008

Nature of Injury	% total injuries reported	Avg. incurred medical cost	% Avg. Medical Cost
Traumatic injuries to muscles, tendons, ligaments, joints, etc	33%	6,684	44.8%
Open wounds	20	1,300	8.7%
Surface wounds and bruises	15	1,680	11.3%
Multiple traumatic injuries and disorders	10	8,730	58.6%

Source*: Washington Dept of Labor and Industries, found at:*
http://www.lni.wa.gov/ClaimsIns/Insurance/DataStatistics/WorkersCompData/default.asp

For most of these traumatic injuries the diagnosis is clear and the treatment straightforward and uncomplicated. For such injuries, there is small doubt as to the appropriate clinical behavior, and hence less need for influencing behavior

[10] See OSHA website at: http://www.bls.gov/iif/oshwc/osh/os/osh06_28.pdf

via financial incentives. By contrast, where disease is the nature of injury, complexity of physician judgments are much higher. Moreover, the average costs for disease treatment are substantially above the average medical cost—the average occupational cancer case is almost 200 times as expensive as the average "wound" treatment.. Likewise, where the diagnosis is unspecified or unknown, the costs tend to be much higher than average.[11]

This injury mix suggests that the best target for imposing better control on medical costs seem to lie in the infrequent injury types that are difficult to diagnose, involve complex treatments, and involve challenging patient management. These seem to be the cases were incentives are needed the most to shape the behavior of clinicians and injured workers being treated. Yet, experience shows that even minor injuries that are diagnosed a sprains can devolve into long term disability and high medical costs. Thus, guidelines are relevant to the treatment of common low back sprain in that they counsel against aggressive diagnostics and treatment unless indicated by specific indicators.

It would behoove a payer to do more than evaluate physicians 'by the numbers.' Reviewing office notes for evidence of compliance with evidenced based best practices can explain why a provider had some unexpectedly high case costs/durations. They could also create qualifications on otherwise good numbers if the clinician seemed to be taking shortcuts and unreasonably limiting treatments. For these reasons some well accepted, evidence based guideline is an essential tool incentive based payment.

CREATING BAD INCENTIVES

The majority of US jurisdictions have cobbled together a patchwork of fee schedules, managed care arrangements, and fee dispute adjudication mechanisms in an attempt to meet simultaneously the following objectives: 1) control rapidly rising medical costs, and 2) not restrict access to high quality care by injured workers. In most states, these attempts are misguided and counter productive. Over and under treatment of injuries appear to be common, as shown by evidence in general health care, and by virtue of treatment disputes before state administrative law judges and the rapidly escalating costs of medical care per claim.[12]

By richly compensating specialty care, such as surgery and complex diagnostic testing, there appears to be an incentive to perform unnecessary and perhaps risky treatments. A detailed study of the causes of rising medical treatments in workers' compensation claims focuses on surgery as a major cost driver. (NCCI, 2008).

Many treating physicians, especially those without training in occupational medicine, do not appear to be spending enough time following ACOEM guidelines on counseling of patients on return to work, therapeutic regimens, and injury avoidance.

Finally, workers compensation is the target of cost shifting when it stands as the most generous payer in town.[13] This creates an obvious financial incentive for the diagnosis of occupational etiology of injury or disease, sometimes under dubious causal circumstances.

How did WC get into this mess? The principle reason is that workers' comp fell victim to first dollar, fee-for-service medicine (F$FFS), i.e., insurance coverage for charges submitted by patient selected physician without deductible. Many health economists single out the F$FFS mechanism as the root cause of the US health care cost explosion. However, as the general health insurance industry has successfully pulled away from F$FFS, the workers' comp system is still stuck in the 1960s with this style of medical practice. Under most circumstances, an injured worker has absolutely no incentive to seek out a low cost provider, nor is there much incentive to select a provider that is going to dispense "tough love" and push the worker into therapeutic return to work.

---

[11] Unsurprisingly, a claim that is hard to categorize using conventional medical terms is probably more likely to have complicating factors that drive up treatment cost.

[12]Elizabeth A. McGlynn *et al.*, The Quality of Health Care Delivered to Adults in the United States, 348 NEW ENG. J. MED. 2635 (2003). See also Steven M. Asch *et al.*, Who Is at Greatest Risk for Receiving Poor-Quality Health Care?, 354 NEW ENG. J. MED. 1147, 1147 (2006). Dr. Teryl K. Nuckols has shown that medical providers frequently disagree on what empirical evidence dictates to be best practice for treatment, and that over and under treatment by treatment guidelines is common. See Rigorous Development Does Not Ensure Guidelines Are Acceptable to a Panel of Knowledgeable Providers, Journal of Internal Medicine, Jan 2008.

[13]In many geographic areas and practice specialties, workers' compensation pays substantially more than group health insurance. See Shufford, 2010.

States re-enforce the old style F$FFS model by relying on fee schedules as cost containment tools. Fee schedules, especially those based on "usual and customary charges" tend to hard wire in the right of a provider to collect the fee schedule amount for performing a particular medical treatment. By convention, the maximum charge allowable is set at percentile of distribution of charged amounts on some sample of medical bills. The percentile is chosen by political give and take between providers, payers, and policy makers.[14] Medicare based fee schedules are somewhat more rational since the Medicare levels are set by a rigorous, cost-based methodology, and the relative value units and rules of administration are updated and refined annually.

In either species of schedule, the merit or necessity of the treatment is never addressed, nor is quality. The only question is whether the treatment fit the descriptive parameters of the CPT code being charged and whether the treatment was necessarily related to the work injury reported and accepted by the payer. What other market is this 'quality blind' purchasing decisions? Little wonder that workers' compensation medical treatment so often deviates radically from centrist norms of good medicine.

FRAMING NEW RELATIONSHIPS

Having described the status quo of how clinicians are compensated and the deficiencies of fee schedules, we need to look to entirely new frameworks to improve outcomes. Creating networks of select providers to manage care should in principle open up new avenues for introducing quality and desired outcomes into workers' compensation. In workers' compensation, managed care networks have no published track record for improving outcomes or reducing cost. Even in states that nominally permit managed care contracting, the method of payment is still a basically a function of the number and type of treatments. Managed care in workers' compensation is mainly a contract between payer and provider to discount service charges in exchange for more business being directed to the provider or streamlined and faster payment. Rarely, if ever, does the contractual relationship offer payment based on ultimate outcomes of injury treatment, or for a provider's track record over a number of claims.

The degree of management in managed care networks focuses on three things:

1. preauthorization of services
2. prescreening of providers to qualify for inclusion in the network
3. providing feedback to providers on treatment patterns through utilization review by experts.

Preauthorization is a labor intensive process that amounts to looking over the shoulder of the clinician and making sure they don't make a mistake in offering too much or too expensive treatment for a particular claimant. It is expensive to administer for the payer, and an irritant to the clinician.

The second form of management comes in many variations. In its simpler and more common form, it amounts to checking to see if a physician meets objective licensing and certification requirements, e.g., board certified orthopedic surgeon. A less frequent and more powerful version has the network manager systematically assessing individual provider performance and outcomes, and from this cutting out the worst providers from the network.

The third and most challenging management approach is to use carefully collected data on performance to educate, reward, and sanction providers. Rewards may be monetary, public recognition, or reduced administrative costs. Sanctions for chronically underperforming doctors are most often elimination from the network.

What is needed is a fundamental remake of these "managed care networks." More sophisticated measurement, evaluation, and feedback is needed.

DESIGN FEATURES OF GOOD INCENTIVE SYSTEMS

In the US, Medicare is a pioneer in designing innovative payment mechanisms, many of which have been adopted by private insurers. Examples include, Diagnostic Related Groups for hospital treatment, Resource Based Relative

[14]Based on the author's personal experience with fee schedule design and witnessing fee schedule development from the perspectives of insiders, fee schedule payment amounts are often based on a pure political "horse trading" between payers and medical providers without any objective rationale for the chosen payment levels.

Value Systems as a detailed cost based system for determining relative compensation on one treatment to another, and the detailed fair billing rules for coding and submitting medical claims for Medicare services. Currently, CMS is investigating a host of pay-for-performance initiatives. One prominent example is paying hospitals one fee for initial encounter and subsequent readmissions related to complications from the original diagnosis and treatment. For physician incentives, Medicare linked its 2007 payment methods for physicians to the reporting of performance data, the so-called Physician Quality Reporting Initiative. This is a radical departure from quality blind payment and clearly seems to be laying the groundwork for more robust pay for performance methods. State Medicaid programs have also embraced physician incentive payments. Given the number of doctors involved and the resources that the federal government can bring to bear on refining, applying, and evaluating quality indicators, this initiative is extremely important. .

The earliest and most robust models for private insurance performance contracting come from group health insurance, especially by HMOs. A survey done in 1992 found a fifth of the responding HMOs used of performance contracting (Christianson, 2007). In a 2003 survey of health plans in 12 metropolitan areas by the Center for Study of Health System Change, 7 of the 12 communities had instances of pay for performance in their health plans (Trude, 2006). Despite these forays into performance contracting must be regarded as tentative first steps. A 2007 RAND study of performance contracting concluded: "Relatively little is known about the impact of the group health P4P programs or the best way to design these programs, either from the literature or conversations with individual program administrators" (Wynn, 2007). The same conclusion was drawn by Christianson (2007) *et al*

in their 2007 survey article for the Robert Wood Johnson Foundation. Trude and Christianson sum up their findings on health plan performance payment systems as follows: "health plans' customization underscores the lack of consensus across plans regarding the most effective approaches. Furthermore, health plan decisions about program design often reflect local market conditions."

Borrowing from the RAND study, Christianson's work, and conversations with key players in the delivery of medical care to injured workers, we offer five principles to consider in reforming the incentives for the delivery of medical care.

What are the Shared Goals Among Stakeholders for a Good Medical Delivery System?

This begs the question of who is a legitimate stakeholder in the system. If the stakeholders are narrowly construed to be doctors in a specialty practice the answer will be different than if the stakeholder list is broadened to include insurance payers, patients, and employers.

The first big divide in opinion on goals is probably over cost versus quality. The two are related but not necessarily in complete harmony. Indeed, quality does often reduce cost, most clearly through reducing iatrogenic injury. However, quality can also mean superfluous treatment only done to assuage the unfounded anxiety or unreasonable intolerance to pain or delay in treatment or noticeable change by some patients.

Another example of goal conflict that may militate against good control of treatment is choice of provider by the injured worker. Labor representatives in advisory councils, commissions and legislative committees often jealously want to maximize choice for the injured worker. This may produce bad medical and cost outcomes.

Finally, physicians want to maximize annual income from their professional practice, and their professional associations may use a sufficient supply of qualified clinicians as the public policy goal. Payers may not be opposed to higher annual incomes for providers if there a concomitant improvement in aggregate medical claim cost. However, payers would have little sympathy with physician income needs if there was an apparent supply of willing providers.

Metrics

This area raise a large number of very difficult questions:

- What are the conceptual elements of an appropriate measures for incentivizing providers?
- What are the most promising treatment/practice areas to start developing metrics?

- Can metrics be borrowed from non-WC systems?
- How is accountability assigned to individual providers and groups for measurement and reward?
- How is an episode of care attributed to a particular provider
- Define "extra work" i.e. additional quality/value that would merit incentive payments.

Because of these methodological and conceptual difficulties, metrics for compensation are challenging, particularly for workers' compensation payers who have limited points of contact and hence data on the majority of providers caring for their claimants.

Inevitably, broadly stated, ultimate goals like "quality" and "risk reduction" are difficult to use as performance metrics. Medical treatment involves too many dimensions As a result, adherence to treatment guidelines is frequently used to serve as the surrogate for quality care.

To most stakeholders, cost should not be the governing principle in determining whether or not an injured worker needed a specific treatment regimen. Instead, effectiveness and secondary risk of treatment are the primary considerations. Surgery appears to be done before less invasive procedures are tried; to the dismay of many occupational medicine specialists.

Collecting and Sharing Data

For a third party to pay for performance, there must be reliable data to measure that performance. Who is to collect the data and how will it be maintained?

Clearly, the task is too great for small groups of providers, or small payers. A large enough number of cases are needed to overcome small sample variation and to demonstrate tendencies or trends in care and outcomes.

Data must be vetted carefully to maintain quality standards of measurement.

Next there is the problem of collecting enough data about cases to statistically adjust each case for complications, such as diabetes or obesity. Outliers that seem to be errors or gross misfits need to be identified and dropped from the sample or suitably adjusted.

Reward Structure

The reward structure is integrally tied to the data systems available to support metrics and reporting. A primary question to resolve is whether stakeholders want to incentivize clinical behavior or broader claim outcomes. The former can be judged against how treatment follows some accepted guideline, with consideration of the fact situation in the claim, e.g., how long should muscle relaxation be tried for the diagnosis of a low back sprain? The latter requires much different data and a much longer time horizon, e.g., what is the length of disability for a case relative to a hypothetical benchmark of lost time?

It is also conditioned on how providers are associated, i.e., are incentives directed at individual clinicians or group/clinical practices. Finally, the longevity of the relationship between payer and practitioners will shape the reward structure. An out of state provider or one that rarely files workers' compensation claims may be difficult to mold into an incentive system.

One very important tactical decision is whether to use carrots or sticks. Should providers be paid more than historically or than the current average if they achieve high points on a metric scale, or should the providers at the bottom of the scale be punished with reduced compensation. Or, should a symmetrical sliding scale be used?

Rewards that are financed from savings attained by wringing "fat" or wasted effort from the system are win-win situations. But, when all the fat is out of the system, how is superior compensation maintained. Payers may tend to forget the bad old days and assume that the current efficient system is the norm. They may be tempted to cut payments to providers based on what the going market rate is for clinicians generally.

How should financial rewards be combined with other rewards or sanctions? For example, business or clients could be directed from low efficiency to high performing providers (like an insurer managing its outsourcing of litigation). Should low payments be combined with negative feedback and threats of severance of the relationship?

Overcoming Political Resistance

Any across the board change to compensation is likely to peak the attention of all medical providers, who in turn will reach out to their professional associations to protect their interests. There is a wide range of sophistication and clout held by different practitioner groups and industry segments. Witness, for example, the clout of the plastic surgeons in getting the 5 percent surcharge on cosmetic surgery removed from the Senate health care reform bill, while at the same stroke the hapless tanning salon industry was slapped with a 10 percent surcharge on its services.

In workers' compensation, surgeons and radiologists have been most successful in lobbying for special consideration in WC fee schedules. Chiropractor political power seems to be very strong in some states and weak in others.

To overcome political resistance and to avoid the risk of making large systemic mistakes, it may be wise to allow a wide range of flexibility among individual payers in choosing a contract model. If large enough, an insurer or self insured employer could negotiate their own metrics and other contractual terms. Smaller payers could sign onto performance networks negotiated and managed by third parties.

To put these principles into practice, payers need to be allowed to establish networks of high quality providers. Current state laws that require payers to contract with 'any willing provider' and allow injured workers to avoid going to the payer designated network are lethal to the viability of a good network. Payers must be allowed to freely negotiate with providers that meet their standards for quality and to select the number of providers needed to meet the expected demand for services.

Rather than negotiating for cuts from charges or fee schedule amounts, enlightened payers should be awarding substantial bonus payments over market rates to top quality providers (as measured by outcomes, patient satisfaction, and chart reviews). Moreover, payers should incent prompt reporting and more extensive use of counseling and patient education in office visits. Specifically, this means recognizing the need for longer office visits.

SOME OF THE BEST PRACTICES TODAY?

This section reviews some models for contracting with providers that use positive incentives for improving outcomes for injured workers. As with health insurance plans, there exist many variations of performance based payments. The variations can be grouped into four broad classes: 1. Network Screened for Quality and Performance, 2. Contracting with Organization, 3. Public Quality Data, and 4. Employing doctors to deliver care to a given worker population. While the lines of distinction are sometimes fuzzy, it will serve to organize a description of key elements in the structure of how doctors can be organized for purposes of incentive payments.

Network of Unaffiliated Providers

There are many different ways a workers compensation payer can avail themselves of a network of doctors to provide care to their claimants. Most of these networks are developed by third parties and "rented" to an insurer or self insured employer for treating injured workers. The basic product offering purports to reduce payment through a discount from standard charges. This is an extremely weak form of network contracting, and provides no real incentive for quality, as measured by treatment behavior, outcome metrics, or improvements in the administration of claims and payment. Even adding utilization and bill review to the network management services does little to create incentives for quality treatment. In many cases, utilization and bill review encourage gamesmanship between the provider and the payer.

Their most sophisticated offering is called an "Outcomes Based Network (OBN)"

"...the Outcomes-Based Network program is aimed at identifying workers' compensation providers who have been statistically shown to contribute to quality patient outcomes and controlled claims costs. The Outcomes-Based

Network was developed in response to the market's desire for smaller occupational health focused networks whereby clients can increase utilization with doctors who are associated with their most desirable outcomes. The Outcomes-Based Network differs from other focused network offerings as it addresses the importance of identifying providers based on total claims outcomes.

Some workers' compensation insurers have negotiated their own networks, and market it as a value added feature they bring to their policyholders, For example, Travelers Insurance is described on their website as follows:

Our expansive medical network is an integral part of **TravComp®**. With presence in all 50 states and the District of Columbia, Travelers' preferred provider network (PPN) covers the working population with discounts averaging almost 20% below fee schedules and reasonable and customary charges. The network adheres to strict credentialing and medical guidelines designed to return the injured worker to productive employment. The network was constructed by medical and claim professionals to treat workers compensation-specific illnesses and injuries to achieve early return-to-work at the fairest cost. Travelers' medical management services division uses the following mechanisms to encourage injured employees to use the preferred provider network unless specialized medical services are not available.

To date, PPO networks have not received high marks from objective researchers or the payers that "rent" them from the organizer. The PPO providers seem to be settling for basic standards for admission to the network and negotiating the best possible discounts from standard charges. These two steps fall are woefully inadequate in bending the curve on medical inflation and improving the quality of care to injured workers.

Contracting with Occupational Clinics

Throughout the US there are clinics that specialize in treating occupational injury and offering workplace health, safety, and testing services for employers. Perhaps the largest nationwide model of this sort is Concentra. Concentra is a very large health service delivery corporation with 300 locations in the US. While founded by physicians, ownership is now in the form of a closely held corporation. Their doctors are employees. Concentra has its own internal treatment guidelines and a culture for reinforcing the delivery of a style of medicine that the company believes is efficient patient care and responsive to the needs of employers. Integrated in Concentra services are employer health and safety and return to work support.

Smaller and more localized versions of the Concentra model are found in most large cities throughout the US. Often they comprise a few occupational medicine or orthopedic specialists and possibly some occupational therapists. The hallmark of this model is physician ownership and management control, with a focus of clinical practice on occupational medicine, including ancillary services like employee pre-hire screening and drug testing.

These local or regional occupational medicine clinics should be fertile ground for performance contracting. Advantages include a high proportion of workers' compensation claims, familiarity with the rules of workers' compensation, and enough management independence to negotiate performance contracts that are customized to workers' compensation. Such clinics would understand the need for prompt medical reports and the type of office notes and attachments claims adjusters routinely request.

Public Quality Metrics

Sharing data and developing it into statistically meaningful measures of individual physician performance (treatment behaviors or outcomes) would be an ideal method of creating the right alignment of incentives.

In a sense, this is what Medicare is attempting to do with its performance data. One unique feature of the Medicare program is that the data will not be shared publicly but will be used in private communications with providers and individual payments.

The Integrated Healthcare Association (IHA) is the primary example of collaborative information sharing on performance metrics. It was developed by an alliance of California employers, health plans, and physician organizations developed to stimulate improvement in patient satisfaction and clinical quality. IHA covers seven health plans and 225 physician groups representing 35,000 California physicians. Physicians can earn bonus payments for individually attaining evidence-based performance goals in three areas: clinical measures, patient experiences, and investment in IT (IHA, 2007; Wynn, 2007).

While states are beginning to collect massive amounts of workers' compensation medical treatment data, no state has yet to publish a comprehensive list of performance metrics for doctors that treated injured workers within their systems. California medical data has been extensively analyzed by the California State Fund and California Workers' Compensation Institute with great success. They have developed methods to fairly rate individual providers for outcomes in workers' compensation. But these ratings are not publicly available. The benefit of using state workers' compensation agency data is that: 1) it would amass more observations than any single insurer could, and 2) it could be linked to indemnity data to show the length of time the injury claim was open and the duration of lost time. The latter data would be vital to measuring outcomes of treatment.

Good public data on the performance of providers treating injured workers would be one means of responding to the declining numbers of occupational medicine providers. Presumably, the physicians at the top of the performance rankings would have a flood of business and enhanced income. Raising the income of specialists in occupational medicine is the only way to reverse the exodus from this specialty.

Employing Providers

There are many fine examples of firms that have set up company owned clinics to provide a broad spectrum of medical care services for both occupational and non-occupational conditions. Prominent business users of this model include Toyota, Nissan, Pepsi, QuadGraphics, Perdue, Disney and Pitney Bowes. Hospitals and large clinics have long used this model for their employees. A study by the National Business Group on Health and Watson Wyatt (2008) reports that more than 23 percent of self-insured companies have on-site medical care delivery facilities (LaPenna, 2009).

While company doctors still care a bad reputation in some circles for poor quality, the aforementioned corporations offer full service medical clinics with very high quality standards. In many cases they treat both occupational and non-occupational needs of employees and covered dependents. Naturally, they excel at return to work and in-house therapy.

These in-house clinics are organized in a variety of ways. They may have contractual relationships with local non-employee providers. They may be implemented and managed by professional management firms that specialize in this sort of delivery system.

Two clear advantages of employee clinicians is that they do not have an incentive to generate treatments to boost their income and that other incentives can be freely built into their compensation package. Such delivery system should presumably base compensation on more than a straight salary and include rewords for outcomes.

To date, the published data shows that these in-house clinics have low medical cost inflation and get high marks from employees for quality and access. Presumably these positive results have fostered the growing interest in implementing such delivery stems.

To summarize the situation in workers' compensation, despite some promising activity in workers' compensation payment systems, the number of doctors that are seriously motivated by objective standards of good treatment and financial incentives to reinforce good behavior seems to be a small fraction of those treating injured workers. If on the basis of doctor surveys one could accept that 25-30% of all physicians have some kind of incentive payment in their compensation. We believe that the proportion of doctors treating occupational injuries under an incentive payment system is far less. This is because most state laws weaken the ability of payers to build and effectively use good networks like those more commonly found in health plans.

SUMMARY

This paper tries to show that workers' compensation medical treatment is heavily burdened by high cost and uneven quality of medical care for injured workers. These problems are far worse than those plaguing the general health care delivery system and other insurance types. This is predominantly—though not exclusively-- due to poor incentives for both medical providers and patients. In fairness, though, insurer and employer shortsightedness and zeal to avoid loss payments with careless regard for the injured workers contribute to the problem.

The vast majority of workers' compensation medical treatments are done without any financial incentives to motivate the provision of high quality care in conformance with the best medical evidence on effectiveness. Despite this medical care is generally good, especially for routine traumatic injuries. Inherent professionalism, risk of lawsuit, and the potential from negative feedback from claims adjusters are likely to be the forces motivating any good care to injured workers.

It is clear from the brief review presented here that pay for performance is already an entrenched force in general health plans and other privately delivered medical systems. By one survey, 30 percent of physicians report that incentives for quality care are build into their compensation schemes (Williams, 2007). With the added muscle of Medicare's Physician Quality Reporting Initiative there should be continued growth in the size and sophistication of payment systems to incent quality and good outcomes.

Workers' compensation payment systems must be overhauled to participate in this movement toward incentive based payment. This paper has laid out principles for designing positive financial incentives for workers' compensation medical care. These principles suggest that good incentive structures require enormous effort to build information systems to support the incentive application. They also require state government to support the use of incentives, even if it means banning bad providers from practicing medicine for injured workers and limiting the choice of providers by workers.

Finally, there are several variations of performance contracting now being used in workers' compensation. Unfortunately for payers of workers' compensation medical claims, there is no rigorous evaluation of the success of these different systems. Anecdotal evidence would suggest that weak networks that profess to offer quality care without real effort at screening and communicating with clinicians are not effective in controlling either cost or outcomes. Networks that produce low cost and good outcomes require a heavy investment in screening and selecting quality providers; they also must excel in communicating standards of conduct, the reward structure, and performance feedback to clinicians. Clearly, there is a strong need for more objective, rigorously developed information on which models seem to work best.

Because they are easier to direct and reward for their ongoing performance, staff models offer advantages. Yet, the some burden of selecting and communicating with employed physicians is equivalent to that of a network. The difference being the volume of cases that one can use to evaluate an individual clinician and the ability to impose rules on treatment practice.

Which variation of these models will bubble to the surface as best? The future will probably find workers' compensation, like health plans, following different paths depending on the community that the care is being given and the state laws that limit or promote incentive contracting. Also, the weaknesses of existing types of provider networks will encourage large self insured companies to continue to develop company owned in-house clinics. .

In order to foster the right incentives for treating injured workers with high quality medicine and promoting early return to work, state would need to empower and encourage payers to develop, or rent, networks of providers with desired training and background and with demonstrated performance in delivering good care. Such networks will only be successful if the organizer of the network can:

1. assure network providers of a large stream of business;
2. select only those providers that it wishes to contract with;
3. eliminate providers based on objective failure to perform according to the network manager's criteria;
4. pay providers according to negotiated incentive plans regardless of other fee schedule amounts.

To be fair to injured workers, these networks would have to meet minimum standards for choice of doctor within the network, allow for medically necessary referrals to specialists, place no limits on the extent of care for non medical reasons (to save expenses), and have a complaint procedure for resolving worker dissatisfaction. If done correctly, strong, quality driven provider networks can be a triple win: injured workers reliably get top quality care; payers save on both medical and indemnity costs per claim; and physicians that deliver quality medicine have substantially higher income and better job satisfaction.

REFERENCES

American Accreditation HealthCare Commission/URAC 2000, *Measuring quality in workers' compensation managed care organizations: Technical manual of performance measures*, URAC, Washington, D.C., viewed August 7, 2007 http://www.urac.org/savedfiles/WorkersCompPerformanceMeasures.pdf

Anastakis, DJ, Beaton, DE, Katz, J, Novak, CB 2009, 'Evaluation of pain measurement practices and opinions of peripheral nerve surgeons', *Hand,* vol. 4, no. 4, pp. 1558-9447.

Christianson J, Leatherman S, Sutherland K 2007, *Paying for quality: Understanding and assessing physician pay for performance*, Robert Wood Johnson Foundation, Princeton, NJ, viewed May 2010 at: http://www.rwjf.org/files/research/no13synthesisreport.pdf .

Darves B 2004, *Physician compensation models: The basics, the pros, and the cons*, viewed 14 July 2010 http://www.nejmjobs.org/career-resources/physician-compensation-basics.aspx .

Groopman, J.2010, 'Health care: Who knows best?', *New York Times Review of Books*, vol. 57, no. 2.

Greenfield, W 1998, 'In search of an effective physician compensation formula', *American Academy of Family Physicians Journal,* viewed Apr 2010 http://www.aafp.org/fpm/981000fm/cover.html .

Frolich A, Talavera JA, Broadhead P, Dudley RA 2007, 'A behavioral model of clinician responses to incentives to improve quality', *Health Policy*, vol. 80, no. 1, pp. 179–193.

Gawande A 2009, 'The cost conundrum: What a Texas town can teach us about health care', *New Yorker,* 2009 Jun 1, pp. 1-15.

Generous provider incentives deliver dramatic returns', *Disease Management Advisor*, vol. 12, no. 4, pp. 40–44.

Haddad, GH 1987, 'Analysis of 2932 workers' compensation back injury cases: The impact on the cost to the system', Spine, vol. 12, no. 8, pp. 765-769.

Integrated Healthcare Association 2007, *Integrated healthcare association announces new efficiency measure in pay for performance to improve healthcare quality and reduce cost*, Integrated Healthcare Association (IHA) Press release, Los Angeles, CA, viewed Mar 2010 at: http://www.iha.org/021507.pdf .

Jellinek P, Isaacs S 2008, *The state of independent medical practice. Report for Physicians Foundation for Health Systems Excellence*, viewed April 2010 at: http://www.mag.org/pdfs/jellinek_report_independentpractice_2009.pdf

Kaiser Family Foundation 2007, *Health care spending in the United States and OECD countries*, viewed Apr 2010 http://www.kff.org/insurance/snapshot/chcm010307oth.cfm .

LaDou, J 2002, 'The Rise and Fall of Occupational Medicine in the US', *American Journal of Preventative Medicine*, vol. 22, no. 4, pp. 285-295.

LaPenna M 2009, 'Workplace clinic: Employer redesign of "the company doctor', *Journal of Healthcare Management,* viewed 14 July 2010 http://www.entrepreneur.com/tradejournals/article/197664735.html .

Lipton B, Robertson J, Corro D 2010, *Medicare and workers' compensation cost containment*, viewed March 2010 at: https://www.ncci.com/documents/Medicare-Research-Brief-Jan10.pdf .

Lipton, B, Laws, C, Li, L 2009, *Narcotics in workers' compensation,* NCCI Issues Brief, viewed 14 July 14, 2010 https://www.ncci.com/documents/Narcotics_in_WC_1209.pdf .

Mealy, D 2009, *State of the workers' compensation line*, NCCI Annual Issues Symposium, Boca Raton, FL.

CHAPTER 11

Closing the Nightmare Claim: Practical Approaches for Ending the Most Difficult Workers' Compensation Cases

Richard W. Lenkov

Bryce Downey & Lenkov LLC; E-mail: rlenkov@brycedowney.com

Abstract: This chapter reviews the proverbial "nightmare claim," that is claims that are problematic because they are old, complex, or perhaps involve difficult claimants, judges or attorneys. Thankfully there are ways in which to successfully manage such cases. Various closing strategies, medical strategies and legal strategies will be presented along with some key investigation steps to take from the first notice of a workers' compensation claim. The author concludes with methods in which to manage expenses and settlement tactics as well.

INTRODUCTION

Every workers' compensation professional has them: the nightmare claim. Whether because they are old, deal with complex issues, have difficult claimants, judges or attorneys, these cases seem to linger forever and can literally keep you up at night.

This article will provide real, hands-on, practical techniques on how to turn these cases around, and how to close them quickly and cost-effectively.

WHAT IS "A NIGHTMARE CLAIM"?

Workers' compensation claim costs are skyrocketing nationwide. Despite the fact that statistics show that the Great Recession of 2008-2010 has actually resulted in fewer overall workers' compensation claims filed, the same statistics show that the cost of defending these claims has gone up. A possible explanation for this dichotomy is an adage that has been around a while but still rings true: workers' compensation claims do not get better with age. While fewer claims are being filed, those that are active seem to linger on longer than ever. This seems counter-intuitive, as one would think that the recent economic downturn would result in claimants wanting to resolve their cases quickly to obtain their settlements or awards.

Nightmare claims cost money. Whether due to complex issues, multiple parties, obstinate opponents or expensive experts, they represent a significant reason why workers' compensation costs are exploding across the country. Closing these claims requires tenacity, focus and aggressive techniques.

The following are some factors that can turn a typical workers' compensation claim into a nightmare.

1. Complex Injury

The more serious the injury, the more likely it is to become a nightmare. Complex injuries are ones that require a lot of time and money to defend. On a very basic level, the more involved the injury, the more expensive the claim is going to be because you are going to deal with a significant number of medical providers and bills. Any time a claim has a significant number of medical bills, the potential exists for progression into a nightmare.

2. Multiple Injuries

The more injuries a claimant has, the more likely that the claim will become a nightmare. While single injuries can certainly become difficult to defend, a claimant who is alleging that multiple body parts have been injured as a result of a work-related accident is going to present different, unique problems. This situation has become more pronounced with the willingness of treating physicians to link conditions like complex regional pain syndrome and post-traumatic stress disorder to routine injuries, despite questionable causal relationships.

Chris E. Stout, Matt Kruger and Jeffrey Rogers, (Eds)

The more claims that an injured worker has open, the more difficult that case will be to close. The "repeat offender" will be one of the most difficult claims to end, for the simple reason that this type of claimant tends to file a brand-new claim as soon as the old one has ended. This recidivism is frustrating and expensive, and runs contrary to the goal of closing claims and allowing both the employer and the employee get on with their lives.

3. Multiple Treaters/Experts

The more treaters and experts that are involved in a claim, the more likely it is that the claim is going down the nightmare path. Every time the claimant sees a doctor and every time the employer hires an expert, the costs of the case can only go up.

4. Difficult Opponents/Claimants

One of the foremost reasons why these cases cannot be resolved quickly is that the claimant is belligerent, difficult, obtuse, unresponsive or just plain slow. These claimants put roadblocks between you and your goal of closing the case quickly, efficiently and inexpensively. They drag the case on forever and bog down an already glacial system.

The same can be said about many claimants' attorneys. It seems strange that an attorney who makes his or her money on collecting fees would not respond to your attempts to pay him or her money to close the case. Yet one of the biggest impediments to closing a case quickly is the unwillingness of opposing counsels to simply return a call.

5. Difficult Treating Physicians

Nightmare claims are often complicated by medical professionals who do not seem to understand or care about the costs or implications of having employees off work for extended periods of time. By failing to aggressively encourage a claimant to return to work, they are enabling that claimant to sit home and remain unproductive, rather than return to gainful employment.

6. Difficult Judge/Venue

We all keep our own lists of venues and judges that are difficult to deal with. A case that is a dream in front of one judge in fact can be a nightmare in front of another. The problem is generally that you do not get to choose the venue in which your case will ultimately be heard, and there is therefore often little you can do to ameliorate this factor.

7. Subrogation

While getting workers' compensation money back in a third-party action is one of the best things that could happen to your claim, subrogation does present some unique challenges that can quickly turn into nightmares if not handled properly. Dealing with spoliation of evidence, statute of limitations, comparative fault, strict liability, pleadings and discovery are all issues that the standard workers' compensation claim does not involve. Sometimes a workers' compensation claims handler does not have much or any experience handling these issues, and therefore special care and attention are needed on these claims.

8. MSA

A Medicare set-aside inherently makes the case more complex and difficult to close, because of the additional time and expense required in the process.

CLOSING STRATEGIES

Nightmare claims do not get better with age. They need to be closed as quickly as possible. There are real-world, practical techniques that employers and claims handlers can use right away. While many of them are basic, they are easy to overlook and, if not done effectively and promptly, can turn a straightforward case into a nightmare in short order.

1. Accident Prevention:

First, to state the obvious, the best way to prevent a claim from turning into a nightmare is to prevent the claim from happening in the first place. By employing the following techniques, an employer can reduce the likelihood of a work injury resulting in a claim and that claim possibly becoming a nightmare:

- Create an environment of safety in the workplace: make safety a priority by establishing a dedicated safety manager, requiring early and ongoing safety training and incentivizing safety.
- Examine the workplace to determine factors that are causing injuries and fix them.
- Create wellness programs to foster an environment of healthy and safe living.
- Make sure that all safety rules are clearly worded, well circulated and generally understood.

2. Early and Thorough Investigation:

There is no substitute for knowledge, for finding out as much information on the claim as possible, and doing so early on. The longer cases go on, the more difficult it is to investigate, interview defense witnesses, obtain recorded statements and preserve evidence. If the investigation is not conducted early and thoroughly, a claims professional is missing a golden opportunity to close a nightmare case.

By the time a case goes to trial or is ready to settle, it is often several years after the initial accident. At that late time, it is generally too late to conduct a thorough investigation, as it is likely that much crucial evidence and key witnesses are no longer around. Accordingly, conducting early and thorough investigations will help to stop claims from becoming nightmares.

Some key investigation steps to take from the first notice of a workers' compensation claim:

a. Conduct an on-Site Investigation:

it is important to be on the scene of an injury as early as practical, especially in larger and more significant injuries. While it is impractical to conduct an on-site investigation on every workers' compensation claim, doing so either yourself, through your defense counsel, or through an investigator is crucial on larger cases. There is no substitute for having eyes and ears on the ground quickly after a significant incident.

One of the primary reasons to conduct an on-site inspection is to interview key witnesses as soon as possible. The longer you wait to do so, the more likely it is that these individuals' testimony may turn the entire case around. They may depart your employment, forget key facts or simply be unwilling to cooperate.

While it may be difficult for a claims handler to get out to the scene of an accident within a reasonable period of time, it can be very efficient, and even economical, to retain an investigator or attorney to conduct the inspection on the employer's behalf. Another benefit of retaining counsel to do so is that privilege can apply to the investigation and therefore protect crucial evidence from disclosure.

b. Lock in the Employee's Story:

One of the key reasons to conduct an early and thorough investigation is to lock in the claimant's version of accident. It will not shock any reader to hear that injured workers often give inconsistent histories of accident. Locking the claimant into an accident history early on can literally turn a nightmare case into a defense finding. If a claimant gives one history on the day of the accident, and another one a week later, it is very persuasive to argue to a judge that the claimant's inconsistent histories demonstrates a lack of credibility and therefore should prevent recovery. Claimants often try to negate the harmful effect of their inconsistent histories by arguing that they forgot, or that minor discrepancies in their histories are not critical. However, workers' compensation judges are generally persuaded by the (common sense) argument that the earliest version of accident is the most reliable, as it was communicated at a time and in a manner when the accident was fresh in the claimant's mind. If a subsequent history differs from that initial recollection of accident, the claimant's credibility is questioned.

It is important to not only interview the claimant as soon as possible, but to memorialize the conversation in a recorded statement. If the claimant later gives a different history, a useful technique in turning a nightmare claim around is to use the claimant's very own words to impeach them.

Another reason to interview a claimant as early as possible is that once they retain an attorney, the chances of you ever talking to them again are slim. No competent claimants' attorney is going to allow you free access to interview their client, and even if they do, they will not allow you to obtain any information that may harm their client's case. Once the claimant "lawyers up," you can be sure that all communication will be through the attorney, and the opportunity to obtain any information that can be used to impeach the claimant will be lost.

The nature of the injury may dictate that you get investigative assistance as early as possible. In fatality claims, for example, you might very well need to have your attorney and your investigator on the scene as soon as possible before crucial evidence is rendered inaccessible or unusable. It is very important in such circumstances to have partnerships with experts who are able to assist you in such complex claims on very short notice.

Key to early and thorough investigation as a means to reducing your workers' compensation exposure is teaching your ground-level first responders on the basic tools of investigating workers' compensation accidents. Accumulating evidence, filling out an accident report, taking photographs, dealing with early medical issues and preserving evidence are all crucial early tasks. While it is often very difficult to have ground-level managers buy into the need to conduct early and thorough investigations, it is important that they do so. While we understand that they are not in the business of litigating workers' compensation claims, but rather selling and manufacturing products, they will almost certainly pay attention when they realize the cost to them and their employer when a simple case turns into a nightmare because of the failure to perform these basic, early tasks.

c. Preserving Evidence.

Preserving crucial evidence is yet another reason to perform a thorough and early investigation into potential nightmare claims. Failing to preserve crucial evidence such as accident reports or surveillance films can be devastating to the defense of a workers' compensation claim. An equally damaging result of failing to preserve evidence can be exposure for a spoliation of evidence claim in a third-party lawsuit. As an example, consider an employee who injures himself using a forklift. He files a workers' compensation claim against his employer. While he cannot sue his employer for civil damages under the exclusive remedy theory, the claimant can file a third-party products liability suit against the forklift manufacturer. In defending itself, the forklift manufacturer seeks to have the forklift tested, only to find out that the employer has either replaced it or altered it or kept using it in the two years since the initial accident. The manufacturer argues that without the primary piece of evidence in the same condition as it was when the accident occurred, it is deprived of its ability to defend itself in the products liability action, and as a result, files a spoliation of evidence action against the employer. The basis of the action is that the employer knew or reasonably should have known that the forklift would be a crucial piece of evidence in a third-party action, and as a result, had a duty to preserve that evidence. The manufacturer would argue that the employer should have taken the forklift out of circulation and kept it in a secure place until it would be needed for the third-party action, or at least until the statute of limitations to file that action ran out.

This is a very real scenario, and one that plaintiffs' attorneys across the country are aggressively pursuing and that courts are allowing. In order to avoid the harmful effects of a spoliation of evidence action, it is vital to have someone conduct a timely, careful investigation so that significant evidence can be identified and preserved.

MEDICAL STRATEGIES

As mentioned above, a difficult injury or difficult treating physicians can be fatal to your defense. On the nightmare claim, employ some tried and true medical strategies in order to turn the case around:

1. Communication:

Good and thorough communication is vital to your medical defense. Obviously, if you don't have enough information, it will be difficult for you to monitor the claimant's treatment and be pro-active, rather than reactive, in bringing medical treatment to an end. Accordingly, your ability to obtain updated medical records and information from the employee's treating physicians is key. Therefore, establishing good relationships with treating physicians and knowing how to get them to respond to you is crucial.

Unfortunately, in many states, an employer's ability to communicate with an employee's treating physicians is limited by law. In those situations, it is vital to obtain an authorization at the beginning of the case that allows the employer to communicate with the treating physician. Hiring a nurse case manager to assist in the communication and information-gathering is also helpful.

2. Company Clinics:

If an employer directs injured employees to company clinics, it is important first and foremost that these clinics concentrate on getting the injured employee to maximum medical improvement and back to work. You want to use clinics that are objective, and if an injured employee needs more treatment, they obviously need to say that. At the same time, however, it is helpful if the clinic is familiar with your workplace, making it easier for them to recommend that the employee return to work.

3. Prior Medical History:

On the nightmare claim, it is important that you have as much information as possible in order to defend the employee's claim. Towards that end, you must obtain as much medical information about the claimant as possible. This is especially true the more complex the case is, as the likelihood that the claimant had a prior medical history that is relevant is extremely high. Moreover, the injured employee may very well deny a prior medical history, at which point a thorough knowledge of their prior medical history is crucial. The bottom line is that in a nightmare claim, information is power, and the more information you have about the claimant's prior medical history, the better.

With this in mind, be aware that in many states there is no formal discovery in workers' compensation. Accordingly, your ability to obtain information from prior medical providers rests on your opponent's veracity in telling you about prior treaters. In order to obtain as much information as possible about the claimant and their history, it is always a good idea to canvass the employee's zip code to determine where they might have been treated beyond the providers that you are aware of. This is a relatively inexpensive endeavor, but one that will potentially yield huge dividends.

4. Direct Medical Care:

The longer medical care goes on, the more expensive it is going to be and the more likely you are to be sitting on top of a nightmare claim. Direct the care and treatment of the injured employee whenever possible. One way of doing so is to take an active role in where the treatment takes place, how much treatment takes place and how much you will pay for it. While some states judiciously govern the degree to which the employer can direct medical care, there is always some room for the employer to become involved. Keeping a close eye on the medical treatment sends a message to the injured employee that this is not going to be a typical claim that spirals out of control, but rather one that is going to be closely watched.

5. Terminating Medical Benefits:

Don't be afraid to terminate medical benefits where appropriate. Typical of a nightmare claim is an injured worker who sees the claim as an opportunity to treat forever and with whomever he chooses. It is imperative that you change this mindset early on. If the employee is going beyond the recommended treatment, is not complying with treatment, or is purposely retarding your efforts to have him reach maximum medical improvement, discontinuing ongoing or medical benefits is generally allowed. Of course, you ought to go through the proper channels before terminating benefits, but doing so can be extremely effective in the right circumstances.

6. Hire the Right Expert at the Right Time:

The proper use of independent medical examinations can be a chapter in and of itself. Suffice it to say that a good opinion from a notable independent expert examiner will help turn your nightmare case around. However, you must make sure that you retain the right medical expert and that you hire them at the right time.

How do you know who the right expert is and when to hire them? Here are some thoughts:

a. Hire an IME physician who is at least as qualified, but preferably more qualified, than your opponent's doctors. If the claimant is relying on an internist to opine on his back condition, make sure that you have an orthopedic surgeon or neurosurgeon supporting your perspective.

b. Hire an expert who specializes in the specific injury involved. There is no better way to lose credibility with a judge than hiring an expert who has no expertise in the specific body part involved. The more specific the injury, the more important it is to have a specialist in that area examine the claimant.

c. Make sure that the doctor actually practices medicine. Be certain that your expert devotes the greatest percentage of his practice to actually treating patients, as opposed to litigating. A doctor who spends an inordinate amount of their practice serving as an expert will have little credibility.

d. Make sure that your doctor has seen the claimant recently. A simple way to win the treater vs. hired expert conflict is to argue that your IME physician saw the claimant more recently, and accordingly, is in the best position to opine on issues like current condition and need for future treatment. More often than not, by the time you get to trial, the treating physician will not have seen the injured employee for months or even longer. Accordingly, the argument that the IME physician's opinions should be followed because they are closest in time is a strong one.

e. Make sure your expert is "independent." The "I" in independent medical examination stands for independent. You need to be sure that your expert truly is objective, and is not seen merely as a puppet. Cultivate a wide range of experts, and don't use the same ones too often.

f. Consider a records review. As discussed throughout the course of this article, nightmare claims are characterized by large expenses. IMEs are no different and can indeed be expensive. It may be more efficient to obtain a records review rather than an IME, which will cost less. Moreover, a records review will often get you a chance to "preview" your expert's opinion without committing to a full-blown IME. Generally, you have to live with the IME report, no matter how harmful, as your opponent will find out about it. With a records review, however, if you don't get the opinion that you are seeking, you can move on to another doctor without being accused of doctor shopping.

LEGAL STRATEGIES

The chances of a claim becoming a nightmare are greater once either the employee or the employer hires counsel. Accordingly, one of the best ways to avoid a nightmare is to keep the case out of the hands of counsel. That said, however, there are strategies to close the case once attorneys do get involved.

A significant impairment to closing a nightmare case is the fact that the claimant has likely been receiving benefits for a long time, and has become comfortable being off work. Accordingly, their attorney has little motivation to move the case forward, and so the case languishes. One way to change that is to make sure that the case is moving forward in the court system. Given the literally thousands of cases that are in the docket in any given state's workers' compensation system, there are significant obstacles to moving the case forward. Without the court's involvement, these cases often sit around for years. In Illinois, for example, there are still cases with 1981 file dates. These old cases need to be closed.

If the courts are not assisting, it is the responsibility of the claims handler and defense attorney to get their attention. One way to do so is to file motions for trial dates. Often claimants' attorneys will simply not respond to your phone calls or letters, and therefore literally bringing them into court is the only tool that you have to pursue the case. Even if the case is not really ready for trial, getting your opponent to meet you face to face at court will help move a dormant case along.

Another tool is a motion to dismiss. If you are not getting a response from your opponent, and a case appears to be ready to resolve, ask the court to dismiss the case for want of prosecution. While not every jurisdiction allows this motion in workers' compensation claims, doing so will at the very least alert the judge to your opponent's recalcitrance and potentially enlist his support in pushing the case forward.

Another successful litigation technique is a pre-trial. A pre-trial is simply an informal hearing before your judge in which both parties present very condensed versions of their case or issues in dispute, and the judge offers his or her opinions. Pre-trials can be accomplished in as little as five minutes, but very often they result in settlement. Sometimes the issues that prevent a nightmare case from closing are those where another set of eyes, particularly by the trier of fact, affords clarity. Other times, one of the parties simply wants to "have their day in court" and have an impartial hearing officer listen to them. A pre-trial provides an efficient and economical way to do so.

Where allowable, discovery is a very effective means to move a case forward. Serving interrogatories and requests for production as early in the litigation process as possible assures that your opponent understands that this is not going to be a typical case that drags on forever. Claimants typically take much longer to answer discovery than the time limits imposed by the court, so even with the most compliant claimants, it is going to take a while to finish discovery. Accordingly, starting the process as early on as possible will diminish delay.

Using discovery to limit the number of issues in dispute is also a good way to keep the case moving forward. It is worth discussing with your opponent the issues that are in dispute as early as possible, in order to focus your time and expense on the things that you truly disagree about. A formal means to do so is through a request to admit, a discovery device for asking your opponent to admit to the veracity of certain issues in dispute. If they do so, those issues are no longer in dispute, and therefore, the discovery process will go much quicker.

SETTLEMENT STRATEGIES

While it is certainly acceptable, and often advisable, to draw a line in the sand and take a case to trial, most workers' compensation claims settle. The trick, especially with nightmare claims, is to settle as quickly and as inexpensively as possible. Closing a nightmare claim hinges on a basic principle: if the players do not communicate, they do not settle. It is important to open a line of communication, one that includes your express desire to settle, with opposing counsel at the beginning of the case. It is equally vital to maintain open communication with your opponent throughout the course of the case. While often there is little choice but to have adversarial and sometimes hostile relations with your opponent, it is best to try to avoid this unfortunate situation. Simply put, angry lawyers and claimants are more litigious and stubborn. To the extent that you are able to foster good relations with your opponent, you improve the chances that the case will not turn into a nightmare. Of course, good relationships are not always in the cards. In some cases, you may realize from day one of the claim that you will not be able to avoid locking horns with your opponent on every issue. Those toxic relationships happen, but the better approach is to make every effort early on to create and maintain a good relationship with opposing counsel to avoid expensive and time-consuming discovery and motions.

One aspect of a claim that often holds up settlement is waiting for a demand from your opponent. Conventional wisdom holds that the case can only be settled when the claimant's attorney makes a demand and the employer responds. That is simply not true. If you want to settle a case, there is no reason to wait for a demand. While it is often preferable to let the claimant make that first step in order to set the ceiling in negotiations, if you always wait for opponent to make the first move, you may be waiting forever and the case will never close. Don't be afraid to make a pro-active offer to get the ball rolling. Claimant's counsel is duty-bound to report any offers to their client. Moreover, don't be afraid to make the first offer on the low side of the range of value. Claimants' attorneys are certainly not shy when making outrageous first demands, so there is no reason not to start low.

Another very effective tool to resolve "old dog" cases and many of them at the time is to hold a settlement day. This is a process whereby you invite many claimants and their attorneys to a single site with the goal of settling their case that day. Crucial to this process is having a decision-maker from the employer present, with the authority and willingness to pay some money to resolve the case. Getting the parties face to face with the ability to discuss issues and resolve them immediately can work wonders in closing nightmare cases.

Structured settlements are often employed to close difficult claims. Putting together an alternative means of paying out benefits offers a creative way to resolve the case.

MANAGING EXPENSES

As stated throughout the course of this article, nightmare claims are distinguished by spiraling costs. In order to close these cases, you must get a handle on all expenses and work constantly to minimize them.

One significant driver of costs in complex cases is attorney fees. In order to control them, require that your attorneys present budgets from day one, and that they update the budgets as the case develops. Your attorney should not only report back on significant developments, but explain how those developments impact litigation expenses. Don't be afraid to question your attorney's projected budget, and ask for revisions if you feel it is unworkable. It is important to set reserves accurately, and in order to do so, you must have accurate budgets from your attorney. No claims handlers want to go to their boss on the eve of trial or settlement and tell them they are under-reserved and under-budgeted.

Also apply these same requirements to other vendors: require an early and accurate budget, and that vendors update it throughout the case. Do not hire any expert without having a written budget in advance. Experts and other vendors should understand and agree that they will take no action without your advance written consent. Providing vendors unlimited freedom will result in skyrocketing costs.

CONCLUSION

Nightmare claims will always exist. By employing some of these tactics, you can turn these claims around and end your nightmare.

CHAPTER 12

Practical Application of Outcomes-Based Networks

Gregory Moore

Harbor Health Systems, LLC

Abstract: The California MPN provides an excellent legislative model for managing a health-care medical network in workers' compensation. This managed care model provides payers with the control to create and certify a medical network from which all injured employees must select physicians and medical services. This containment of patient traffic ensures higher rates of compliance in the use of approved providers than typical healthcare and workers' compensation models.

MPNs that select providers based primarily on fee discounts may generate higher total claim costs if they provide poor quality care that results in more numerous treatments and delays returns to work. Harbor Health Systems, LLC has been engaged in a nine-year effort to develop the tools, systems, and data needed to identify providers that truly reduce total claim costs by providing superior medical care which reduces the number of treatments required for recovery and enables employees to return to work more quickly. Many practical lessons have been learned about identifying, building and managing outcomes-based network of quality providers through a pilot implementation that has produced significant positive results.

INTRODUCTION

Harbor Health Systems, LLC (Harbor Health) was founded in 2001 with the goal of making quality a practical and effective tool for managing a healthcare delivery system. The strategic vision was to use historical claims and billing data to select physicians for an outcome based medical network solution. We believed that creating a network centered on the providers who scored well would save money through a reduction in complications, improvement in care decisions, and higher quality patient management.

For the past nine years, Harbor Health has worked to develop analytical tools and methods for identifying the best providers, as well as web based network management tools to assist payers and employers with building and managing networks that focused on these providers. Over these years we have identified hurdles and opportunities that have resulted in a proven solution for managing an outcomes-based medical network.

CURRENT LIMITATIONS IN MEDICAL NETWORKS

One of the more popular network models for cost containment is the use of Preferred Provider Organizations (PPOs). The PPO model is a network of physicians, medical providers, medical services, and medical facilities contracted to provide care at discounted rates. The payer controls its costs by keeping as much traffic as possible with discounted providers. The effect of the PPO is measured by penetration rates (how many providers accessed by patients were under contract) and savings (how much did the contract reduce the cost of a bill). These measures can be misleading, and result in what we refer to as a

PPO Paradox

The PPO Paradox is twofold: performance of the network improves with increases in expenditure and by contracting as many providers as possible.

To illustrate the first component, consider the following example:

Two patients go to two different physicians with the same injury. MD 1 is under contract to provide care at a 10% discount; MD 2 gets reimbursed at full price. Let's set the cost per visit at $100, for which MD 1 gets paid $90 based on their contract discount and MD 2 gets paid $100. As a result of complications, the patient at MD 1 had to have 8 visits; MD2 was able to resolve the case without complications in 5 visits.

Chris E. Stout, Matt Kruger and Jeffrey Rogers, (Eds)

Under the PPO measures, MD 1 resulted in a savings of $80, and MD 2 resulted in a savings of $0. The problem is that MD 1 cost $220 more in medical charges to treat the same injury as MD 2.

The second aspect of the PPO Paradox is the incentive to contract with as many providers as possible. It is unreasonable to assume that medical care is consistent regardless of the treating physician, as there will always be variance between human providers. It is simply a mathematical fact that 50% of MDs are better than the other half. With that fact established, it becomes intuitive that a network that includes all providers is only half as good as a network that includes only the top 50%. A network built based on volume will inevitably dilute any quality effect of including better performing providers.

Typically, when payers of care shop for a network, they send their bills over the past year to the vendors and have the networks identify how many are 'in-network'. It seems like a simple math problem – if you received a 10% discount on 50% of the bills under your current PPO agreement, and a new network would have provided 10% discount on 60% of the bills, the new network will save you money. But in fact the total cost of claims may be higher if the system has characteristics that drive greater frequency of visits and/or inferior medical outcomes. Insurance companies are not getting a better product simply because company 2 has more contracts than company 1. In the end, the patient does not automatically have access to better care and the care delivered is not superior just because one company has more contracts than the other.

At Harbor Health, we measure a factor called an Outcomes Quotient (OQ) ™ that scores a network based on the total composition of provider outcomes scores, with each provider's outcomes score weighted based the use of the specialty for the health market serviced (meaning in workers' compensation the primary care providers and orthopedic surgeons affect OC more than most other providers.) A higher OQ means that the average experience of patients accessing the network should be better with respect to outcomes than a network with a lower OQ. As a PPO expands its contracting to include more providers, it is inevitable that the network's OQ will go down over time.

The PPO is effective at reducing the unit price for care, but as a stand-alone solution the model inevitably fails to deliver better care as a result of the PPO Paradox. Harbor Health does not compete with the PPO model and in some cases has successfully partnered with PPOs to create a combined solution that leverages the strength of the contracting and provider management aspects of the PPO. The key to these solutions is managing a clear quality program for managing the inclusion of providers in the final network.

DEFINING A QUALITY GOAL

It is hard to find fault with the statement that quality is a good prescription for all stakeholders in healthcare. Quality medicine is not a new concept, and most forward-thinking healthcare companies incorporate aspects of quality into the design of their model. The problem isn't whether quality matters, but understanding how it matters. If you ask stakeholders throughout the workers' compensation or healthcare system to define quality, you should expect widely varied responses. Defining a 'Quality Goal' is a process of determining the measure(s) that will drive all aspects of selection and management of providers in a quality network.

Different Quality Goals will render different results. For example, if quality is defined by the extent to which providers follow clinical pathways, you can build a simple model that measures historical compliance with UR pathways and predicts the likelihood of a provider following evidence-based medicine. It is a reasonable assumption that claims will go well when the physician is making reasonable decisions on the level and direction of treatment. But, is that the whole picture? What about the patient's trust of the provider? Patients that don't trust that their physician are more likely to bounce between physicians for the same services, are less likely to comply with follow-up, and are less likely to believe they are healed when the physician says they are ready to go back to work. Is a better doctor the one who treats the most consistently with guidelines or the one who gains the confidence of the patient? Chances are it is both, but if the Quality Goal of a program is too narrow it will fail to identify providers based on material factors.

The quality goal for Harbor Health is to identify providers who heal the patient effectively, treat the patient with respect, work well with the claims team to manage the case, and do not financially abuse the system. With a quality goal defined, Harbor Health designed its first measurements as a four-point scorecard as follows:

- Outcomes measures that look at the claim as a whole by measuring factors like duration, disability (TTD, TPD, and PD), and costs (medical and indemnity).
- Abuse measures that look at the results of bill review edits (rejection / reduction reasons) to identify patterns that demonstrate a repeated process for improperly maximizing reimbursement.
- Claims satisfaction that measures the provider's compliance with report writing, ease for scheduling and follow-up, and the perception of whether the provider is working for the best outcome for the patient.
- Patient satisfaction that surveys patients in areas like the office environment, staff professionalism, and the confidence in the physician's diagnosis and treatment.

THE CHAINSAW VERSUS THE SCALPEL

Real world factors lead to errors that are mathematically unavoidable. A successful program must address these factors and design solutions accordingly. When considering the challenges of designing a healthcare scorecard, consider the standard deviation of the population's health. If you measure a large population's use of the healthcare system, the average patient is about as easy to define as the average person. How much of the population is the average weight? How much of the population engages in the average amount of exercise? Any effort to measure outcomes has to be sensitive to the fact that few people are actually average, few injuries happen in the average way, and people's perceptions of their injury are rarely average. People have a large standard of deviation, and as a result so do the measures of the population's health.

In workers' compensation there are only two inclusion criteria – was the patient employed and was the cause of the injury or illness work related? Whether patients are obese, diabetic, or otherwise healthy, they are all going to be treated in the same system. As a result co-morbidities will inherently influence the accuracy of the scoring and the ability to predict a provider's performance based on historical data. Unfortunately, workers' compensation insurance companies do not typically have access to information on degenerative diseases or psychological disorders. A perfect model would adjust for co-morbidities, confounding variables, and risk weighting. Imperfect data means that there will always be a margin of error in the results.

The analogy of the chainsaw versus the scalpel describes the type of decision that a network developer would need to consider regarding the sophistication of the inclusion or exclusion criteria. A chainsaw is capable of cutting a large quantity far more effectively than a scalpel, but with a significantly different level of accuracy. The tolerance for accuracy depends heavily on the size of the task and the impact of inaccuracy on the outcome.

A network that covers a sizable population and geography will involve thousands of physicians and medical professionals. In most markets, there are enough providers available that cutting deeper than necessary is the best approach to ensuring that the final product contains only trusted providers. As an example, the acceptable providers may be the top 50%. If the calculated error is $\pm$ 12%, then setting the inclusion level at 38% will mean that anyone that falls on the lower end of the error will at least be in the top 50%.

This also means that a provider who is in the top 27% may have been excluded as a result of the accuracy of the data.

In this example, we can achieve a high rate of confidence that the providers selected for a particular network are from the top 50% in spite of a large margin of error in the tool used to select providers. Because the tool is more similar to a chainsaw than a scalpel, both above average and below average providers were cut from the final network. As long as we have significantly more providers available than the minimum number necessary to serve the intended population, we can be successful with the chainsaw approach.

Depending upon how the available providers were stratified, there will most likely be situations in which too few providers remain after the initial cutting to meet the needs of the covered population. In these circumstances it is necessary either to have a measurement tool that is more like a scalpel to identify providers, to develop alternative access plans, or to accept that in some areas and specialties limited available will result in less confidence in the selected providers.

SETTING THE TOLERANCE FOR ALPHA VERSUS BETA ERRORS

Because any practical measure for selecting providers will have a margin of error, there will always be false negative readings and false positive readings (alpha and beta errors).

The California MPN allows the payer to define a list of approved providers that all injured workers must use for care unless they have previously designated a personal physician. The managed care control for this model is 'containment', not direction of care. Because this list is defined by the payer, the state reduces the ability of the payer to challenge the care provided in-network. For this type of model, inclusion should be set to exclude false positives as it is far more damaging to include a poor performing physician than to exclude a high performing physician.

In Harbor Health's data there are over 50,000 physicians that have seen at least one workers' compensation case in California in the last two years. A California MPN is capable of covering most employed populations in the state with less than 10,000 physicians when all likely specialties are included. This means that even the largest network can provide sufficient access to care with only 20% of the available providers.

Over time, outcomes-based models that continue to evaluate performance prospectively become more accurate. As patient traffic becomes more focused on fewer providers, the network management can become more selective. Higher case volume (N) will mean smaller errors that will result in more accurate decisions on inclusion or exclusion.

PROVIDER PARTNERSHIP

After almost a decade focused on finding the best physicians to include in medical networks, there are some trends that stand out with almost every provider that scores well in Harbor Health metrics:

- For these providers, quality is not a result of external pressure, but rather a personal pursuit. Consistently, I hear the best providers describe their efforts to be the best regardless of whether anyone was paying attention or giving accolades.
- For these providers, quality is a way of living. Almost every provider I speak with that scores well in our metrics describes things they think of every day in order to improve their practice. It is interesting to note that across four or five different metrics, providers that score well in one metric tend to score well in most metrics. It seems clear from practical experience that the best providers are good in many different areas because they work to improve in all aspects of their practice.

The core concept behind the outcomes-based network is provider performance. To be successful this must extend beyond the selection process into a partnership with the providers. Aspects of this partnership include fair processes for inclusion or exclusion, education, and collaboration.

As explained in the analogy of the chainsaw versus the scalpel, measures will not be perfect for several reasons. If a network is to be fair in its partnership with physicians, there needs to be recourse if a physician feels they are excluded as a result of errors inherent in the system. A well rounded program should include due process for providers to appeal a decision on whether to include them in a network. The end goal of the solution, after all, is to work with the best providers available. While the initial decisions on inclusion of providers may be made with a chainsaw, the network should always be refined with the scalpel. On a case by case basis, exclusion reviews that take into consideration information provided by the physician will be more accurate.

A second aspect of partnership is continuous improvement through collaboration, including the sharing of information on results. Good is a relative term in outcomes, because it is defined as good within a cohort of providers. Average scoring providers today who are committed to quality will become leaders in the future, while physicians who stop working to improve will fall behind their peers over time.

Many physicians are limited in the scope of information they have on the total claim. A patient can leave a physician's office in good shape, but costs for the claim may be inflated by an ineffective report or by the patient restarting their case with a new physician. Getting the complete picture back to the physician will allow the provider to focus their quality practices in the areas that are impacting the patient's total experience and the outcome of the total claim. When providers are given sufficient data and measured over time, the outcomes-based network will refine participation to the providers who will be the best tomorrow. Providing evidence feedback will assist in improving the Outcomes Quotient of a network by ensuring that providers have the tools they need to improve their personal results.

Operationally, it is also important to have processes that assist underperforming physicians and medical groups that are making responsible efforts to improve. When a provider's performance falls below an acceptable relative measure, there has to be a process of intervention. Harbor Health's approach to managing a network over time weights the physician's or medical group's responsiveness to issues. A provider who rated three stars yesterday, but four today is more valuable to the overall network than a provider who fell from five to four. Accordingly, it is imperative that an outcomes-based network have a mechanism to reach out to providers whose performance is lagging and provide the opportunity to improve performance.

While the accuracy of Outcomes Scores is limited by even the best sources of data, an organized physician partnership program greatly improves the likelihood that the outcomes-based network will perform better not only the payer, but also for the injured worker and the physician.

CASE EXAMPLE

In 2008, Harbor Health and Sedgwick Claims Management Services (Sedgwick CMS) began an intensive partnership to implement an outcomes-based network solution that leverages the strengths of both organizations. After significant investments in new analytics, data cleansing, and operational optimizations, the advanced solution, the Sedgwick CMS / Harbor EPO MPN, went live on a pilot basis in April of 2009. In the first year, this model provided medical care for roughly 3,500 injured workers in California from three *Fortune* 500 companies. Outcomes of these cases were compared to the outcomes of the same employers' claims from the prior year, when all of the employers had also used more traditional MPN managed care programs. The results were as follows (see Table **1**):

Table 1: Effects of outcomes-based medical networks on high level claims outcomes.

Measure	% Change
Total cost (Med, Indemnity, and Expense) per claim	- 17.5%
TTD per claim	- 29.2%
PTD per claim	- 15.2%

Source: *Sedgwick CMS / Harbor EPO MPN, 2009 Data*

The number of employees and claims only showed slight variation year to year, and in both years the employers had consistently aggressive return to work and employee management programs in place. Overall industry data and results from Sedgwick CMS clients that did not participate in the pilot program suggest that average costs in these areas increased in California during that same time period.

It is still too early to measure the full impact of the outcomes-based MPN, but these initial results are encouraging and suggest that the investment in the new network model provides significant ROI opportunity. We look forward to evaluating the program's performance compared to two-year industry results when that data becomes available.

Sedgwick CMS Managed Care Practice Lead Kimberly George provided the following input on the outcomes-based model and its impact on their client's workers' compensation programs:

"The first-year results of our California pilot implementation of the Sedgwick CMS/Harbor EPO MPN provide strong evidence that this common sense healthcare delivery model is having a positive impact. We are seeing that in both the quality and timeliness of care received by injured workers, and in reductions in the total cost of workers' compensation claims, including combined medical and wage replacement expenses, for participating employers. We are actively developing similar options for our clients in other jurisdictions, subject to state laws and the availability of compatible medical infrastructures."

CONCLUSION

Outcomes Based Networks are still at an early stage of development as a potential solution to healthcare as a whole. An effective implementation requires significant data feedback and aggressive management, as is the case with the Sedgwick CMS / Harbor Net program. The investment into the program by the companies was justified by retrospective analysis that projected and 8.5:5 ratio reductions in claims outcomes such as duration and cost. The results of the first year are consistent with these projections, giving us a high level of confidence in both the retrospective and prospective models. It will take at least another year and the addition of a broader spectrum of employers to truly prove the model, but the preliminary results have been consistent.

The measures utilized to select providers were based on performance measures, not lowest cost. Additionally, the network discounts for the case study were replaced with full fee schedule contracts for the highest scoring providers. This suggests the cost savings measured in the first 12-months shows a correlation between claims savings and quality.

CHAPTER 13

The Ethics of Clinical Guidelines and Other Tales of Evidence-Based Practice: Points and Counter-Points*

Joseph Paduda

Health Strategy Associates, LLC.; E-mail: jpaduda@healthstrategyassoc.com

Abstract: Chris Stout's earlier chapter herein addresses issues of evidence based-practice and evidence-based medicine as applied to workers' compensation situations, and additionally offers a model of a practice's work-in progress in the active application of such approaches. This chapter will delve into related issues, in particular, the relatively new (to workers comp) area of comparative effectiveness, and the somewhat less sophisticated but much more common process of clinical guideline development.

THE ETHICS OF CLINICAL GUIDELINES - THE PAYER'S ETHICAL DILEMMA

Comparative effectiveness involves examining the outcomes of two different treatment options and determining which is more successful in addressing the underlying condition. There is precious little real comparative effectiveness research conducted in this country; most research merely looks at whether or not a treatment, drug, therapy, or procedure has any impact at all on the designated condition. As a result, many medications are approved for sale that demonstrate little improvement in outcomes over already-established drugs.

In contrast, most clinical guidelines merely assess the ability of one treatment methodology to affect the underlying condition. Whether considering comparative effectiveness or clinical guideline development, the point of these studies is as obvious as it is important. Healthcare providers and patients should make their treatment selections based on two fundamental issues—what is the best way to cure (or if incurable and chronic, control) the problem, and what is the impact of the selected treatment on the patient's quality of life. It is not until more recent times that this latter point has come into consideration. Some of this newer focus is the result of studies indicating that 80% of a person's healthcare spending is during his or her last 24 months of life – often while vegetative, in pain, or with little hope of survival, much less improvement (Appleby, 2006).

In workers' comp, a 35 year old man with a lumbar injury wants not only to be pain free, but also to be able to go back to the job that he left and not be forced into one of lesser "quality" (i.e., perceived status/prestige, pay rate, etc.). Unlike in group health, Medicare and Medicaid, the 'right' outcome in workers comp is to fix the injury AND get the person back to the SAME level of functionality (i.e., job/work).

I'm fascinated by this issue as it strikes at the heart of the problems with, and perhaps solutions for, the health insurance crisis. If we are to solve the access and cost problem, payers, providers, and patients must be comfortable with the decision process and methodology. Today, there's precious little 'comfort' with the current 'system'. And that's understandable.

THERE'S A LOT OF 'ART' IN MEDICINE

Physicians diagnose conditions and recommend specific treatments based on what they think will help, often without much in the way of peer-reviewed research supporting their views. Much is based on their own training and experience and the knowledge passed on to them by their medical school professors and colleagues, provided in specialty society and other medical journals, passed on by medical device and pharmaceutical firms, and learned at conferences and symposia.

Most of the time this knowledge delivers the "right" outcome; the patient gets better. But in many instances there are at least a couple different treatment options for the patient's condition. Physicians recommend what they think will work based on the patient's unique characteristics (physical, emotional,, medical history), and these

Chris E. Stout, Matt Kruger and Jeffrey Rogers, (Eds)

'recommendations' may be several. For example, chronic lower back pain treatment options may include rest, surgery, physical therapy, medications, chiropractic, some of the above, all of the above, and variations of each of the above.

Sticking with the back pain issue, think of this from the payer's perspective. The wide variation in back surgery rates is well-documented, with Medicare data indicating a 500% variation between Ft Myers and Miami Florida. We don't know why there's such a wide difference, but it is safe to assume that the rate is too high in Ft Myers, too low in Miami, or perhaps both.

When a physician in Ft Myers recommends surgery for a patient with a back condition, it is understandable why payers would have concern over the appropriateness of the procedure. To address this concern, payers may utilize clinical treatment guidelines in an effort to determine if the recommendation is "appropriate." In some cases, the guidelines provide clear and convincing support for or against the procedure, but in many others the finding is not so clear cut. The patient may have some but not all of the clinical findings that are 'necessary' to support surgery; there may be other medical conditions present that complicate treatment determination; the patient may want one type of treatment for their own reasons, and/or the jurisdiction's laws and regulations may not support the use of clinical guideline in the medical management process.

The result is the payer - and the physician - are functioning in a somewhat grey area. There are obvious financial factors in play as well. The physician gets paid to do the procedure, the pharma company gets paid if the patient takes their meds, the device company gains revenue for each device sold, the payer saves money if expensive procedures aren't performed, the patient may want drugs for inappropriate reasons.

The ethical issues are apparent. While we would hope that decisions would be based solely on the evidence, there often isn't enough of the right type of evidence to arrive at a clear cut decision. When that occurs, what other factors affect the decision? How are disagreements resolved, and what is that resolution? When there's strong disagreement, what factors, evidence, criteria are 'used' to support the parties' different positions?

CLINICIANS' PERSPECTIVES

Critical to understanding the use of clinical guidelines is in understanding their limitations. Payors' medical directors typically use clinical guidelines as just that, "guidelines," not as rigid and absolute truths. The claimant's history and other factors must be considered, by the payor and treating physician, and the guidelines used as a basis for discussion of the optimal treatment plan for that specific individual. Guidelines do tend to rule out medical treatment labeled as "experimental and investigational"; while experimental treatment may be efficacious for that specific patient, there is a paucity of scientific information the provider and payor can examined to make that determination. In fact, experimental treatment, as well as some types of treatment long ouyt of the experimental stage, may be detrimental for that specific claimant. Many of the ethical issues that you reference are bridged by peer to peer discussion during informal reconsiderations. The Utilization Review process wherein clinical guidelines are employed should be interpreted less as a primary medical cost savings program and more as a vehicle to ensure that the patient receives best-in-class care. It is this optimal quality of care that helps promote rapid recovery and return to work.

According to the Institute of Medicine, there is clinical evidence to support roughly half of what we do in medicine. This does not mean that the other half is wrong; much of what we think works really does, but the studies to prove it have not been done. Evidence based guidelines only speak to the 50% that has been studied, and so can be very misleading.

Worse, the guidelines do not help us address the errors of omission, the most common problem in medicine by far, the high value things that should have been done, but aren't. For example, a brief discussion about smoking cessation is a well recognized high value intervention, but is not reimbursed and in our time pressured practices is ignored by many.

The bottom line: we need to look at the aggregated outcomes of each physician's care in terms of value. Good outcomes require many inputs, the majority of which cannot yet be measured by guidelines, especially for complex problems like back pain. Yet there are wide differences in outcomes that individual doctors and individual clinics get. Those who get patients back to full work quickly and cheaply ON AVERAGE should be rewarded with additional business, immunity from most insurer "oversight" and ideally a share of the savings.

While guidelines are a worthwhile place to start the quality process, medicine should adopt the statistical process control methods that have made manufactured goods so much more reliable; look at the outcomes in aggregate, and learn from the outliers, both the good and the bad. Do "run charting" and don't waste oversight resources looking at random variations, rather at care that is statistically above or below the norm. Insurers need to collaborate with employers to look at both the short and long term disability as well as the costs of care to define the outcome measures to reflect the entire value proposition.

A GUIDELINE DEVELOPER'S PERSPECTIVE

There is an apparent and long-standing conflict between the "art" and "science" of practicing. Presumably, if enough quality information were available (and in a usable format), the "art" could be displaced in favor of the "science." Making guidelines practical, while aligning with the incentives and cultural influences that drive physician behavior, is obviously an immense challenge.

Perhaps the biggest challenge facing developers is the expense, ethical issues, and time-consuming nature of the ideal research tool – randomized controlled trials, or RCTs. The randomized controlled trial is considered to provide the most reliable evidence because the processes used during the RCT minimize the risks of confounding variables and bias influencing the results. Moreover, and RCT uses a control group, a group of subjects who do not receive 'no treatment', a "usual" or "standard" treatment, or a placebo and serves as the basis of comparison.

Although RCTs occupy the top of the medical research hierarchy, they are not infallible but rather should be considered as better than the alternatives. While many valid approaches to research exist, they are uasually ranked below the RCTR. 'Hierarchies' have been developed and promulgated to address other aspects of research that may effect validity.

There are even differences within RCTs, with multi-center RCTs considered to provide the best evidence for the effectiveness of an intervention because the the research is based on a range of different populations, settings and circumstances. A well-conducted single-center RCT also produces results that are at a slightly higher risk of error or bias, and are considered valid evidence on the effectiveness of an intervention.

Next on the ladder are findings from a meta-analysis, a systematic review of pooled RTCs generated in a similar manner, and thus can be considered rigorous enough for most purposes.

An observational study, one in which the investigator(s) merely observe and don't seek to intervene. Observational studies include case series, case-control or cohort studies are considered inferior to RCTs sapecifically due to concerns that they are at greater risk of error than RCTs. Obaervational studies are more subject to selection bias which can distort the treatment effects, making those effects appear smaller or larger than they really are.

Ideally, guideline organizations will utilize the 'most senior' research methodology and explicitly describe the risks and potential biases of the research used in their guideline development process. This rigorous approach will ensure all parties are well-aware of any potential biases or concerns, reducing the opportunity for inappropriate usage while ensuring stakeholders can compare 'competing' guidelines on the basis of their underlying research.

Implementing guidelines on a day to day basis requires careful consideration of the purpose, potential background of users, and possible risks and downsides of guidelines.

Ideally, medical management efforts will incorporate appeals processes and staff to quickly resolve disagreements between payers and providers. IN addition, treating providers should be provided with documentation of the clinical guidelines used in adverse determinations, along with any back-up materials relevant to the specific case. Importantly, too, on the out-put end, is the collection of outcomes for ongoing development of the guidelines.

In some ways, occupational health is outside the mainstream in modern medical practice. Non-'work comp' physicians are often poorly trained in the "work" part of the work/life balance and as such, often fail to consider the critical importance of the patient's productivity to their health. Return-to-work can be thought of as a proxy for effective health care; When a patient is too ill to work, that is the beginning of a health care episode. When she is healthy enough to return to work, then there is a positive outcome marking the end of the episode. Anyone interested in the "big picture" of measuring outcomes in health care should take a strong interest in return-to-work data.

By definition "guidelines" will not fit every patient or situation. When this occurs, medical managers should have a process in place to address the situation. One approach is contained within the Official Disability Guidelines (or ODG); process called "Documenting Exceptions to the Guidelines" in Appendix D of ODG Treatment in Workers' Comp. The purpose of this section is to outline a process for providers within states and provinces that have adopted ODG for healthcare provided under workers' compensation to ensure appropriate medical treatment for their patients in the rare instances where a procedure is not covered; necessary care falls outside of the recommendations; comorbidities dictate another course of therapy; or the patient's personal circumstances mandate a deviation from the otherwise scientific remedy. Therein comes the "art."

Medical treatment guidelines, employed appropriately, help ensure the needs of the patient are addressed with the best medical treatment available. Guidelines that are too restrictive may control costs in the short term, but, by limiting potentially-necessary medical care to injured workers, lead to unnecessary suffering and potentially higher ultimate costs due to litigation and adversarial relations. Non-productive utilization review costs skyrocket when denials and friction clog the system, as good providers stop taking workers' comp patients because they can't get necessary medical care approved.

Guidelines that are too vague or lack credibility due to a shaky research basis can also cause more harm than good. When employed these guidelines can prevent appropriate medical management as they are too broad and allow too wide a range of treatment in some instances. The result is payers fees for utilization review go up with no appreciable impact on the medical care delivered to claimants.

Finally, the ethical issues around use of clinical guidelines can only be resolved with the understanding that all of the stakeholders need to have access to the same information. This leads to more consistent and responsible care and better outcomes. Guidelines should be used as a communication tool between physician, employer, insurer, and patient. This allows for a more transparent and better-planned recovery process where "hidden agendas" and one-sided interests and incentives can be minimized, and the physician-patient relationship can be emphasized. In the era of the internet, this collaborative approach to outcomes-driven medicine is realistically within reach.

TEXAS' EFFORTS TO ADD SCIENCE TO THE ART OF WORK COMP MEDICINE

As anyone who has studied physician practice patterns is only too aware, there is wide variation in how physicians practice; the kinds of tests they order, whether they admit patients to the hospital or treat on an outpatient basis, the drugs they prescribe and the outcomes they deliver. If we are to gain control over health care costs and ensure patients receive the right treatment and payers get value for their dollars, we have to force more science into the art of medicine.

Texas' Division of Workers Comp's push to publish data on work comp physicians' compliance with clinical guidelines is a step in the right direction. While only in the formative stage, and pretty limited at that, the effort is long overdue but nonetheless a critical step in reforming the dysfunctional mess that is our health care system.

HOW MANY DOLLARS ARE WASTED ON PHYSICAL THERAPY?

Obviously, there are a number of healthcare providers involved in the care and treatment of workers comp patients—orthopedists, radiologists, pain management specialists, interventional radiologists, plastic surgeons, athletic trainers, psychologists, pharmacists, occupational therapists, sports medicine physicians, chiropractors, and physical therapists.

This latter most group of professionals is arguably the most frequently seen healthcare professional used in workers compensation.

Managing PT is challenging. The clinical guidelines for physical therapy (PT) that do exist (with one exception we'll get to in a minute) usually say something like "two visits a week for four weeks," without describing what is to be done during those visits, who's supposed to do what gets done, and equally important, what shouldn't be done – all of which should be driven by the patient's diagnosis and physical condition.

That's the primary reason physical medicine (PT and chiropractic) accounts for about one out of every five dollars spent on medical care in work comp, and would account for big bucks in group if it weren't for tightly written benefit limits (x visits at a 50% copay).

Please note, however, this author is a believer in the ability of appropriate PT to make a significant clinical impact in patients, and have seen a significant amount of data that support the use of PT in helping injured individuals return to functionality. But this author has also audited many work comp claims where the claimant had been to PT hundreds of times. Hundreds.

In once particular case, the claimant had over five hundred visits over a three year period, with each PT note looking identical to the previous one. The payer couldn't cut off the treatment because the treating physician had ordered it, and the clinical guidelines weren't robust enough to force the issue in court.

In a 2010 New York Times article on just this issue, by Gina Kolata said:

"My doctor at the Hospital for Special Surgery in New York, Joseph Feinberg, seems to share my opinion [that much of PT is waste]. 'Very often, I think the hot packs, cold packs, ultrasound and electrostimulation are unnecessary,' he said, adding, 'For sure, in many cases these modalities are a waste of time.'"

James J. Irrgang, a researcher in the department of orthopedic surgery at the University of Pittsburgh and president of the orthopedic section of the American Physical Therapy Association said "There is a growing body of evidence that supports what physical therapists do…You can waste a lot of time and money on things that aren't very helpful."

The lack of credible evidence-based clinical guidelines can make it difficult for payers to contest unnecessary treatment, especially in those states where regulations make it tough for payers to stop paying for unnecessary treatments.

There are credible, thoroughly researched clinical guidelines specific to PT, with the best focused not only on how many visits over how many weeks, but what should be done during those visits. I've reviewed all of the guidelines used in work comp for PT, and the most thorough are published by Expert Clinical Benchmarks, a subsidiary of MedRisk. (NOTE: MedRisk is a client of this author).

Guidelines can't be developed in six months; rather they must be carefully researched, assessed by acknowledged experts in the field, tested against claims and medical billing data, and reviewed periodically. There are far too many companies touting their "utilization review" programs which are based on little more than the "same old same old" guidelines that have never worked in the past, or quickly-assembled amalgamations of journal articles, neither of which will be of any help in front of a work comp judge.

What does this mean? If you're serious about managing PT, start with science.

A PHYSICAL THERAPIST'S PERSPECTIVE

As noted, there are good PTs, and bad PTs. There is good PT management, and bad PT management. Some PT is quite useful, appropriate, and necessary, and some is not. When payers don't use solid clinical guidelines it makes it very difficult for adjusters, case managers, peer reviewers, and hearing judges to differentiate between appropriate and inappropriate PT. And there's lots of inappropriate PT in work comp.

In the course of my consulting practice, there have been dozens of cases where claimants received more than a hundred PT visits over a year, and many where the total number was well over two hundred. This type of utilization is simply indefensible, and unfortunately often results in adoption of regulatory control mechanisms.

Some states have chosen to use caps on visits as proxies for utilization management, with 24 appearing to be the most common limit. This is at best a blunt instrument, but nonetheless it appears to have resulted in lower costs for physical medicine in the jurisdictions that have adopted the "24 visit rule."

CONCLUSION

Clinical guidelines, based on solid research and used transparently, can and do help ensure claimants receive the right medical treatment for their condition while preventing therapies and services that have marginal benefits or might actually harm the patient.

* ***Editor's note:*** I have enjoyed Joe Paduda's Managed Care Matter's blog (www.joepaduda.com) ever since I was first told about it. Joe has an elegant way of cutting to the proverbial chase, but does so with plenty of support for his arguments and perspectives. That is not an easy balance. He does not go on rants, but he nevertheless has a defined and unambiguous point of view. And honestly, while I don't always agree with every blog posing, I very much respect is work and I enjoy his writing style. So, I obviously wished to have his perspective and content in this work—selfishly, because I like it so much—but also because I wanted to do what I could to help grow his already large following of readers (like me) who look forward to his postings by exposing the audience of this book to his writing. The result is the content herein this chapter from his website that is an amalgam that deals with the treatment guidelines/evidence-based practice/ comparative effectiveness as applied to workers compensation in particular. Joe has generously allowed this content be published herein, but I highly recommend you become a subscriber to his Managed Care Matters blog wherein you can get frequent intelligent updates on issues that matter to you. In fact, you can also see that his skills are not limited to solely workers compensation, but also General Insurance Issues, Health Care Issues, Health Policy, Health Wonk Review (love it!), Manage Care - Group Health, Managed Care – Auto, Medicare and Medicaid, Pharmacy, PBMs, and Pharma costs, Property and Casualty, Providers, and Research. Joe is amazing, and we appreciate not only his work, but his willingness to share his perspectives herein. This volume is better for it.—CES

REFERENCE

Appleby, J, 'Debate surrounds end-of-life health care costs', 2006, *USA TODAY*, 18 October, viewed 21 July 2010 http://www.usatoday.com/money/industries/health/2006-10-18-end-of-life-costs_x.htm.

CHAPTER 14

The Anatomy of a Disaster Workers' Compensation Case, How Defending a Claim Turns a Small Case into a Monster

Kim Edward Presbrey

Presbrey & Assoc PC; E-mail: kim@Presbrey.com

Abstract: The complexity of workers' compensation cases can result from manifold causes—the nature of the injury and the circumstances of the injury are obvious, however there can be additional factors less obvious, like mutual suspicions of the worker and his/her employer, poor case management, misinformed expert witnesses and a myriad of other culprits that can conspire to prolong a case and maximize an untoward outcome for all parties involved. This chapter will delve into various, true-life case examples that illustrate such problems and result in so-called "nightmare cases."

INTRODUCTION

The vast majority of files fall within a few well-defined categories. There are medical only files that require the employer or its carrier to simply pay the medical bills incurred in a timely fashion which causes the claimant to not seek counsel to collect unpaid bills.

The medical plus permanent injury files are also quite predictable for the most part. The injuries that occur are obvious and witnessed and needing immediate medical care. The permanent injuries that result from these injuries are expected and well categorized by the past decisions decided by the Workers' Compensation Commission. Examples of these types of cases are repetitive trauma resulting in carpal tunnel syndrome, lifting heavy objects that result in immediate low back pain and disc injuries or falls that result in broken wrists and broken ankles.

Not every one of the described cases is simple or straight forward, but most of them are resolved within limits that both sides end up believing fall within reason. Unless there is some completely unforeseeable medical event, these cases do not become nightmares as a result of the litigation\adjuster decisions.

The following scenario is a true story with the names changed to protect the innocent. However if you are a student of workers compensation case law, it will probably become apparent to you what case is being discussed.

INTERVIEW WITH THE PETITIONER'S ATTORNEY

Ron Rover appears at his attorney's office for an initial interview. He is a 48 year old man, who is morbidly obese, diabetic, and appears older than his stated age. He was a maintenance man for a local school district and gave a history of moving a large table used in the auto body shop at the high school when he noted the onset of numbness in his right arm. He stated to the petitioner attorney that he reported this incident and then went to the local clinic that had been treating him for a large number of medical maladies throughout the years, but most notably, diabetes.

The petitioner told the lawyer that his treating doctor had assumed that the numbness in his arm was the result of diabetic peripheral neuropathy and did not prescribe any tests which would have noted any orthopedic or neurological abnormalities.

The next question posed to the petitioner was his reporting of the "accident" to his employer because at this point in time the 45 days had long past on the notice to the employer. The petitioner assured the attorney that such a notice had been given and the attorney responded that he would only file the case if the petitioner could get a signed statement from his supervisor.

ATTORNEY COMMENTS

At this point, I am presented with a cloudy case on all fronts. I have a man who has a numb arm which could be from his unrelated diabetes. Causal connection becomes a huge issue at this point. No matter how clean the case is, I know that the other side is not going to have any problem clouding these waters with an IME. Besides the diabetic issue, I believe from the interview that the accident is unwitnessed and the best I will do with proving accident is that it was reported immediately and that he was doing the type of work he says he was doing at the time of the event. Medical testimony, medical bills, and medical treatment while getting some type of benefits started are going to be critical to the management of this file.

SECOND INTERVIEW

The client comes to the attorney's office and presents him with a signed statement by his supervisor that Rover reported the accident to him on the date previously stated by Rover. He also stated that his treating doctor with his HMO had ordered a cervical MRI. The MRI showed a disc herniation and that the orthopod, to whom he was referred, has recommended surgery.

The attorney advises the client of several avenues to pursue. Because the petitioner has group insurance, the attorney advises the client that he can simply go ahead and have the surgery under his group plan and wait to see what the Workers Compensation Commission decides to do after he has had the surgery. The client points out that this is a viable solution from the standpoint of the payment of the medical bills, but that his group insurance has no short term or long term disability benefits and that he could starve waiting for a decision on his case. The attorney then advised the client that he can do nothing until after the case has been heard and decided, but that it is possible that he could wait several years for the case to conclude and because the petition would only be asking for prospective medical and temporary total disability benefits, the case would have to be tried a second time after his surgery for an award on permanency.

The client concludes that neither scenario is perfect, but that if he is going to have to wait for justice to occur, he will have the surgery and wait with his pain alleviated. At this point, the client believed that his employer was being vindictive and was prepared to respond in a similar manner. He scheduled his surgery with the HMO doctor and prepared to wait out the process. He was not provided any medical management. He was not provided any alternative opinions as to what might cure or mitigate his physical condition. He was being dragged into the litigation process with a serious medical condition and a handful of dice to roll. His employer and the claim adjuster did not realize it, but they would have to watch the dice roll.

THE DEPOSITIONS

In the state of Illinois the depositions of the experts are taken prior to trial. Even though I practiced prior to the advent of depositions in workers' compensation cases, I am uncertain as to why this particular procedure came into existence. I believe that it occurred because of the length of time it was taking to schedule doctors' depositions. The hearing officers would find themselves with cases pending for months after they had heard the evidence of the lay witnesses and found this to be somewhat of a scheduling nightmare. The problem with this from a due process standpoint is that it greatly disadvantages the employer because the testimony of the claimant is not in evidence and as a result of this the defense doctor's testimony is not based upon the history of the accident given by the claimant under oath. It frequently renders the defense doctor's testimony superfluous.

In this case the deposition of the treating doctor was taken first. He was not a doctor who testified regularly in front of the workers compensation commission. He did testify that in his opinion the surgery was necessary based upon a reasonable degree of medical and surgical certainty and that the surgery was necessitated by the accident as described to him by the claimant, i.e. moving a table in the auto body shop. He admitted on cross examination that some of the claimant's symptoms were probably related to his diabetes and that he had degenerative changes in his neck prior to the accident. However, he reiterated that the cervical MRI showed a disc herniation and that in his opinion the herniation had been caused by moving the table. He stated the delay in diagnosis was simply the result of the confusion caused by the peripheral neuropathy caused by the diabetes. The deposition was otherwise uneventful.

The next deposition taken was of the examining physician. This doctor is a well-known doctor to the workers' compensation commission. He does numerous independent medical examinations on behalf of employers and has authored hundreds of reports denying benefits to claimants. He is clearly biased in his opinions however he is a practicing spine surgeon whose skills as a surgeon are acknowledged.

In this case the doctor drafted a report, as required by case law, prior to his deposition. In this report, he stated that he found a pre-injury MRI report that showed that the claimant had a disc herniation in his neck. He stated that the report was contained in the voluminous treating medical records from the clinic where the claimant was initially treated for his neck condition and where he was treated for many years with his general practitioner and many other doctors at this clinic employing over 100 other doctors. Illinois law requires that the doctor's report be furnished to the opposing counsel at least 48 hours prior to the deposition. Suffice it to say, a comprehensive search was made of the treating medical clinic records that had been furnished pursuant to subpoena. No such MRI report was found in the treating records. The only MRI report that could be found was post-injury.

The examining doctor's deposition proceeded as normal. His direct testimony confirmed the existence of the pre-injury MRI report and his reliance on that report in his opinion that the injury to the claimant's neck was not caused by moving the table. As a cross-examination the doctor was again questioned about his certainty regarding the importance of the MRI report. He was asked again if that was the basis of his opinion. He was then asked to find the pre-injury MRI report in the treating medical records. He began looking through the records. He looked for over ½ hour. He then asked for a recess. He then came back into the room and admitted that he was mistaken and that the MRI report did not exist.

At this point, the employer's insurance company should have made every effort to commence settlement discussions. The employer had no defense to the issue of causation regarding the accident as their expert doctor's opinion was without weight. This means that there would never be an issue as to the manifest weight of evidence on this issue because the employer had no evidence on this issue. Unless the employer could prove that accident did not occur or that the claimant had injured himself somewhere else, it was highly unlikely that the employer could prevail in this case. No offer was made.

THE EMERGENCY HEARING

In Illinois there exists an emergency hearing process referred to as a "19(b) hearing". This hearing can be requested by the claimant at anytime when he/she is owed either medical or weekly benefits. The emergency aspect of this hearing is greatly slowed by the deposition and independent medical examination process. It can take months to schedule depositions with busy surgeons and it can even take months to schedule the independent medical examinations that occur prior to the deposition. Of course the common insurance company mantra of "deny, delay, defend" works very effectively in many instances. However it can be a very expensive practice if it turns out that a seriously injured claimant has a compensable case. The reason for this is that the entire time the employer is defending the case the claimant is accruing benefits and receiving medical treatment in a completely unreviewed manner. No medical management occurs, no vocational rehabilitation occurs, no utilization review occurs and basically the employer gets stuck with any medical bill that the claimant incurs while the case is pending.

At this point, the defense counsel realized that he was going to have an impossible task of proving that the claimant's accident did not cause the claimant's injury. The treating doctor had supported causation and the examining doctor had based his opinion on a non-existent report. Therefore, his defense of the case became the notice. He was defending this case based upon the employer stating that the claimant had not given the employer notice of the accident within 45 days of the accident occurring. The notice provision can be satisfied by giving notice to any supervisory person including a foreman.

The trial commenced with the testimony of the claimant. He testified that he had given notice of his accident to his foreman. He also testified to how the accident occurred and otherwise covered the elements necessary to prove a prima facie case before the hearing officer. Unpaid medical bills were put into evidence in the amount of about eighty thousand dollars along with testimony that the claimant had not worked since the accident and had not received any weekly benefits.

The defense then called their first witnesses. The first witness they called was the foreman that the claimant testified to whom he had given notice of the accident. The witness stated that he knew nothing of the accident and that the claimant had never given him notice. On cross-examination, the foreman was confronted with the signed, written statement secured by the claimant prior to the filing of the case. He admitted that it was his signature but continued to try to say that he did not know about the accident but only that the claimant was moving the table. This was devastating to the defense.

Following the hearing and prior to the hearing officer's written award, a demand was made to the employer for one hundred thousand dollars and the payment of all medical bills. The claimant was destitute and badly in need of money and although he was not working, would have accepted the sum of money to resolve his case. The defense made no offer.

The hearing officer awarded the back weekly benefits and all of the medical bills. The defense appealed the decision to the full commission. The full commission affirmed the decision of the hearing officer and the defense appealed the case to the circuit court. The circuit court affirmed and the defense appealed the case to the appellate court. The appellate court affirmed the decision of the circuit court and remanded the case back for further proceeding concerning whether the claimant was entitled to further interim benefits and or permanent disability. This process took over 2 years and the claimant continued to go without weekly benefits or oversight of his medical care.

REVIEWS AND APPEALS

One of the biggest and most frequent mistakes that claim adjusters, TPAs, and employers make is riding the ship to the bottom of the sea. If the ship is sinking, jump into a lifeboat and live for another day. Riding the ship to the bottom seldom ends well. Reviewing a case after it has lost at arbitration generally ends the same way. Small cases become big ones, and big cases become nightmares.

Unless the arbitrator has made some horrific error regarding the facts of the case, the facts will stand as determined at arbitration. The arbitrator was in the room when the witnesses testified. He saw their demeanor. He saw the look on the attorney's faces as their own witnesses said that they did not like. Being in the room carries a lot of weight with the Commission, even if they are uncertain about the outcome of the case. In Illinois the Commission hears the case "de novo" or new. It means that they are not bound by the evidentiary decisions of the arbitrator and can make their own findings of fact and conclusions of law. In practice, the arbitrator's decision is much stronger than simply a recommendation and this is especially true if the Commission knows the arbitrator to be experienced and competent.

If the case is reviewed, six to nine months of time will elapse before the case is heard and another couple of months will pass before a decision is rendered. Briefs are required during this process and the adjuster/TPA should be required to read both briefs before letting the case be argued in front of the panel. It is usually quite clear from the briefs which side is going to win. Bad facts and bad law generally make good brief writing a very difficult experience. If you read your side's brief and don't like it, it is probably a bad case to have argued. There is still time to jump in the lifeboat. Jump.

Once the case is lost at the Commission level, the chances of winning with a further appeal are less than 5%. I don't have any empirical data to back up that statement, but I have handled over 80 cases at the appellate level, and have seen very few cases reversed either in person or in reading the cases that are decided. It is a time consuming and expensive process. Defense attorneys make a lot of money writing briefs and attending hearings. Claimants continue seeing doctors without any oversight and weekly benefits continue to accumulate.

Why is the process so ill-advised? The Commission finds the facts. The Circuit and Appellate Courts must accept their facts or find that the facts the Commission found were against the manifest weight of the evidence. This is a huge burden. There must be literally no evidence that supports the findings of the Commission. It is a rarity because the briefs at the Commission make such an event very obvious to the Commission. It should also make it very obvious to the parties. In the above described case, the employer's doctor made a critical error in his report; the issue of causation was never going to be won by the employer. They had no evidence and could never win on the issue of manifest weight.

The other basis of reversal at the appellate level is reversal as a matter of law. There are very few legal questions outside of the amendments of 2006 that have not been decided. It is rare that the Commission makes a legal error.

They hear the same types of cases every day. How much they award is not a legal question. Which doctor they believe is not a legal question. These two questions dispose of 95% of all cases. The Appellate Court has probably heard close to 3000 cases in the last 20 years. Most of the legal questions have been answered.

The appellate process in the above described case lasted three years. A lot can go wrong in three years. One of the things that went wrong in this case is that the employer decided to pay the medical bills that were awarded at the 19(b) hearing before there was a final order. The bills were approximately $85,000. When the final award was made it included those bills. The claimant wanted full payment of the award plus the statutory 9% interest. The employer wanted credit for the partial payment on the award. The case went back to the Circuit Court for enforcement of the award. The employer was assessed all of the claimant's attorney's fees from the beginning of arbitration. The employer was assessed additional penalties. This decision of the Circuit Court was also appealed to the Appellate Court. It was summarily affirmed and remanded back to the Circuit Court for enforcement. The money owed was taken from the employer's checking account pursuant to a turnover order.

A case that could have been settled prior to trial for $100,000 was now going to cost more than $500,000 to settle. The claim adjuster was fired. The defense attorney was fired. The defense firm lost the account. The account lost the employer as a customer.

CONCLUSION

One critical mistake that is made by the parties to litigation is that the process is fluid. Smart adjusters watch trials. They assess how the case is going and make their decisions as the case progresses. Very few adjusters ever attend trials anymore. I am sure it is a cost issue. They could have paid for a lot adjusters' time if they could have saved the $400,000. Once the sides become entrenched, there is always a good chance that disaster will follow. Smart defense attorneys and smart claim adjusters never let themselves get set up for the big hit.

CHAPTER 15

Advances in Laser Therapy for the Treatment of Work Related Injuries

Brian A. Pryor, PhD

LiteCure, LLC.; E-mail: brianp@LiteCure.com

Abstract: Laser Therapy has been used as a therapeutic modality for many years and has yet to become a standard of care. This modality has great potential to be used in the clinic for the reduction of pain, inflammation and to aid in the healing process. For years many studies have been done showing the benefits of laser therapy but implementation of this technology into clinically successful products has been lagging behind. This chapter will briefly review the science behind laser therapy, the traditional systems which were used and new technologies, Class IV lasers, now being used to treat injuries seen in the work place. New advances in this technology are being made which are leading to improved and consistent clinical outcomes. The mechanisms of action for pain relief, reduction of edema and tissue healing will be presented as well as important parameters to use in order to succeed when choosing this exciting therapeutic modality. Included are brief reviews of laser therapy when treating epicondylitis, carpal tunnel syndrome, neck and back pain as well as in post surgical rehabilitation applications. Laser therapy is a tool which can have great benefit when treating both acute stage injuries as well improving some chronic conditions.

INTRODUCTION

Lasers have been used for many years for a variety of medical applications. Applications such as laser hair removal and vision correction have aided in popularizing this high tech innovation in the field of medicine. Surgical lasers are also now being used to perform surgeries which previously would have been very difficult with traditional techniques. Lasers also have been used in rehabilitation and occupational therapy clinics for many years, especially in some European counties. This technology is now getting integrated more and more into everyday practices in the United States, as good products with sound science are being introduced to the marketplace.

Over 30 years ago, Andre Mester first observed that a very low level of laser energy was causing cellular changes in mice (Mester 1967). Since that first observation there have been thousands of studies done on using lasers to influence cellular repair, reproduction or inhibition (Hode & Turner 2002). Many of these studies have utilized very low output power, laser systems.

For the past 10 or more years, the lasers used in physical therapy and occupational therapy have been low power devices, typically between 5 mW to 500 mW of output power. These devices have been called "low level lasers" or "cold lasers." These terms arose to differentiate these types of therapeutic applications from more powerful laser systems which are used to ablate tissue for surgical or cosmetic applications. Most of these terms have been inspired more by marketing than by science. The term cold laser was first used by the early scientist in this field performing *in vitro* studies since many skeptics claimed that heat and not laser light was the cause of the cellular changes they were reporting. Being diligent scientists, they measured the insignificant temperature changes during their experiments and proved that the laser light was causing cellular changes. The entire field then took on the term, cold laser therapy. In fact almost all lasers when used clinically for any significant amount of time will produce a small temperature change in tissue. The important thing to acknowledge is that the rise in temperature is not the cause of the cellular changes. The stimulation of cellular activity is caused by a photochemical response to the laser light.

The reservation of many therapists to integrate laser therapy into their clinic has resulted from conflicting findings in the literature. Often times these studies have been done with very low dosages which have shown inconsistent or even poor results. The studies performed on more superficial conditions such as wounds have shown very good clinical results. The challenge has been with more complex conditions or those with a deep tissue component. Newer laser systems with higher output power are now available and gaining acceptance in the market due to the ability to treat deep tissue such as a hamstring injury. Results are more consistent and due to the ability to deliver a larger amount of energy, broad areas can be treated in a short time assuring a therapist won't "miss" the troubled area.

Chris E. Stout, Matt Kruger and Jeffrey Rogers, (Eds)

New scientific studies are proving positive outcomes on challenging conditions using these higher powered laser systems (Alaskym *et al* 2010; Charles *et al* 2010).

MECHANISM OF ACTION

Photochemical effects can occur when laser light is absorbed by a chromophore and a biochemical change is inspired. Photobiomodulation, which is the term the industry has decided upon, is an example of a photochemical process in which photons from a laser source interact with cells and cause a stimulation or a biochemical change. The mechanism of action of laser therapy or photobiomodulation has been debated for some time. To this day there are various thoughts to the exact mechanism. In fact there may be several potential mechanisms and even slightly different mechanisms depending on the type of cell being stimulated. The most supported mechanism is that cytochrome c, which is found in the mitochondria inside the intercellular membrane, acts as the photoreceptor. Cytochrome c absorbs light from 500 nm to 1100 nm due to specific properties of this large molecule (Karu 1995). Once light is absorbed cytochrome c is excited and can more readily bond with oxygen and become cytochrome c oxidase which is critical to the formation of ATP. ATP is critical for energy production in the cell and leads to host of biologic responses or secondary mechanisms. These mechanisms lead to the reduction of pain, inflammation and healing of tissue.

REDUCING PAIN

Pain management has been one major indication for laser therapy. How does this work? There have been extensive studies looking various mechanisms resulting from photobomodulation and resulting pain relief (Hode & Turner 2007; Faegapani *et al* 2008).

Upon laser interaction with cells the following processes have been seen to occur. There is an increase in serotonin (5-HT) levels (Cassone *et al* 1993; Walker 1983; Cassone *et al* 1990). Serotonin acts as a chemical messenger that transmits nerve signals between nerve cells. Serotonin levels impact mood.

There are also increases in Beta Endorphins, which decrease pain sensation.

These increases (Montesinos 1988; Labajos 1988; Cramond *et al* 1994), can act to abolish pain at the receptor site.

Nitric Oxide which is critical for normal action potential in impulse transmission activity in nerve cells is also increased upon laser stimulation (Mrowiec 1997). NO also has an effect on vasodilatation which enhances oxygenation.

Bradykinins which can be prevalent in injured tissue, induce pain sensation by stimulating nociceptive afferents. Laser therapy has been shown to decrease these peptides reducing pain levels (Jimbo *et al* 1998).

Therapeutic lasers have also shown the following positive effects:

Normalization of Ion Channels, Ca++, Na++, K+ proven to reduce pain levels (Alvarez-Leefmans *et al* 2005; Friedman & Lubart 1911).

Blocked Depolarization of C-Fiber Afferent Nerves (Wakabayashi 1993): Therapeutic lasers can suppress the excitation of these fibers, particularly in low velocity neural pathways from nociceptors (Kawatani *et al* 1993).

Increase Nerve Cell action potential: Injury or trauma can impair the resting potential of nerve cells leading to a very low threshold for pain. Laser treatment has shown to increase the resting potential closer to the norm of ~70 mV(Blom *et al* 2000).

Increase release of Acetylcholine(Lupyr & Sergienko 1986; Mester *et al* 1977): Acetylcholine helps normalize nerve signal transmission in the autonomic and somatic pathways.

Axonal Sprouting and Nerve Cell regeneration: Several studies have shown the lasers positive effects in nerve repair which can have a dramatic effect in pain relief (Anders *et al* 1993; El-Ani *et al* 2009; Anders *et al* 2005).

All of these proven cellular responses contribute to pain relief upon therapeutic laser treatment. These mechanisms, together with the anti-inflammatory and the tissue healing benefits make the laser an integral modality in both making patients feel better and get better.

Reducing Inflammation

In addition to the above mentioned mechanisms for reducing pain, laser treatments have been shown to reduce inflammation. The following actions have been proven to produce key elements which aid in the reduction of edema.

- Enhancement of ATP (Friedman & Lubart 1911; Cui *et al* 2002; Casanassima *et al* 1984)
- Stimulation of Vasodilatation (NO) (Gladwin & Shiva 2009)
- Reduction in Interkeukin-1 (Albertini *et al* 2005)
- Stabilization of the Cellular Membrane (Greco *et al* 2001)
- Acceleration of Leukocytic Activity (Greguss *et al* 1978)
- Increase Prostaglandin Synthesis (Abiko *et al* 2000; Harada *et al* 2004)
- Enhanced Lymphocyte Response (Karu 1991)
- Increased Angiogenesis (Krispel *et al* 2002; Belkin *et al* 1994)
- Temperature Modulation (Kurokawa *et al* 1991; Maeda 1990)
- Enhanced Superoxide Dismutase SOD levels (Eichler *et al* 2003; Eichler *et al* 2005)

PROMOTING HEALING

Wound healing has been the area where most of the traditional laser therapeutic studies have been completed. The results in these studies have been very encouraging and the mechanisms of tissue healing are important for other injuries; such as tears and contusions, as many of the same mechanisms are needed to promote tissue healing.

Below is a list of important physiological changes upon laser treatment along with references to the studies which measured these modifications.

- Enhanced Leukocyte Infiltration (Karu 1991)
- Increased Macrophage activity (Bansal *et al* 2003; Qin *et al* 1992; Bolton *et al* 1990)
- Increased Neovascularization (Gladwin & Shiva 2009)
- Increased Fibroblast Proliferation (Cagnie *et al* 2003; Abrahamse & Hawkins 2006)
- Keratinocyte Proliferation (Graves *et al* 1990)
- Early Epithelialization (Bayat *et al* 2005)
- Growth Factors Increase (Benayahu *et al* 2005; Abrahamse *et al* 2008)
- Greater wound tensile strength (Mester *et al* 1967)

The combined effect of pain relief, reduction of edema and promotion of tissue healing makes laser therapy a valuable tool in all aspects and stages of treatment of injuries. Treatments can be performed soon after an injury and help with both pain relief and healing.

HOW MUCH LASER LIGHT IS NEEDED?

Certainly there is a threshold, or an optimal amount of light which is needed to turn on the therapeutic effects listed above. Hundreds of the scientific studies have been done *in vivo* and have characterized the optimal dosage or range of dosages need to achieve a cellular response (Hode & Turner 2007).

These studies are imperative, since they give a baseline for the amount of laser energy we need to deliver in a given area to achieve results at the cellular level. However, if we were to use this same dosage which had an effect when exposed in a Petri dish, on the surface of the skin, we would get considerably less dosage at the tissue in which we want to achieve therapeutic results.

When using a therapeutic laser *in vivo*, we need to consider many additional parameters. If most of the laser light is absorbed in the dermis, for example, then we cannot achieve an optimal effect. When laser light hits tissue, it can be absorbed, scattered (including reflection), or transmitted. The main components in tissue that we need to consider are: melanin, oxyhemoglobin, deoxyhemoglobin, and water. We can get light into the body with wavelengths from 600 nm (red end of the spectrum) to 1100 nm (near infrared end of the spectrum). The range is often referred to as the "therapeutic window" for laser applications.

Although these wavelengths can penetrate, each wavelength has unique penetration characteristics.

If we put an ordinary white light source, a flashlight, into the palm of our hand, we will see a red glow out the other side. Longer wavelengths such as red penetrate deeper. The amount of red light visibly seen through the hand is dependent on the color of the skin. Melanin absorbs light strongly, so dark skin will absorb more light, especially wavelengths from 500 nm to 800 nm. Wavelengths longer than 1200 nm absorb in water very strongly and therefore it is difficult to get much penetration in tissue. These longer wavelength lasers are typically used in ablative procedures such as surgery or skin resurfacing.

The important parameter for a therapy laser system to have is the appropriate wavelength to allow penetration to deep tissue. Wavelengths longer than 800 nm can typically achieve appropriate depths to treat most musculo skeletal conditions. When dealing with wounds or more superficial conditions shorter wavelengths such as 635 nm can be used effectively, since penetration is less important.

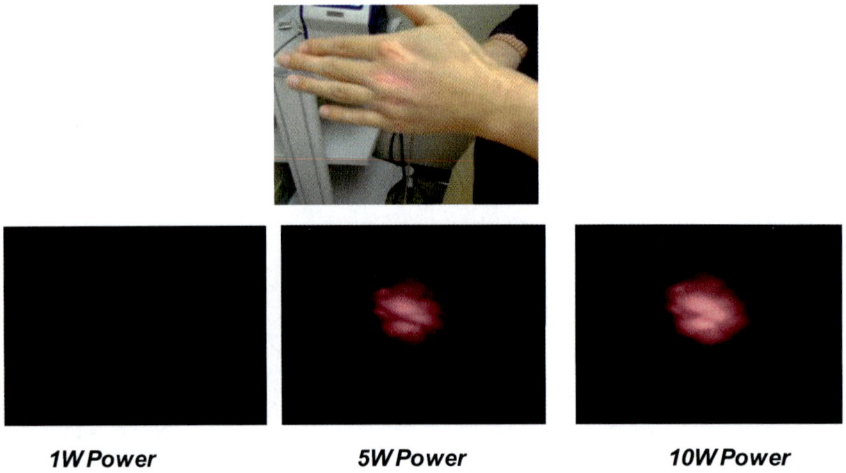

Figure 1: 980nm/810 nm laser output penetrating though a hand as a function of output power. Images were taken at a fixed exposure rate using an Infrared sensitive camera. This figure shows that high output power penetrates deeper as a function of exposure time.

Since all wavelengths have a probability of scattering, absorbing, or transmitting, the more power, or the greater number of photons you have, the greater depth of penetration as a function of time. (See Fig. **1**) Let's assume that we get 2.5% of the total laser light delivered to the skin actually reaching the patella tendon. If we use a 250 mW laser source, we are only getting 6.25 mW at the tendon or.00625 J per second of exposure.

If we use a 10 W laser source, we will get 250 mW at the tendon or 0.25 J in a second. By using a lower powered laser source for a longer time you can potentially achieve a large dosage to deep tissue. Using the example above, for the 250 mW laser to achieve the equivalent amount of energy as the 10W laser puts out in 1 second it would take almost 1 minute. (See Table **1**)

Table 1: Treatment time for various output power laser systems

Output Power	Dosage	Size of treatment area	Treatment Time
5 mW	4 J/cm^2	5 in x 5 in	35 hours
100 mW	4 J/cm^2	5 in x 5 in	1 hour 47 min
250 mW	4 J/cm^2	5 in x 5 in	43 min
500 mW	4 J/cm^2	5 in x 5 in	21.5 min
5 W	4 J/cm^2	5 in x 5 in	2 min 9 sec
10 W	4 J/cm^2	5 in x 5 in	1 min 5 sec

In principle a lower power unit with the appropriate wavelength for good penetration (800nm to 1000nm) used for a long period of time, ultimately will be able to get to the same depth and yield therapeutic results. However, one study showed that results were not the same by using a very low power density. It was shown that under 10^{-5} W/cm^2 even when exposed for a long period of time, had no measurable results (Andreichuck *et al* 1993).

Many conditions are very hard to diagnose to a very precise afflicted area, or often times conditions have other involved muscles contributing to the pain. Therefore it is important to treat as broad of an area as possible. This is where newer, higher power laser units can have a great advantage. Since you can get a therapeutic dosage of light deep into tissue, in a short treatment time, it is possible to treat a very broad area. This enables the affected area and satellite areas of pain to be effectively treated.

A good example of this, is when treating a patient with carpal tunnel syndrome. Carpal tunnel is typically associated with an impairment associated at the carpus/wrist. Often times the pain may be associated with a nerve impairment in the area around the elbow, or possibly at the cervical spine. As discussed previously, a typical range for effective dosage is on the order of 4 to 10 J/cm^2. Since the target area is not extremely deep, in the case of carpal tunnel we would use approximately 5 J/cm^2. If we assume we want to treat the entire wrist area (3"x 6" or 116 cm^2) it would take approximately 580 J (5 J/cm^2 * 116 cm^2). When treating with a typical lower power laser with 250 mW output, it takes approximately 38 minutes. Treating the same area using a higher power, 10 W, laser would only take 58 seconds. The older, lower powered laser systems make it very hard to treat a broad enough area to get consistent results in an everyday clinic. Treating carpal tunnel effectively and consistently, takes a treatment protocol which can address the possible involvement of the nerve route all the way to the cervical spine area. (see Fig. **2**) This type of comprehensive approach is not practical when using a lower power laser system. If using a 10 W laser, treating this entire area will take 4 to 6 minutes depending on the size of the patient and there will be positive and consistent outcomes.

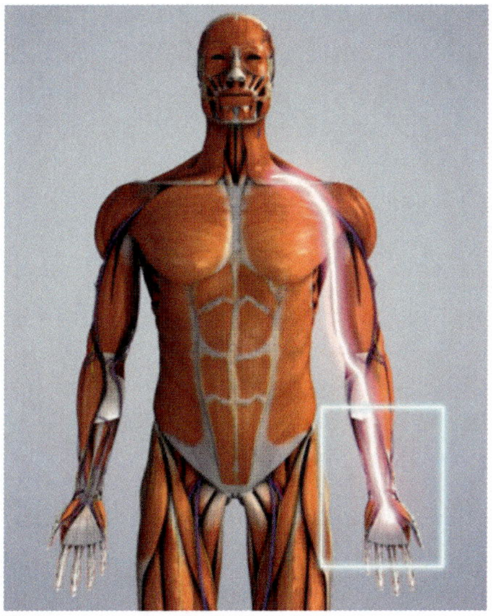

Figure 2: Nerve route to treat when treating carpal tunnel syndrome

THE FOLLOWING SECTIONS WILL GO OVER SOME TREATMENTS AND STUDIES DONE ON SEVERAL OF THE MOST COMMON, WORK RELATED INJURIES.

Epicondylitis

Laser Therapy can be a very effective modality in treating epicondylitis. Some of the early studies done using laser therapy showed negative to moderate results (Haker *et al* 1987; Haker & Lundeberg 1990; Basford *et al* 2000).

All of these studies used very low dosages and only treated small, very select areas. Other studies using a more comprehensive treatment area, with a larger dosage, show significant results in blinded studies (Simunovic & Trobonjaca 2001; Simunovic *et al* 1998; Adamek *et al* 1997; Terashima 1990; Damjanova & Manolov 2000).

One study compares the treatment of laser, corticosteroid injections, and a combination therapy of laser and injections. The combined treatment had a significant higher analgesic effect over the other two (Konstantinovic 1997). This study reminds us that using appropriate adjunctive therapies can often lead to much enhanced outcomes.

A summary of studies on the effect of laser therapy on tendonitis was done by Bjordal (Bjordal 1997). This review concluded that laser therapy was an effective treatment both at reducing the inflammation, as well as stimulating tendon regeneration. Optimal dosages were between 0.2- 4 J/cm^2 for regeneration and 3-8 J/cm^2 for reduction of inflammation. A recent double blind study using a higher power class IV laser has shown significant results at 3 month follow up of the laser treated group over a sham group, when measuring grip strength, pain with grip and lateral palpation. The treatment technique used a very comprehensive protocol and relatively short treatment times (Alaskym *et al* 2010).

With a comprehensive treatment approach, laser therapy is an effective modality in treating medial and lateral epicondylitis with long lasting results.

Carpal Tunnel Syndrome

Carpal Tunnel syndrome is another very common work related condition which can be improved by treatment with laser therapy. The key to getting success when treating this condition is to use a broad approach to treatment. Just treatment of the carpal area may not yield results, as often this condition can stem from irritation of the cervical spine region. One study showed by treating the spinous processes, the pain and tingling was alleviated (Chermanz *et al* 1997).

A very nice study showing long term results was done by Neaeser, *et al.* This study showed significant decreases in Melzack pain score, median nerve sensory latency, Phalen sign and Tinel sign, post-real treatment series but not seen post-sham treatments. Patients were able to perform prior work (computer typist, handyman) and their condition remained stable for 1-3 years (Naeser 2002).

As with many conditions, laser treatment of carpal tunnel syndrome, should be complimented by exercise and other standard protocols. Conditioning and changes in work habits are imperative to success and full resolution. As mentioned earlier, treating a broad area and including the nerve route, when treating carpal tunnel will ensure rapid and consistent results.

NECK AND BACK PAIN

Neck and back pain are very common, often difficult to find a specific cause to the pain and always difficult to treat. The pain can often be nonspecific, making both diagnostics and treatments very challenging. Lasers have been shown to be effective when used in the treatment regime for these areas (Barnsley *et al* 2006; Bjordal *et al* 2003). A recent meta-analysis of clinical studies using lasers, concluded that laser therapy reduces pain immediately after treatment in both acute and chronic neck pain and pain relief lasted up to 22 weeks after treatmentBjordal *et al* 2009).

A recent pilot study, being done by the Health Sciences Department of Colorado University, Denver, compared the pain relief obtained for nonspecific lower back pain between manipulation with Class IV laser therapy versus manipulation alone. The manipulation + laser group had significantly less pain at week 4. With both neck and back pain it is important to use a laser system which has appropriate penetration to reach deep tissues.

Since laser therapy can relieve pain and increase blood flow it will help to increase mobility for neck and back patients. Acute neck and back pain will respond to laser treatments very quickly, many times a positive response is seen after the first treatment. For more chronic conditions, it can take longer to see an effect, 3 to 5 treatments to even see a small benefit and it may take up to 12 treatment sessions, in order to see a significant improvement. Working soft tissue while delivering therapeutic laser will also help to improve outcomes in these challenging cases. (See Fig. **4**) This treatment approach is the key to having prolonged results. The combination of laser treatments, stretching and exercise can have a major effect when treating patients with neck and back pain.

POST SURGICAL APPLICATIONS

Integrating laser therapy into post surgical rehab can lead to much quicker and better overall outcomes. By using the laser immediately post surgery, you will be able to reduce inflammation and pain. Since the laser also has tissue healing effects, the surgical site will improve faster, and there may be less scarring from the surgical incisions. Post rotator cuff repair and post anterior cruciate ligament repair, are two procedures which adding laser therapy to the post surgical rehabilitation plan, can dramatically improve the healing rate.

Patients will be more compliant to exercise, stretching, etc. since after the laser treatment they will have much better range of motion and less pain. Most surgical rehab programs can benefit greatly by adding laser therapy.

TREATMENT BASICS

When treating patients, it is critical to understand the overall diagnosis and work laser therapy into the rehabilitation program. A broad area should be treated as well as treating any potentially contributing muscle or joint. Fig. **3** shows a typical area which would be treated in the case of epicondylitis. When using a laser with output power of greater than 4W, or anytime the patient feels any warmth, a scanning method should be used. The patient should feel soothing warmth during treatment, this sensation should never be more than a pleasant warmth. If the temperature is uncomfortable, the output power should be reduced. These higher power laser units will allow for a broader and faster treatment.

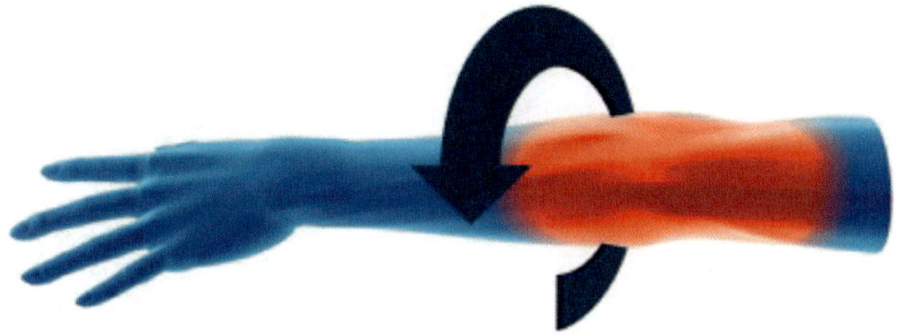

Figure 3: Comprehensive treatment area for laser treatment of epicondylitis

Scanning of the area with the laser should be done in a grid type pattern in order to ensure comprehensive coverage of the affected area. Some laser systems allow the handpiece to be placed in contact with the patient's tissue. In this case some manual manipulation or massage can be done while delivering therapeutic laser treatment (see Fig. **3**). This can be a very effective approach when treating deep tissue conditions such as muscle or tendon tears or strains. Slight passive range of motion should be used when possible, during the last few minutes of treatment. Treatment of any associated trigger points with the laser is also a very effective way to enhance therapeutic results. Many therapists will combine soft tissue work after laser therapy. Another common adjunct therapy is to use TENS or e-stim after completing laser therapy.

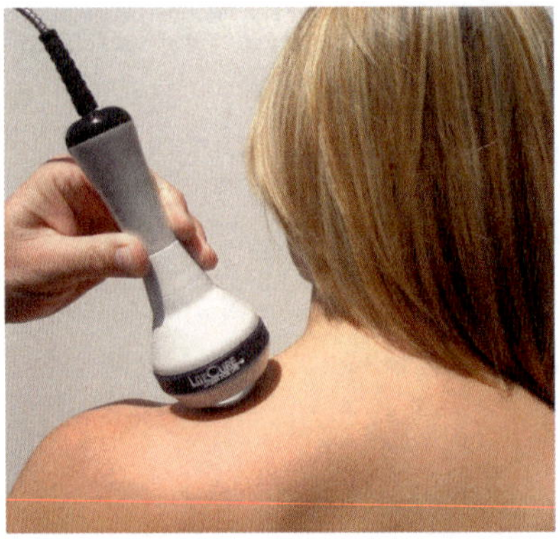

Figure 4: Example of a laser therapy handpiece allowing tissue massage/manipulation while delivering laser energy.

It is typically recommended that laser therapy be done every other day for a three week period, for a total of 6 to 9 treatments, depending on the condition, and if it is acute or chronic. When appropriate, laser treatments can be given on a daily basis. If patients are in an environment where treatment is given every day, then it is recommended to treat with the laser on a daily basis. Acute conditions will respond very quickly to laser treatment and a significant benefit may be realized after the initial treatment. Typically a total of 6 treatments will be needed to see major improvement. Chronic conditions will take longer to respond and may take up to 3 treatments to realize any benefit and as many as 12 treatments to see significant outcomes.

Another advantage of using laser therapy is that there are very few contraindications. The contraindications which most manufacturers lists are, don't treat pregnant patients, don't treat patients who are taking any photosensitive medication; don't treat patients with cancer, don't treat over open growth plates, don't treat the eyes, don't treat the testicles, don't treat over any active hemorrhaging. Eye safety is the biggest precaution when performing laser therapy. Appropriate eye wear supplied with the laser should be worn by the clinician and the patient when treating. The eye should never be treated and when treating conditions around the face, specific eye wear, like metal eye shields must be utilized. Most contraindications listed for laser therapy are based on prudence and not on the results of studies. For comparison, cosmetic lasers such as skin resurfacing or hair removal systems, are very powerful, hundreds of times more power than even the most powerful therapeutic lasers. Even at these high powers and large dosages used in these types of ablative procedures, there have been very few side effects out of millions of treatments.

Laser therapy treatments are very easy to administer, and depending on the power level of the laser being used, treatment times take less than 10 minutes for most peripheral conditions and less than 15 minutes when treating a large area like the back or hip. The laser is easy to integrate into standard treatment protocols in a clinic. Uniform administration is achieved without requiring a high level of technical skill. Patients enjoy treatments, and will mostly respond very quickly, leading to faster more effective outcomes and enhanced compliance.

CONCLUSION

The future of laser therapy will be an exciting one. Preliminary studies are showing promising results when treating conditions such as peripheral neuropathies, strokes, and many other debilitating conditions. Fundamental studies in laboratories are continuing to refine our understanding of the mechanisms of action of laser therapy. The results of these laboratory studies need to be followed up with the appropriate animal models and then followed through to good scientifically sound, clinic based studies with measurable outcomes. As we learn more, we will be able to refine device specifications and protocols for clinicians to have the appropriate tool for treating specific conditions. The field of biophotostimulation is growing, and will continue to find new applications where lasers and other light devices can be used to address a variety of medical issues. Multidisciplinary collaboration will lead to faster discoveries and better therapeutic tools.

When implementing laser therapy in the clinical environment, you need to make sure you use the right tool for the right job. You need to take into account the types of conditions you are treating and the time you can afford treating those conditions. Lasers can be an integral tool for treating the majority of rehab and workman's compensation related conditions. This tool, like all others, must be used appropriately in your treatment regime to maximize overall outcomes. As discussed above, the laser will help compliance with other parts of your treatment program, helping to expedite positive outcomes and getting people back to in the game and back to work. Laser therapy can be an important modality when treating both acute and chronic work related injuries.

REFERENCES

Abiko, Y, Sakurai, Y, Yamaguchi, M 2000, 'Inhibitory effect of low-level laser irradiation on LPS-stimulated prostaglandin E2 production and cyclooxygenase-2 in human gingival fibroblasts', *European Journal Oral Sciences*, vol. 108, no. 1, pp. 29-34.

Abrahamse, H & Hawkins, D 2006, 'Effect of multiple exposure of low-level laser therapy on the cellular responses of wounded human skin fibroblasts', *Photomedicine and Laser Surgery,* vol. 24, no. 24, pp. 705-714.

Abrahamse, H, Mathope, T, Moore, T, Mvula, B 2008, 'The effect of low level laser therapy on adult human adipose derived stem cells', *Lasers in Medical Science*, vol. 23, no. 3, pp. 277–252.

Adamek, M, Cieslar, G, Laitl-Kobierska, A, Sieron, A, Zmudzinski, J 1997, 'Effect of low-power laser radiation in the treatment of the motional systems overloading syndromes', *Proc SPIE,* vol. 3198, no. 76, pp. 76-82.

Alaskym, P, Kiefer, J, Druse, R, Petznick, M, Roberts, D, Stoll, S, 2010, 'A randomized controlled trial for the efficacy of therapeutic class IV laser treatment for tendinosis', *Proceed ACSM,* vol. 1108, no. 1780.

Albertini, R, Bjordal, JM, Faria Neto, HC, Lopes-Martins, RA, Martins, PS 2005, 'Spontaneous effects of low-level laser therapy (650 nm) in acute inflammatory mouse pleurisy induced by Carrageenan', *Photomedicine and Laser Surgery*, vol. 23, no. 4, pp. 377-381.

Alvarez-Leefmans, FJ, Arguelles, CF, Granados-Soto, V 2005, 'Peripheral and central antinociceptive action of Na+-K+-2Cl- co-transporter blockers on formalin-induced nociception in rats', *Pain*, vol. 114, no. 1, pp. 231-238.

Anders JJ, Borke RC, Van de Merwe, WP, Woolery, SK 1993, 'Low power laser irradiation alters the rate of regeneration of the rat facial nerve', *Lasers in Surgery and Medicine*, vol. 13, no.1, pp. 72–82.

Anders, J, Byrnes, K, Ilev, I, Waynant, R, Wu, X 2005, 'Low Power Laser Irradiation Alters Gene Expression of Olfactory Ensheathing Cells *In Vitro*', *Lasers in Surgery and Medicine*, vol. 37, no. 2, pp. 161–171.

Andreichuck, T, Karu, T, Ryabykh, T1993, 'Supression of human blood chemiluminescence by diode laser irradiation at wavelengths 660, 820, 880 or 950 nm', *Laser Therapy*, vol. 5, pp. 103-109.

Barnsley, L, Chow, RT, Heller, GZ 2006, 'The effect of 300 mW, 830 nm laser on chronic neck pain: A double-blind, randomized, placebo-controlled study', *Pain*, vol. 124, no. 1-2, pp. 201-210.

Bansal, H, Dube, A, Gupta, PK 2003, 'Modulation of macrophage structure and function by low level He–Ne laser irradiation', *Photochemical and Photobiological. Sciences*, vol. 2, pp. 851–855.

Baranauskas, V & Parizotto, NA 1998, 'Structural analysis of collagen fibrils after HeNe laser photostimulated regenerating rat tendon', in *2o Congress World Association for Laser Therapy; Sep 2-5. Kansas City*, Proceedings, Kansas City, pp. 66.

Basford, JR, Cieslak, KR, Sheffield, CG 2000, 'Laser therapy: a randomized, controlled trial of the effects of low intensity Nd:YAG laser irradiation on lateral epicondylitis', *Arch Phys Med Rehabil*, vol. 81, no.11, pp. 1504-1510.

Bayat M, Rakhshan, M, Razavi, N, Taheri, S, Vasheghani, M 2005, 'Effect of low-level laser therapy on the healing of second-degree burns in rats: a histological and microbiological study', *Journal of Photochemistry and Photobiology B: Biology*, vol. 78, no. 2, pp. 171-177.

Belkin, V, Bibikova, A, Oron, U 1994, 'Enhancement of angiogenesis in regenerating gastrocnemius muscle of the toad (Bufo viridis) by low-energy laser irradiation', *Anatomy and Embryology,* vol. 190, no. 6, pp. 597-602

Benayahu, D, Maltz, L, Oron, U, Stein, A 2005, 'Low-Level Laser Irradiation Promotes Proliferation and Differentiation of Human Osteoblasts *in Vitro', Photomedicine and Laser Surgery*, vol. 23, no. 2, pp. 161-166.

Bjordal, JM 1997, 'Low level laser therapy in shoulder tendonitis/bursitis, epicondylalgia and ankle sprain. A critical review on clinical effects', Masters Thesis in Physiotherapy Science, Div Physiotherapy Science, University of Bergen, Norway.

Bjordal, J., Chow, R Couppe, C, Ljunggren, E Tuner, J 2003, 'A systematic review of low level laser therapy with location-specific doses for pain from chronic joint disorders', *Australian Journal Physiotherapy*, vol. 49, no. 2, pp. 107-116.

Bjordal, JM, Chow, RT, Johnson, MI, Lopes-Martins, RAB 2009, 'Efficacy of low-level laser therapy in the management of neck pain: A systematic review and meta-analysis of randomised placebo or active-treatment controlled trial', *The Lancet*, vol. 374, no. 9705, pp. 1897-1908

Blom, K, Cambier, D, De Muynck, M, Ollevier, G, Vanderstraeten, G, Witvrouw E 2000, 'The influence of low intensity infrared laser irradiation on conduction characteristics of peripheral nerve: A randomized, controlled, double blind study on the sural nerve', *Lasers in Medical Science*, vol.15, no. 3, pp.195-200.

Bolton, P, Dyson, M, Young, SR 1990, 'Effect of light on calcium uptake by macrophages', *Laser Therapy*, vol.5, pp. 53–57.

Cagnie, BJ, Cambier, DC, Cornelissen, MJ, Declercq, HA, Vinck, EM 2003, 'Increased fibroblast proliferation induced by light emitting diode and low power laser irradiation', *Lasers in Medical Science,* vol. 18, no. 2, pp. 95-99.

Casamassima, E, Catalano, IM, Cingolani, A, Molinari, S, Passarella S, Pastore D, Quagliariello E 1984, 'Increase of proton electrochemical potential and ATP synthesis in rat liver mitochondria irradiated *in vitro* by helium-neon laser', *FEBS Letters*, vol. 175, no. 1, pp. 95-99.

Cassone MC, Lombard A, Rolfo PM, Rossetti V, Urciuoli R, 1993, 'Effect of *in vivo* HeNe laser irradiation on biogenic amine levels in rat brains', *Journal of Photochemistry and Photobiology B: Biology,* vol.18, nos.2-3, pp. 291-294.

Cassone MC, Lombard A, Rossetti V 1990, 'Neurotransmitter content and enzyme activity variations in rat brain following *in vivo* HeNe laser irradiation', *Proceedings,Round Table on Basic and Applied Research on Photobiology ad Photomedicine* Bari, Italy November 10th and 11th.

Charles, F, Kim, J, Kingsley, JD, Mathis, R, McMillan, V, Mojock, C, Panton, L, Simonavice, E, Williams, K 2010, 'Effects of Class IV Laser Therapy on Disease Impact and Function in Women with Fibromyalgia', *Proceed ACSM,* vol. 1108, no. 1081.

Chermanz, Z, Lee, W, Mason DA 1997, 'Carpal Tunnel Syndrome Treated with a Diode Laser: A Controlled Treatment of the Transverse Carpal Ligament', *LASER THERAPY,* vol. 9, pp. 131- 136.

Cramond, T, Galligan, JP, Laakso EL, Richardson C 1994, 'ACTH and Beta-Endorphin levels in response to low level laser therapy for myofascial trigger points', *Laser Therapy*, vol. 6, no. 3, pp. 133-142.

Cui, Y, Kataoka, Y, Mochizuki, ON 2002, 'Effects of near-infra-red laser irradiation on adenosine triphosphate and edenosine diphosphate contents in rat brain tissue', *Neuroscience Letters*, vol. 323, no. 3, pp. 207-210.

Damjanova, J & Manolov, V 2000, 'Therapeutic influence on patients with epicondylitis and myotendinitis of upper extremities by the means of low-intensity laser', *Fizikalna Kurortna i Rekhabilitatsiona Meditsina*, vol. 39, no. 1, pp. 15.

Eichler, M, Friedmann, H, Kaplan, D, Lavi, R, Lubart, R, Rickover, O, Shainberg, A, Shneyvays V 2003, 'Low energy visible light induces reactive oxygen species generation and stimulates an increase of intracellular calcium concentration in cardiac cells', *Journal of Biological Chemistry*, vol. 278, pp. 40917-40922.

Eichler, M, Friedman, H, Lavi, R, Lubart, R, Shainberg, A 2005, 'Low-Energy Laser Irradiation Promotes Cellular Redox Activity', *Photomedicine and Laser Surgery*, vol. 23, no. 1, pp. 3-9.

El-Ani, D, Nevo, Z, Rochkind, S, Shahar, A 2009, 'Increase of Neuronal Sprouting and Migration Using 780nm Laser Phototherapy as Procedure for Cell Therapy', *Lasers in Surgery and Medicine*, vol. 41, no. 4, pp. 277–281.

Fregapani, P, Matos de Oliveira, M, Neto, N, Pozza, D, Sobrinho, JB, Weber, J 2008, 'Analgesic action of laser therapy (LLLT) in an animal model', *Med Oral Patol Oral Cir Bucal,* vol. 13, no. 10, pp. E648-52.

Friedman, H, Lubart, R 1911, 'Nonlinear photobiostimulation: the mechanism of visibleand infrared laser- induced stimulation and reducation of neural excitability and growth', *Laser Therapy*, vol.3, no. 1, pp. 15-18.

Gladwin, MT, Shiva, S 2009, 'Shining a light on tissue NO stores: near infrared release of NO from nitrite and nitrosylated hemes', *Journal of Molecular and Cellular Cardiology,* vol. 46, no. 1, pp. 1-3.

Graves, PJ, Haas, AF, Isseroff, RR, Rood, PA, Wheeland, RG 1990, 'Low-energy helium-neon laser irradiation increases the motility of cultured human keratinocytes', *Journal of Investigative Dermatology*, vol. 94, pp. 822–826.

Greco M, Marra, E, Moro, L, Passarella, S, Perlino, E, Petragallo, VA, Vacca, RA 2001, 'Helium-Neon laser irradiation of hepatocytes can trigger increase of the mitochondrial membrane potential and can stimulate c-fos expression in a Ca2+-dependent manner', *Lasers Surgery and Medicine,* vol. 29, no. 5, pp. 433-441.

Greguss, P, Haina, D, Mester, A, Mester, E, Nagylucskay S, Tisza S Waidelich W 1978, 'Effects of direct laser radiation on human lymphocytes', *Arch Dermatol Res*, vol. 263, no. 3, pp. 241-245.

Haker E, & Lundeberg T 1990, ' Laser Treatment applied to acupuncture in lateral humeral epicondylalgia: A double blind study', *Pain*, vol. 43, no. 2, pp. 243-247.

Haker, E, Lundeberg, T, Thomas, M 1987, 'Effect of laser therapy vs placebo in tennis elbow', *Scand. J of Rehab Med*, vol. 19, pp. 135-138.

Harada, T, Kobayashi, T, Mizutani, K, Musya, Y, Taira, K, Tobe, M, Wakae K 2004, 'A clinical study on serum prostaglandin E2 with low-level laser therapy', *Photomedicine and Laser Surgery*, vol. 22, no. 6, pp. 537-539.

Hode, L & Tun'er, J 2002, *Laser Therapy Clinical Practice and Scientific Background,* Prima Books AB, Grangesberg, Sweden.

Hode, L & Turner, J 2007, *The Laser Therapy Handbook,* Prima Books AB, Grangesgerb, Sweden.

Jimbo, K, Noda, K, Suzuki, K, Yoda, K 1998, 'Suppressive effects of low-power laser irradiation on bradykinin evoked action potentials in cultured murine dorsal root ganglion cells', *Neuroscience Letters*, vol. 240, no. 2, pp. 93-96.

Karu, T 1991, 'Low-Intensity Laser Light Action Upon Fibroblasts and Lymphocytes', in Calderhead, RG &
Ohshiro, T, *Progress in Laser Therapy*, J. Wiley and Sons, Chichester, New York, Brisbane, Toronto, Singapore, pp.175-180

Karu, T 1995, 'Mechanisms of interaction of monochromatic visible light with cells', *Proc.SPIE,* vol. 2630, pp. 2-9.

Kawatani, M, Matsumoto, I, Sato, T, Takeshige, C, Tsuchiya K 1993, 'Diode laser irradiation selectively diminishes slow component of axonal volleys to dorsal roots from the saphenous nerve', *Neuroscience Letters,* vol. 161, no. 1, pp. 65-68.

Konstantinovic, L 1997, 'Combined low-power laser therapy and local infiltration of corticosteroids in the treatment of radial-humeral epicondylitis', *Vojnosant\it Pregl,* vol. 54, no. 5, pp. 459-463.

Krispel, Y, Maltz, U, Mirsky, N, Oron, U, Shoshany, Y 2002, 'Promotion of Angiogenesis by Low Energy Laser Irradiation', *Antioxidants & Redox Signaling*, vol. 4, no. 5, pp. 785-790.

Kurokawa, Y, Ohara, I, Ouchi, H, Taguchi, T 1991, 'Thermographic Changes Following Laser Irradiation for Pain Relief', *J Clin Laser Med Surg*, 1991; vol. 9, no. 2, pp. 143-146.

Labajos M 1988, 'Beta-Endorphin levels modification after GaAs and HeNe laser irradiation on the rabbit: A comparative study', *Investigacion Clinica Laser*, Vol. 1-2, pp. 6-8.

Lupyr, VM, Sergienko, NG 1986, 'Cholinesterase and norepinephrine activity under the laser irradiation of accupuncture points', *Fiziologicheskii Zhurnal*, vol. 32, pp. 297-303.

Maeda T 1990, 'Histological, thermographic and thermometric study *in vivo* and excised 830 nm diode laser irradiated rat skin', *Laser Therapy*, vol. 2, no. 1, pp. 32.

Mester, A, Mester, E, Tisza, S, Vizi, E 1977, 'Acetylcholine releasing effect of laser irradiation on Auerbach's plexus in guinea-pig ileum', *J. Neural Transmission*, vol. 40, no.4, pp. 305-308.

Mester, E, Szende, B, & Tora, JG 1967, 'Effect of laser on hair growth of mice', *Kiserl Orvostud,* vol. 19, pp. 628-631.

Montesinos M 1988, 'Experimental effects of Low Power Laser in Encephalon and Endorphin Synthesis LASESR', *Journ Eur Med Laser Ass*., vol. 1, no. 3, pp. 2-7.

Mrowiec J 1997, 'Analgesic effect of low-power infrared laser radiation in rats', *Proc SPIE*, vol. 3198,no. 83, pp. 83-89.

Naeser, M 2002, 'Low-level laser therapy (LLLT) plus microamps TENS applied to acupuncture points significantly reduces pain in carpal tunnel syndrome (CTS)', *Archives of Physical Medicine and Rehabilitation*, vol. 83, pp. 978-988.

Qin, JZ, Xin, H, Xin, SY, Zeng, H 1992, 'The activating action of low level helium-neon laser irradiation on macrophages in mouse model', *Laser Therapy*, vol. 4, pp. 55–58.

Simunovic Z & Trobonjaca, T 2001, 'Comparison between low level laser therapy and visible incoherent polarized light in the treatment of lateral epicondylitis- tennis elbow [Supplement]', *Lasers in Surgery and Medicine*, vol.13, no. 9.

Simunovic Z, Trobonjaca T, Trobonjaca, Z 1998, 'Treatment of medial and lateral epicondylitis- tennis and golfer's elbow with low level laser therapy: a multicenter double blind, placebo controlled clinical study on 324 patients', *Journal of Clinical Laser Medicine & Surgery*, vol. 16, no. 3, pp. 145-151.

Terashima H 1990, 'Low energy laser irradiation for lateral humeral epicondylitis and de Quervains disease [ILTA Okinawa Congr Abstr Issue]', *Laser Therapy*, vol. 2, no.1, pp. 27.

Wakabayashi, H 1993, 'Effect of irradiation by semiconductor laser on responses evoked in trigeminal caudal neurons by tooth pulp stimulation', *Lasers in Surgery and Medicine*, vol. 13, no. 6, pp. 605-610

Walker, J 1983, 'Relief from chronic pain by low-power laser irradiation', *Neuroscience Letters* vol. 43, nos. 2-3, pp. 339-344.

CHAPTER 16

Persistent Problems in Clinical Practice

Peter Rousmaniere

Consultant and Journalist; E-mail: pfr@rousmaniere.com

Abstract: Medical care accounts for 60% of the total cost of workers compensation claims. Claims that payers under invest in medical intelligence, thereby allowing medical errors and sub-optimal treatment to happen more than they need to be. However, structural, system-wide factors are behind some of the persistent problems in clinical practice. Systemic problems persist in making assessments of work causality of injury and in estimating permanent impairment. States have since the early 1990s erected a complex structure of managed care practices, however, they are flawed in a number of ways, and claims payers fail to implement them as comprehensively as they could. Claims are in a position to invest more in medical intelligence to encourage and facilitate improvements in clinical practice.

INTRODUCTION

There were in 2008 3.7 million OSHA recordable work injuries and illnesses, of which 1.1 million required at least one day away from work (Bureau of Labor Statistics, US Department of Labor 2009). Virtually every one of these injuries involved a medical response, as ephemeral as a temporary bandaging or as momentous as a lifetime of treatment, rehabilitation and maintenance. Each one tests the resilience of not only the injured worker herself, but also the medical community and those who arrange for medical care.

One would expect that medical response to work injuries had over the decades become highly routinized, with the roles of the various players finely etched into careers of practice. In large measure, this is true. Yet in very important respects, the foundation of medical care for injured workers is fragile or unstable. Persistent challenges exist for clinical practice in evaluating and treating work injuries. In varying ways these challenges affect medical doctors, chiropractors, physical and occupational therapists, and clinic-based and worksite-based nurses.

This chapter explores four important dimensions of clinical practice within the workers compensation system: how clinicians evaluate the work causality of an injury or illness; how medical expertise for treating injured workers is defined; how managed care operates, with a focus on medical provider networks and use of treatment guidelines; and how permanent impairment is evaluated. For each of these dimensions problems have persisted over time.

ESTABLISHING MEDICAL CAUSALITY

At the bottom of every work injury or illness is an explicit finding by a medical professional that the condition is work-related, that is, it arose out of and in the course of work. Not very many clinicians who make these decisions have to defend their decisions to a skeptical audience. Their reasoning may be lazy and vital information to make a sound decision may not be available. The clinician, pressed for time, may rely on rules of thumb that oversimplify the issues. Often the personal attitude of the physician plays a significant role, especially in the realm of overuse or repetitive stress disorders. Some physicians view themselves as patient advocates, some as industry advocates.

But the clinician does not decide on causation in isolation. Her reasoning has to be harmonized with legal reasoning to arrive at a decision on causality ready for a workers' compensation court, if called upon, to review. Causality reasoning is a joint act of medicine and law, and can be rickety, arbitrary, and subject to strong biases.

In assessing the worker, the clinician is expected to take a complete medical history, study evidence of workplace exposure, conduct a clinical examination, and through differential diagnosis arrive at a decision on causality. Both a correct diagnosis must be made (20% of diagnosis in worker injuries may be in error) and causality must be established. The clinician must analyze the information based upon current medical literature and epidemiological data. She must consider if the condition is an aggravation or exacerbation of a prior condition, or the sole cause of the present medical condition.

Chris E. Stout, Matt Kruger and Jeffrey Rogers, (Eds)

With these impressions and information, the clinician is then expected to decide on causality according to a statutorily established threshold of confidence. Most jurisdictions have mandated one of the following thresholds: more probable than not, with reasonable degree of medical certainty, and with reasonable degree of medical probability.

Consider the difficulty of establishing causality when multiple factors play into the analysis, including prior work conditions and non work related health conditions, both of which a fresh work injury can aggravate to the extent that treatment of the fresh condition might not be effective unless these other conditions are treated.

The fragility of this form of medical reasoning is readily apparent when one considers the lack of formal training of many physicians in causality analysis, particularly for physicians outside occupational medicine practice. Written guidance that includes useful practical instruction is hard to come by. The American College of Occupational and Environmental Medicine (2008) is a source of training on causality analysis.

Where medical reasoning is poorly articulated and documented, it can lead to misadventures in legal reasoning where there is a legal dispute. Lawyers have already an inconsistent grasp on medical evidence. An example is provided by a Long Island, New York attorney specializing in workers compensation claims defense. He is experienced in disease claims, including asbestosis claims. New York State has precise requirements for proving the extent of disability from the pulmonary function tests, but few defense attorneys, or the claimants' attorneys, knew how to read or use the test results, according to him.

DEFINING MEDICAL EXPERTISE

There is no consensus in the medical community and among workers compensation professionals about what makes a clinician particularly proficient in treating injured workers.

At the 30,000 foot level, the expert is viewed as proficient in returning the injured workers back to maximum functional restoration at the earliest time, at the lowest cost, and with assistance provided to the employer for early return to work. But what does this operationally mean for the clinician? Absent a consensus, it is difficult to train clinicians to be proficient and difficult to agree how to select a clinician over others to treat an injury. And absence of consensus cripples any serious effort to align state laws to encourage the use of "better" clinicians.

One way to define expertise is to define the kind of errors which clinicians make in treating injured workers. A clinician who performs with no or virtually no errors might be deemed to be an expert.

Clinicians make three types of errors (Rousmaniere 2007). The first error type is a mistake in diagnosis or treatment. Workers compensation professionals such as adjusters recoil from the reality that serious mistakes occur often. But this is the dark side of medicine. The problem is created in part, but only in part, by changes in best practice and in the high level of specialization required. An example is the very inconsistent quality of electro-diagnostic tests. In part due to the relatively low cost of testing equipment, many clinicians are doing these tests. The level of training of testers is inconsistent. Roughly 40% of electro-diagnostic tests for wrist and hand conditions have been reported to be erroneous.

One of the most frequent serious clinical mistakes is what is called poor patient selection. Will this particular patient benefit or be harmed by spinal fusion, or pain treatment? A highly respected orthopedic surgeon in Boston, who has reviewed hundreds of proposed spinal fusions, estimates that half the time surgeons fail to take into account behavioral aspects of patients that forebode poor post-surgical prognosis.

The second error type is ineffective vocational assessment and counseling, including return to work planning and vocational coaching with the patient. Every time a clinician discusses possible treatment with an injured worker, that patient has a largely incoherent but momentous interior dialog about her or his work future. Fear of future pain is a strong predictor of delayed recovery. The clinician may effectively ignore the most important end result of treatment, which is not medical recovery but functional restoration and return to gainful employment.

The American College of Occupational and Environmental Medicine promotes the competences in vocational assessment and counseling through its various programs, including its initiative in preventing needless work disability.

The third error type runs through the other types errors but deserves it own label: co-morbidity misadventures. The majority of high cost claims involve organic (such as diabetes and cardiovascular conditions) or psychological (such as depression) problems along with the primary diagnosis. Co-morbidities crush coping capacity and sharply reduce recovery odds. Co-morbidities, particularly if left unaddressed, are associated with very high healthcare utilization. Depression and smoking are strongly associated with chronic pain and even early childhood sexual abuse has been proposed as associated with chronic pain.

Perhaps medical expertise is hard to define because much of the clinician's work involves addressing the non-medical issues of patients. The medical community is expected to treat conditions which are only partly medical in nature, and in reality include both medical issues and non-medical psychosocial predicaments of the injured workers. One noted hand surgeon in Boston was known to say that most carpal tunnel syndrome is located in the head.

Clinicians are also expected to be reasonably fluent in the language of claims adjusting. Examples of communication breakdowns include not explaining why a recommended treatment is medically necessary and related to the claim; not clearly defining work restrictions, and failing to provide medical reports in a timely manner. It is worth noting that with the exception of Washington State, no state provides encouragement or mandates to payers to compensate clinicians for these special communications.

However expertise is defined – by competencies, avoidance of errors, training, certifications, etc. – the lack of consensus about expertise makes it difficult to find common ground about what the community of healthcare providers for injured workers should look like. Regulators and payers have not shown much commitment to seriously study and define expertise in clinical practice.

ADAPTING MANAGED CARE STRATEGIES

Managed care – strategies to influence the delivery of medical care – has evolved in the workers compensation field in response to two waves of rapid increases in the cost of claims, creating financial crises. The first, seminal wave occurred in the late 1980s and early 1990s; the second wave in the early 2000s.

Despite over twenty years' of experience in trying to "fix" medical care, there has never been a satisfactory resolution to a core challenge, which is how to arrange for medical care in a way that delivers appropriate functional recovery for patients at appropriate utilization and cost. Critics of regulatory and private sector practices have never failed to argue that regulators and insurers (which include third party administrators) are doing too little, or the wrong thing. Every spike in the cost of medical care has triggered declarations that a crisis is at hand. There have been plenty of spikes, sometimes with average medical cost per claim rising more than 10% from one year to the next.

The workers compensation community has not so much created managed care strategies as it has absorbed and adapted strategies that have been developed in the group health insurance community. The process, attenuated over years and now decades, can result in mal-adaptations. There is no reason to expect that a strategy used in the group health insurance community will be assured of success, partly because it may not have worked anyway in the original setting, partly because the unique demands of treating injured workers were not taken fully into account.

During the late 1980s, workers compensation claims costs were rising in many states. At the time many states tightly regulated the price of workers compensation insurance. Some of these states refused to pass on the rising claims in the form of insurance premium hikes. This was in a time when other industries such as airlines and telephone service had already been deregulated. Where premiums were allowed upwards, increases on rates of well over 10% a year for multiple years were not uncommon.

States responded to these financial trends in a headline-creating mode by enacting major changes in their workers compensation laws. Some states created publically sponsored insurance companies – state funds – to restore stability in the insurance markets and, as a second thought, to introduce a channel for innovative ideas in how to manage injury prevention and claims.

Out of this period of crisis arose several of the major innovations in managed care in workers compensation. Interestingly, the states which were the most innovative, which included Oregon, Massachusetts, and New Hampshire, also had relatively greater experience in managed care in the group health insurance community through high penetration of health maintenance organizations. At that time, HMOs appeared to possess the best ideas for preventive care and organization of medical care. It was logical to think that their ideas could be successfully borrowed.

One type of innovation was the medical reimbursement fee schedule. The rationale of fee schedules is not uniform, but at least appears to focus on containing medical costs at the unit of service level, and placing small payers on a level playing field with large payers, who presumably have greater negotiating power. Presently only six states remain without a fee schedule (Indiana, Iowa, Missouri, New Hampshire, New Jersey, and Virginia). Most fee schedules are expressly linked to Medicare fee schedules, and/or adjusted to match prevailing commercial insurance rates. These schedules ignore the unique demands placed on clinicians when they treat injured workers, and are an example of mal-adaptation. This problem is addressed more fully in another chapter.

MEDICAL PROVIDER NETWORKS

A principle innovation in the early 1990s was the medical provider network that restricts worker choice of provider. Oregon legislated an ambitious program; New Hampshire a more modest one; Massachusetts a nominal one. Other states followed suit in the mid 1990s. During the next financial crisis among insurers, in the late 1990s and early 2000s, more states showed interest. California, then by far the most costly state in terms of workers compensation premiums, enacted a law in 2004 which authorized the use of restricted networks. So did Texas at about that time.

As is the case in every aspect of workers compensation managed care, insurers and self-insured employers (represented by their third party administrators or self-administered), reacted variably to legislative mandates for restricted provider networks.

Provider network legislation incented the payer to recruit medical providers whom they deemed as superior into the network. But many payers failed, and continue to fail, to seize the opportunity. Rather, they use provider network legislation to seek to negotiate deeper insurance model for a provider network: one which encourages the most inclusive possible reimbursement discounts from medical providers. In effect, they made no sustained commitment to promote medical expertise. Many have been ready to use a group health recruitment approach and which ignores the special needs of workers compensation, such as provider competence to address vocational recovery issues.

On the other hand, some payers have sought to aggressively search for and recruit providers they deem superior in quality. And – this is particularly the case with large self insured employers – some have initiated the development of "quality" provider networks even where restricted network legislation was not in place. In other words, they began to design and use networks which the injured worker is encouraged to voluntarily use on the grounds of ease of access and perceived quality.

Careful studies of the effect of provider networks on quality of care and functional outcomes are rare. With extremely few exceptions, payers do not build up sufficient medical intelligence, either internally or in partnerships with outside parties, to monitor providers to document which were delivering superior results. The Workers Compensation Research Institute conducted some studies which showed that medical care within provider networks cost less; but it did not report whether functional recovery was any better, such as would be measured by duration of disability.

One recent study has documented the wide variance in proficiency among physicians to affect vocational outcomes and economize in medical expense. This study exists only because an insurer invested heavily in medical intelligence so that it would more deeply understand patterns of care. The Louisiana Workers Compensation Corporation in the 2003 partnered with a team of medical practitioners and researchers affiliated with Johns Hopkins University to refine its pre-existing provider network (Louisiana is a "worker choice" of provider state) and to analyze its claims performance.

Out of this partnership a study was published in 2010 (Bernacki et al 2010). The authors looked at claims that occurred over a five year period, from 1998 through 2002. They classified claims according to how they were initially valued. They made note of claims which migrated during the course of their lifetime from low to high reserves. And they isolated those doctors – 77 in number – who were responsible for at least five of these upwardly migrating claims. They tracked these doctors and compared them to hundreds of other doctors for all types of claims, for instance even those claims which were initially reserved and eventually closed for a low sum.

For most of the claims these 77 doctors touched, duration of disability was on average longer, in most case much longer, and medical expenses were much larger, sometimes by a factor of two or more. The greatest discrepancy was in the claims with initial low reserves. The high intensity doctors were far more likely to double or triple the costs of these claims.

In sum, less than 4% of treating doctors caused *entire* claims costs to the insurer to increase by 50% without any evidence that that this increase was due to higher medical severity of the cases they took on.

Until more payers and regulators undertake more studies at this proficiency, the rationale for provider networks as a vehicle for better outcomes will remain poorly documented.

TREATMENT GUIDELINES

Another important managed care initiative was the introduction of medical treatment guidelines. During the financial crisis of the late 1980s and early 1990s, some states began to draft treatment guidelines which, when applied through utilization review (another innovation of that period) were intended primarily to discourage treatment which was excessive and/or not based on carefully documented justification. Some states, such as Massachusetts and Colorado, launched task forces to promulgate their own guidelines.

The popularity of guidelines, either formally endorsed by states or applied through private sector initiative, grew after the second financial crisis of the late 1990s and early 2000s. The American College of Occupational and Environmental Medicine and the Official Disability Guidelines published competing versions in the mid 2000s. These and other published guidelines have been widely disseminated throughout the workers compensation community.

Guideline development is a continuous process of culling from the medical literature which itself produces upwards of several hundred journal articles a year that pertain to treatment of the most common work related conditions. Analysts identify a pertinent article, rate it on its quality, that is credibility; summarize it; and construct brief assessments of the level of literature endorsement for specific treatments, which range from surgical procedures to medication to physical therapy.

Guidelines have met their most challenging test of effectiveness in the subject of chronic pain. The two major publishers of guidelines, noted above, have issued publications which address specifically chronic pain related treatment.

In the latter part of the 2000s, medical cost inflation in workers compensation, which had been high for over a decade, continued to climb even as medical costs in the group health community appears to moderated and even as indemnity costs – compensation to the worker to make up for lost wages – rose modestly. As a result, medical costs as a percentage of total claims costs rose nationwide from about 40% of claims costs in 1990 to 60% in the late 2000s. In some states, medical costs are over 70% of total claims costs.

Most of the recent medical cost inflation can be attributed to chronic pain, in the form of steeply rising pharmacy costs and expensive pain-relieving surgery costs. It became not unusual for the expected lifetime costs of chronic pain patients to exceed well over $100,000 in projected drug costs and over $100,000 in surgical costs. Roughly half of total claims costs are associated with claims to which there is a chronic pain component.

This is the archetypal condition today when payers and medical providers wish to cite a condition that bedevils the field of caring for injured workers. To test the effectiveness of treatment guidelines, one can ask how effective they have been in the treatment of chronic pain.

Treatment guidelines have not proven very effective in encouraging best practice for chronic pain. Their lack of success can be traced to two weaknesses in the proposition that guidelines can improve quality of care. One weakness is that while guidelines may be strong in illuminating the clinical rationale for and against a kind of treatment, they are relatively silent on the matter of the question of whether and how to treat based on the behavioral profile of the patient.

Obesity, smoking and depression are signs that a patient is at risk of benefiting from certain treatments such as, for example, lumbar fusion surgery, which is a popular form of surgery. The guidelines do not explicitly guide the clinician through steps to determine prognosis based on behavioral signs. This absence may be attributable to the paucity of journal-based literature on behavioral risk factors. In any event, many workers with these signs receive treatment when they probably should not. Half of lumbar fusion surgeries have been estimated to be inappropriate due to these signs.

A second weakness of treatment guidelines is that payers have been selective about which provisions in treatment guidelines for chronic pain they elect to adhere to. They have often been unwilling to comply with the guidelines where the guidelines indicate initiative by the payer. The payer has the discretion to promote the most effective, less risky care, yet the payer often does not.

How does this happen? Treatment chronic pain can be categorized as medication, non-conservative care which includes injections and surgery, and conservative care such as exercise and counseling. Pain medication for long term treatment almost always involved opioid drugs, such as Oxycontin, which are expensive and bring a risk of inadvertent of deliberate misuse that can result in addiction and even death (roughly 100 injured workers a year die from use of opioids). Opioid medication is difficult for many patients to manage side effects. Surgery and injections are associated with high costs and questionable outcomes. Conservative care is inexpensive and imposes no risk of complications or side effects.

But payer claims staffs often hold deep rooted, even culturally-based, skepticism about conservative care, and they often refuse to pay for treatment. This irony is the more disconcerting in that chronic pain treatment guidelines tend to promote conservative care, the effectiveness of which has been studied and documented for over 30 years.

Payers often refuse to pay for smoking cessation programs for opioid recipients who are addicted to smoking, despite evidence that smoking is associated with becoming dependent on opioids and that smoking is very prevalent among long term opioid patients.

Payers have also resisted addressing patient safety by ordering urine drug tests of patients on long term opioid treatment although these tests are recommended by guidelines and strongly endorsed by medical professional organizations concerned about misuse of drugs. Some 40% of long term opioid patients are typically found to be not adhering to prescribed drug regimes.

In sum, whether through gaps in treatment guidelines, or reluctance of payers to promote them fully, guidelines have not delivered on their promise to set medical care right.

PERMANENT IMPAIRMENT EVALUATIONS

One of the key roles of physicians in medical care for injured workers is rendering estimates of the degree of permanent impairment of the worker. The process by which an "impairment rating" is established is labyrinthine and controversial. Dispute repeated attempts to find a protocol which meets the approval of all parties, impairment ratings remain an unsettled area of clinical practice.

The American Medical Association has published six editions of the "AMA Guides to the Evaluation of Permanent Impairment." The AMA has published guides since 1958. Today, 26 states formally recognize one edition (from the 3rd in through the 6th) as sole protocol for impairment measurement.

In 2008, the AMA published its 6th edition of its guides. This edition strives to make the protocol more logical and less subject to inter-rater variability, which has been a problem with prior editions. Some 80% of impairment ratings have been estimated to be inaccurate. The steps to apply the new edition are as follows: confirm the medical diagnosis specifically related to the work injury; take a clinical history; do a physical exam; perform objective tests; reference clinical studies; and document patient functional history (Rousmaniere 2008). Then the rater uses, step by step, a methodology to arrive at a specific numerical rating.

The reception by the workers compensation community to the 6th edition has been mixed. Claimant bar has assiduously tried, with some success, to convince states to postpone the latest edition or to outright reject it. Its concerns include the somewhat correct perception that the new edition tends to deliver lower impairment scores. Lower scores lead to lower permanent disability awards and smaller settlements.

Advocates for the new edition believe that the edition more fairly takes into account improvements in surgery (such as knee surgery, due to microsurgical techniques) which deliver much improved functional recovery. The 5th edition had said that surgeries were cited as an indication of higher, not lower, impairment. Advocates believe that the methodology is relatively straightforward to learn; critics argue that the learning process is disruptive.

Today, several years after its publication in 2007, the new impairment guide remains mired in dispute.

CONCLUSION

This chapter addresses persistent problems in clinical practice in occupational medicine. These are not the only problems; a fuller examination will treat the torturous handling of many occupational diseases in the workers compensation systems of states. Nonetheless, they show the unsettled, often fragile nature of practice standards and adherence to these standards.

A theme which runs through these problems is the chronically low investment by the workers compensation system in medical intelligence. This under-investment is particularly noticeable among insurers, many of whom can afford the investment and would presumably gain economically by knowing more about the treatments that make up now 60% of their claims payments.

The following initiatives are examples of greater investment in medical intelligence:

- Engaging medical directors who are respected within the pertinent healthcare service CHANGE SERVICE TO MARKET
- Enhancing the influence of medical directors in claims operations
- Developing provider networks with an eye to expertise of the providers.
- Focusing on reducing medical errors.
- Compensating clinicians to recognize their special investment in expertise and practice time for occupational injuries.
- More in-depth analysis of clinical performance.

National healthcare reform, with its emphasis of comparative medical effectiveness research, may spur state legislatures, workers compensation regulators and payers to pay more attention to the quality of clinical practice. Thus healthcare reform, while not expressly addressing workers compensation, may exert a welcome impact.

REFERENCES

American College of Occupational and Environmental Medicine 2008, *Musculoskeletal Exam and Treatment Techniques,* viewed 13 May 2010, http://www.acoem.org/uploadedFiles/Continuing_Education/Courses/Musculoskeletal%20Course%20Details.pdf.

Bernacki, EJ, Tao, X, Yuspeh, L 2010, 'The impact of cost intensive physicians on workers compensation', *Journal of Occupational and Environmental Medicine,* vol. 52, no. 1, pp. 22-28.

Bureau of Labor Statistics, US Department of Labor 2009, *Workplace Injuries and Illnesses – 2008,* viewed 13 May 2010, http://www.bls.gov/iif/oshwc/osh/os/osnr0032.txt.

Rousmaniere P 2007, 'Fixing compensation by fixing errors', *Risk & Insurance,* 1 June.

Rousmaniere, P 2008, 'New edition, new controversy', *Risk & Insurance,* 1 June, viewed 13 May 2010, http://www.riskandinsurance.com/story.jsp?storyId=97683655&query=New%20edition,%20new%20controversy.

Rousmaniere, P In Press, 'When workers fail to claim', *Risk & Insurance.*

CHAPTER 17

How Medical Practice Patterns Vary for Low Back Conditions

Dongchun Wang[1], Kathryn L. Mueller[2], MD, MPH, FACOEM, Dean Hashimoto[3], JD, MD, Sharon Belton[4], PhD and Richard A. Victor*, JD, PhD

*[1]Workers Compensation Research Institute; [2]Professor, Department of Emergency Medicine, School of Public Health, University of Colorado at Denver; [3]Partners HealthCare System and Boston College Law School; [4]Workers Compensation Research Institute and *Workers Compensation Research Institute; E-mail: rvictor@wcrinet.org*

Abstract: Back pain is a common source of disability, both from work-related injuries and from injuries that occur outside the workplace. Annually in the United States, over $15 billion is spent for the treatment of low back pain and disorders, and approximately 15 percent of the costs in workers' compensation medical care are for low back pain cases. This study focuses on care provided or directed by physicians and addresses the following questions: What are the patterns of medical care for workers with common low back conditions in the 16 states studied? How do these patterns vary across states? How do the patterns of medical practice in the study states compare with evidence-based treatment guideline recommendations? Overall, we found that workers with similar low back conditions received very different care, depending on the state. These interstate differences were most noticeable for cases with nonspecific low back pain in the areas of diagnostic services and pain management injections. For disc cases, the interstate differences were most notable in the utilization of nerve testing, pain management injections, back surgery, and physical medicine. Large interstate differences in the timing of care were also seen for both types of low back conditions.

INTRODUCTION

This chapter summaries the results of a study that found large interstate variations in the utilization patterns of medical care for work-related common low back conditions among 16 states (Wang *et al.*, 2008).[1] The study also identified medical practice patterns that deviated from evidence-based treatment guidelines. This chapter highlights the types of care involved and the states where those patterns occurred. It raises, but does not answer, important questions about the appropriateness of such differences across the states and relative to medical practice standards.

Back pain is a common source of disability in the United States, both inside and outside the workplace. Annually Americans spend more than $15 billion to treat low back pain and disorders (Light, 2005), and roughly 15 percent of the costs in workers' compensation medical care are for low back pain cases.[2]

A long tradition of studies has documented the geographic variations in medical practice and has raised concerns about the appropriateness and cost-effectiveness of such variations in care for individuals with similar conditions. Wennberg and his colleagues at Dartmouth have published numerous articles dating back to the early 1970s that document area variations in medical practice in Medicare and group health populations, raising questions about the appropriateness of care in areas outside expected norms (Dartmouth Atlas Project, 2007). Eccleston and her colleagues (2007) found large interstate variations in the costs and utilization of medical services in workers' compensation medical care.

This chapter focuses on two common low back pain conditions: (1) disc disorders with or without radiculopathy and (2) nonspecific low back pain. One might think that two workers with similar medical conditions would receive similar care, regardless of what state each lives in. This study shows that it is often not the case. By highlighting differences across states in the types of medical care provided to workers with work-related low back conditions, the study should be useful to health care providers seeking to improve care for injured workers, to payors looking for

[1] The 16 states are Arkansas, California, Connecticut, Florida, Georgia, Illinois, Indiana, Louisiana, Maryland, Massachusetts, Michigan, North Carolina, Pennsylvania, Tennessee, Texas, and Wisconsin. The 16 states represent approximately 60 percent of the medical benefits paid nationally during the study period.

[2] The figure is estimated based on the Workers Compensation Research Institute's Detailed Benchmarking/Evaluation database for the 16 states in this study. The low back pain cases considered in the estimation are the low back injuries with or without more-serious medical conditions.

Chris E. Stout, Matt Kruger and Jeffrey Rogers, (Eds)

norms for appropriate care, and to policymakers searching for opportunities to improve care for injured workers and reduce costs to employers.

OBJECTIVES AND SCOPE OF THE STUDY

This study addressed the following questions:

- What patterns of medical care are observed for common low back conditions?
- How do the patterns vary across states? In which states are the patterns of care typical, and in which states do they substantially deviate from an observed norm?
- How do the patterns of medical practice in the states compare with evidence-based guideline recommendations?

In conducting this study, we focused on care provided or directed by physicians. Care provided by chiropractors was excluded from the study. Another Workers Compensation Research Institute (WCRI) study provides some information on interstate variations in chiropractic care (Eccleston, Petrova, and Zhao, 2007), and future studies may further examine interstate variations in chiropractic care for common low back conditions.

DATA AND APPROACH

The WCRI Detailed Benchmarking/Evaluation database was the source of data for this study. From that database, we selected claims with more than seven days of lost time that had injuries occurring from late 1999 to early 2003 and received medical care through early 2004. Among these claims, we identified 81,243 cases that had common low back conditions and received care provided or directed by physicians.[3] Those cases accounted for 9.8 percent of the claims with more than seven days of lost time in the 16 study states, representing 7.1 percent of the total medical payments. The detailed medical billing data associated with the low back claims were used to capture medical services during the first year of treatment.[4]

We focused on two groups of specific low back conditions: (1) disc disorders with or without radiculopathy (referred to as disc cases throughout the chapter) and (2) nonspecific low back pain. The disc category includes cases with diagnoses of disc herniations or other disc disorders that may or may not have symptoms of sciatica or lumbosacral neuritis and radiculitis. A small percentage of disc cases may have had degenerative disc conditions that coexist with radiculopathy and/or disc herniations. The nonspecific low back pain category includes cases with sprains and strains of the lumbar and sacroiliac regions, lumbago or low back pain, and unspecified backache. Neither the disc nor the nonspecific low back category includes cases with any "red flag" conditions recorded in the bills, such as tumors, infectious diseases, fractures or dislocations, or spinal cord injuries. Because we classified the low back categories based on the diagnoses assigned and billed by the treating providers in the medical bills, one important limitation for the study is that the categories are not perfectly homogeneous, especially for the category of disc disorders with or without radiculopathy. To ensure the credibility of the key findings, we took a more conservative approach in analyzing the results and performed the sensitivity analysis taking into account the potential impact of classification issues on the comparative results.

For each group of low back cases, we examined the patterns of medical practice with respect to the use, timing, and intensity of specific services like X rays, magnetic resonance imaging (MRI), nerve testing, pain management injections, spine surgery, and physical medicine. For physical medicine services, we focused on patterns of physical medicine care, including passive modalities and active therapy provided by physical therapists or physicians, not by chiropractors.

Comparisons of medical practice patterns and the recommendations of evidence-based treatment guidelines focused on the use and early timing of certain types of services for common low back conditions. For comparison purposes, we

---

[3] We excluded from the analysis any case that ever involved the care of a chiropractor to more accurately capture interstate variations in practice patterns of care among physicians.

[4] We tested the sensitivity of those results using 12 months of care rather than a longer period, especially for surgery. Although a longer period involved somewhat more care, we found that the interstate variations were consistent.

selected several widely accepted evidence-based treatment guidelines in accordance with the Appraisal of Guidelines for Research and Evaluation methodology (AGREE Collaboration, 2001): the American College of Occupational and Environmental Medicine (ACOEM) guidelines (Glass and Harris, 2004); the European spine guidelines (Airaksinen *et al.*, 2006; Van Tulder *et al.*, 2006); Cochrane reviews (Cochrane Collaboration, various years); and the *British Medical Journal* clinical evidence (British Medical Journal Publishing Group, 2007). Of those guidelines, the ACOEM guidelines specifically address work-related injuries; the others have applicability to back conditions in general but do not distinguish between work- and non-work-related injuries. One might question the relevance of using the broader set of guidelines to assess the patterns of medical care for work-related low back conditions, given that workers receiving workers' compensation benefits might have unique characteristics and that some goals of workers' compensation systems, such as return to work, might be achieved through different care. While we recognize this point of view, we believe that the selected guidelines provide an evidence base for more effective care regardless of the payor source, and they should apply to medical care provided to patients receiving workers' compensation benefits. We also recognize that there is a paucity of available studies on whether certain patterns of care (e.g., early MRIs) lead to better outcomes in the context of workers' compensation. This study was primarily aimed at describing what the existing patterns of treatments are and how those patterns compared to existing evidence-based treatment guidelines. Our work was foundational, and future research is needed to determine whether better outcomes can be achieved by some treatment patterns that appear to deviate from these treatment guidelines.

The period for this study is important, especially for California, Florida, Tennessee, and Texas, where major reforms have been undertaken in recent years. Because the current systems in those states are influenced by the reforms and the processes that affect medical care delivery, the results presented in this study, which are largely or entirely pre-reform, may provide a baseline for monitoring relevant aspects of reforms.

The 16 states included in our analysis are those for which the DBE database has representative data. They are geographically diverse and represent differences in fee schedules, choice of provider, and other key aspects of workers' compensation systems. Some of the states have high cost and high utilization, whereas others do not. The claims in our sample represent 22–40 percent of the claims in each of the 16 states over the study period, covering voluntary and residual markets, the self-insured market, and state funds when applicable.

MAJOR FINDINGS

Overall, we found that workers with similar low back conditions received very different patterns of care depending on the state. The interstate differences were most notable for cases with nonspecific low back pain in the areas of nerve testing, pain management injections, and physical medicine. For the disc cases, the interstate variations were most notable in the utilization of surgery, nerve testing, pain management injections, and physical medicine. In addition, we observed large interstate differences in the timing of care for both types of low back conditions.

We also found a number of areas of medical practice in a number of states where care delivered was often inconsistent with recommendations from evidence-based treatment guidelines. The inconsistencies were particularly evident in the rate of use and the early use of radiology services (X rays and MRIs) for cases with nonspecific low back pain and the early use of these same radiology services for disc cases. The early use of injections and surgery in some states was also inconsistent with the recommendations in evidence-based treatment guidelines.

In the next two sections, we discuss the major findings separately for nonspecific low back pain and disc cases. Tables **1** and **2** summarize the extent of interstate variations in medical practice patterns. The last column of each table shows which practice patterns were compared to the recommendations of evidence-based treatment guidelines.

Nonspecific Low Back Pain Cases

Diagnostic Radiology

The use of MRIs among nonspecific low back pain cases was more frequent than what evidence-based treatment guidelines generally recommend. Nearly twofold variation was seen among the 16 states in the percent of cases that had MRIs, ranging from 23 percent to 43 percent. Fewer cases received MRIs in Connecticut, Maryland, Massachusetts, and Wisconsin (23–24 percent), but more in Arkansas, pre-reform Florida, Louisiana,

North Carolina, pre-reform Tennessee, and pre-reform Texas (35–43 percent). When MRIs were provided, they were more likely to be performed early (within four weeks of injury) in Arkansas, Illinois, Pennsylvania, and Wisconsin (45–52 percent of first MRIs compared with the typical range of 27–43 percent among the 16 states). Evidence-based treatment guidelines do not recommend MRIs for nonspecific low back pain, especially not in the first four weeks of conservative care. Thus, the more frequent use of MRIs observed appears to be inconsistent with the guideline recommendations. In Louisiana, 9 percent of nonspecific low back cases had multiple MRIs, much higher than the median of the 16 states (2 percent).

Table 1: Interstate Variations in Utilization Patterns of Medical Services for Disc Cases[a]

	% of Cases with X rays	**% of Cases with X rays that Had First X ray within 4 Weeks Postinjury**	**% of Cases with 2+ Visits for X rays**	**% of Cases with MRIs**	**% of Cases with MRIs that Had First MRI within 4 Weeks Postinjury**	**% of Cases with 2+ Visits for MRI**
Arkansas					++	++
California[b]					– –	–
Connecticut			–			
Florida[b]						
Georgia						
Illinois					++	
Indiana						
Louisiana			+			+++
Maryland						
Massachusetts	–		– –			
Michigan						
North Carolina						+
Pennsylvania					++	
Tennessee[b]						
Texas[b]						– –
Wisconsin			–		+	
Minimum	57%	65%	15%	74%	22%	11%
25th Percentile	72%	70%	29%	78%	35%	17%
16-State Median	75%	72%	33%	82%	39%	19%
75th Percentile	81%	74%	37%	84%	47%	22%
Maximum	85%	77%	45%	90%	56%	32%
Compared to Guideline Recommendations		Yes			Yes	

Note: Included are 2000–2003 cases with more than 7 days of lost time that received medical care provided or directed by physicians during the first year of treatment. The utilization measures of physical medicine services reflect presurgical nonchiropractic practice patterns of physical medicine care.

[a] The disc cases include those with disc disorders that may or may not have symptoms of sciatica or lumbar neuritis and radiculitis. Those cases do not have an ICD-9 code indicating underlying red-flag conditions, such as tumors, infectious diseases, fractures, and dislocations. Although we excluded cases with the primary ICD-9 code indicating degenerative disc conditions, some cases included in the category may have such conditions that coexist with radiculopathy and/or disc herniations.

[b] Major reforms have been undertaken in recent years in California, Florida, Tennessee, and Texas. The results in this table are largely or entirely from the pre-reform period.

Key: ICD-9: International Classification of Diseases, 9th Revision; MRI: magnetic resonance imaging.

Minus signs and plus signs represent percent above or below the 16-state median for the value of a given measure in a state, as indicated.

– – –: More than 60 percent below. – –: 40–60 percent below. –: 20–40 percent below. Blank: Within 20 percent above or below median.

+: 20–40 percent above. ++: 40–60 percent above. +++: 60–80 percent above. ++++: More than 80 percent above.

Table 1: Interstate Variations in Utilization Patterns of Medical Services for Disc Cases[a] (continued)

	% of Cases with Nerve Testing	% of Cases that Received NCV Tests without EMGs	% of Cases with Nerve Testing that Had First Nerve Testing within 4 Weeks Postinjury	% of Cases with 2+ Visits for Nerve Testing	% of Cases with Injections	% of Cases with Injections that Had First Injection within 4 Weeks Postinjury	% of Cases with Injections that Had Injections Initiated after 6 Months Postinjury	% of Cases with 4+ Visits for Injections
Arkansas	–	++		–		++		
California[b]	+	++	– – –	++		– – –	+++	–
Connecticut	– –	+++	++	– – –	–		+	– – –
Florida[b]		+++	– – –	+		– – –	++	+
Georgia		++	– – –	–	+			++
Illinois			++++	+		+++	–	+
Indiana	–	– – –	+	– –	+	++++	– – –	
Louisiana		– –	– – –	++		–		
Maryland	+		++			–	+	+
Massachusetts	–		–	– – –	–	– –	+++	– – –
Michigan	++	– – –	++	++++	–			
North Carolina	–		– –	–		–		
Pennsylvania	+	– –		+++		+		+
Tennessee[b]	–	– – –					–	–
Texas[b]	++	++++		++++		– –	+	
Wisconsin		–	++++			++++	– –	+
Minimum	10%	0%	2%	1%	31%	4%	5%	2%
25th Percentile	17%	3%	4%	1%	41%	6%	14%	5%
16-State Median	21%	5%	8%	2%	47%	9%	17%	6%
75th Percentile	26%	8%	11%	3%	50%	12%	22%	7%
Maximum	32%	13%	16%	5%	62%	23%	29%	9%
Compared to Guideline Recommendations	Yes	Yes	Yes		Yes	Yes		

Note: Included are 2000–2003 cases with more than 7 days of lost time that received medical care provided or directed by physicians during the first year of treatment. The utilization measures of physical medicine services reflect presurgical nonchiropractic practice patterns of physical medicine care.

[a] The disc cases include those with disc disorders that may or may not have symptoms of sciatica or lumbar neuritis and radiculitis. Those cases do not have an ICD-9 code indicating underlying red-flag conditions, such as tumors, infectious diseases, fractures, and dislocations. Although we excluded cases with the primary ICD-9 code indicating degenerative disc conditions, some cases included in the category may have such conditions that coexist with radiculopathy and/or disc herniations.

[b] Major reforms have been undertaken in recent years in California, Florida, Tennessee, and Texas. The results in this table are largely or entirely from the pre-reform period.

Key: EMG: electromyography; ICD-9: International Classification of Diseases, 9th Revision; NCV: nerve conduction velocity.

Minus signs and plus signs represent percent above or below the 16-state median for the value of a given measure in a state, as indicated.

– – –: More than 60 percent below. – –: 40–60 percent below. –: 20–40 percent below. Blank: Within 20 percent above or below median.

+: 20–40 percent above. ++: 40–60 percent above. +++: 60–80 percent above. ++++: More than 80 percent above.

Table 1: Interstate Variations in Utilization Patterns of Medical Services for Disc Cases[a] (continued)

	% of Cases with Surgery	% of Cases with Surgery that Had Surgery Done within 6 Weeks Postinjury	% of Cases with Surgery that Had Surgery Done after 9 Months Postinjury	% of Cases with 2+ Surgical Visits	% of Cases with Physical Medicine	Median # of Days from Injury to 1st Physical Medicine Visit	Median # of Physical Medicine Visits	Ratio of Passive Modalities to Active Therapy
Arkansas	+	++	– –	+			–	++++

California[b]	– –	–	++++	– –			++++	++++
Connecticut				–		–		
Florida[b]	–	– –	++++			+	–	–
Georgia		–	+	+				– –
Illinois						–		
Indiana	+	–	–					–
Louisiana		–	++++			+	+	+
Maryland		– –	++					
Massachusetts						+		
Michigan								
North Carolina	+	+		+++		+	–	–
Pennsylvania			+	–		–	+	– –
Tennessee[b]	++		–	++++			– –	
Texas[b]	–	– –	++++	– –			+	
Wisconsin		+	–	++		–		
Minimum	17%	7%	4%	1%	68%	14	8	0.6
25th Percentile	25%	9%	5%	2%	73%	16	10	0.8
16-State Median	29%	13%	7%	2%	80%	19	12	1.1
75th Percentile	34%	15%	11%	3%	82%	22	13	1.2
Maximum	45%	19%	21%	5%	91%	26	19	2.0
Compared to Guideline Recommendations		Yes						Yes

Note: Included are 2000–2003 cases with more than 7 days of lost time that received medical care provided or directed by physicians during the first year of treatment. The utilization measures of physical medicine services reflect presurgical nonchiropractic practice patterns of physical medicine care.

[a] The disc cases include those with disc disorders that may or may not have symptoms of sciatica or lumbar neuritis and radiculitis. Those cases do not have an ICD-9 code indicating underlying red-flag conditions, such as tumors, infectious diseases, fractures, and dislocations. Although we excluded cases with the primary ICD-9 code indicating degenerative disc conditions, some cases included in the category may have such conditions that coexist with radiculopathy and/or disc herniations.

[b] Major reforms have been undertaken in recent years in California, Florida, Tennessee, and Texas. The results in this table are largely or entirely from the pre-reform period.

Key: ICD-9: International Classification of Diseases, 9th Revision.

Minus signs and plus signs represent percent above or below the 16-state median for the value of a given measure in a state, as indicated.

– – –: More than 60 percent below. – –: 40–60 percent below. –: 20–40 percent below. Blank: Within 20 percent above or below median.

+: 20–40 percent above. ++: 40–60 percent above. +++: 60–80 percent above. ++++: More than 80 percent above.

Table 2: Interstate Variations in Utilization Patterns of Medical Services for Nonspecific Low Back Pain Cases[a]

	% of Cases with X rays	**% of Cases with X rays that Had First X ray within 4 Weeks Postinjury**	**% of Cases with 2+ Visits for X rays**	**% of Cases with MRIs**	**% of Cases with MRIs that Had First MRI within 4 weeks Postinjury**	**% of Cases with 2+ Visits for MRI**
Arkansas				+	++	++++
California[b]			+		– –	
Connecticut	–		– –	–	–	– –
Florida[b]			+++	+		++
Georgia			++			
Illinois					+	
Indiana			–		+	
Louisiana	+		++++	+		++++

Maryland				–		
Massachusetts	–		– – –	–	–	– –
Michigan						
North Carolina			++			++
Pennsylvania			–		++	
Tennessee[b]			+++	+		
Texas[b]			+			
Wisconsin	–		– –	–	++	–
Minimum	42%	78%	4%	23%	13%	1%
25th Percentile	53%	84%	8%	28%	27%	2%
16-State Median	64%	86%	11%	32%	33%	2%
75th Percentile	70%	88%	16%	38%	43%	3%
Maximum	77%	91%	26%	43%	52%	9%
Compared to Guideline Recommendations	Yes	Yes		Yes	Yes	

Note: Included are 2000–2003 cases with more than 7 days of lost time that received medical care provided or directed by physicians during the first year of treatment. The utilization measures of physical medicine services reflect presurgical nonchiropractic practice patterns of physical medicine care.

[a] The nonspecific low back pain cases include cases with sprains and strains of the lumbar and sacroiliac regions, lumbago or low back pain, and unspecified backache. A small percentage of those cases may have had radicular findings that were in the doctor's notes but not assigned to the bills by treating providers. We excluded cases with underlying red-flag conditions.

[b] Major reforms have been undertaken in recent years in California, Florida, Tennessee, and Texas. The results in this table are largely or entirely from the pre-reform period.

Key: MRI: magnetic resonance imaging.

Minus signs and plus signs represent percent above or below the 16-state median for the value of a given measure in a state, as indicated.

– – –: More than 60 percent below. – –: 40–60 percent below. –: 20–40 percent below. Blank: Within 20 percent above or below median.

+: 20–40 percent above. ++: 40–60 percent above. +++: 60–80 percent above. ++++: More than 80 percent above.

Table 2: Interstate Variations in Utilization Patterns of Medical Services for Nonspecific Low Back Pain Cases[a] (continued)

	% of Cases with Nerve Testing	% of Cases that Received NCV Tests without EMGs	% of Cases with Injections	% of Cases with Surgery	% of Cases with Physical Medicine	Median # of Days from Injury to First Physical Medicine Visit	Median # of Physical Medicine Visits	Ratio of Passive Modalities to Active Therapy
Arkansas		–	–	++++				++
California[b]	++	++	–	– –				+++
Connecticut	– – –	++	– –	– –				
Florida[b]	+	+	+			+++	–	–
Georgia			+	++			–	–
Illinois		+						
Indiana	–	– – –	++	++				–
Louisiana	++++	– – –	+	++++		++		+
Maryland				–				+
Massachusetts	– –	– –	– –	– – –		++		
Michigan	++++	– – –		++++				
North Carolina		+	+	++++		++		–
Pennsylvania	+	– –	–					– –
Tennessee[b]			++	++++		+		
Texas[b]	++++	++++		–				
Wisconsin	–						–	

Minimum	2%	0%	3%	0.2%	65%	9	6	0.6
25th Percentile	4%	4%	6%	1%	73%	11	7	0.7
16-State Median	4%	9%	7%	1%	77%	11	8	1.0
75th Percentile	6%	12%	9%	3%	80%	15	8	1.1
Maximum	12%	17%	11%	4%	82%	19	9	1.7
Compared to Guideline Recommendations	Yes	Yes	Yes					Yes

Note: Included are 2000–2003 cases with more than 7 days of lost time that received medical care provided or directed by physicians during the first year of treatment. The utilization measures of physical medicine services reflect presurgical nonchiropractic practice patterns of physical medicine care.

[a] The nonspecific low back pain cases include cases with sprains and strains of the lumbar and sacroiliac regions, lumbago or low back pain, and unspecified backache. A small percentage of those cases may have had radicular findings that were in the doctor's notes but not assigned to the bills by treating providers. We excluded cases with underlying red-flag conditions.

[b] Major reforms have been undertaken in recent years in California, Florida, Tennessee, and Texas. The results in this table are largely or entirely from the pre-reform period.

Key: EMG: electromyography; NCV: nerve conduction velocity.

Minus signs and plus signs represent percent above or below the 16-state median for the value of a given measure in a state, as indicated.

– – –: More than 60 percent below. – –: 40–60 percent below. –: 20–40 percent below. Blank: Within 20 percent above or below median.

+: 20–40 percent above. ++: 40–60 percent above. +++: 60–80 percent above. ++++: More than 80 percent above.

X rays were used more often and earlier than recommended by evidence-based treatment guidelines for nonspecific low back pain cases. Among the 16 study states, between 42 percent and 77 percent of nonspecific low back pain cases received X rays, with Connecticut, Massachusetts, and Wisconsin at the lower end (42–48 percent). When X rays were provided, they were usually provided at the beginning of care; half of the cases with X rays had the first X ray within one week postinjury. The median number of days from injury to first X ray ranged from four to eight days, and 78–91 percent of first X rays were performed within four weeks postinjury. Evidence-based treatment guidelines do not recommend X rays for nonspecific low back pain without serious underlying medical conditions, especially in the first four weeks of conservative care. Across all states, the use and early timing of X rays for nonspecific low back pain substantially departed from evidence-based treatment guidelines, even in the states with lower rates of use of the services.

Nerve Testing

Except in Louisiana, Michigan, and pre-reform Texas, nerve testing was not often used for nonspecific low back pain cases. In most states, only 2–6 percent of nonspecific low back pain cases had nerve testing. However, in Louisiana, Michigan, and pre-reform Texas, 9–12 percent of cases received nerve testing. Evidence-based treatment guidelines do not recommend nerve testing for nonspecific low back pain without suspected radicular conditions. The results in Louisiana, Michigan, and pre-reform Texas might be inconsistent with the evidence-based treatment guidelines.[5]

Pain Management Injections

Fewer workers with nonspecific low back pain in the two New England states received pain management injections; but more workers received injections in some southern states and Indiana. Approximately 6–8 percent of nonspecific low back pain cases received pain management injections in most states. Fewer workers received the injections in Connecticut and Massachusetts (3 percent) but more in pre-reform Florida, Georgia, Indiana, Louisiana, North Carolina, and pre-reform Tennessee (9–11 percent).[6]

Surgery

Surgery was rare for nonspecific low back pain cases but relatively more frequent in Arkansas, Louisiana, Michigan, North Carolina, and pre-reform Tennessee. In 9 of the 16 states, less than 2 percent of nonspecific low back pain cases had spine surgery during the first year of treatment. Surgery was done more frequently in

[5] We say this because a small percentage of cases in the nonspecific low back category might have had radicular findings in the doctors' notes.

[6] In the states with higher rates of injection, the use of injections for nonspecific low back pain may not be consistent with evidence-based treatment guidelines that do not recommend injections for such cases. However, some coding issues may contribute to the result.

Arkansas, Michigan, North Carolina, and pre-reform Tennessee (around 3 percent). At nearly 4 percent, Louisiana had the highest rate of surgery among the states for nonspecific low back pain.

Physical Medicine

Most workers with nonspecific low back pain received physical medicine treatment as part of conservative care. In most states, 72–82 percent of cases had physical medicine services provided by physical therapists or physicians. The percentage was somewhat lower in Arkansas and Massachusetts (65–67 percent). Remember that these are the cases with care directed by physicians, not chiropractors. Not surprisingly, the percentage of cases receiving physical medicine care in pre-reform California and pre-reform Texas, although the highest among the study states (82 percent), was not considerably different from the 16-state median (77 percent).[7]

Nonchiropractic physical medicine care was typically initiated within two weeks postinjury in most states; and the frequency of visits was similar across all states in the study. Among nonchiropractic physical medicine providers (mostly physical therapists), physical medicine services were typically initiated within 9 to 11 days postinjury. However, it took longer in pre-reform Florida (19 days for a typical case); Louisiana, Massachusetts, and North Carolina (16 to 17 days); and pre-reform Tennessee (14 days). Once the care began, workers with nonspecific low back pain typically had six to nine visits for such care in all states studied.

Passive modalities were used more often in some states than active therapy, especially in Arkansas and pre-reform California, which was not consistent with the evidence-based guidelines. In half of the states, workers with physical medicine care received more services for active therapy than passive modalities during the first year of treatment. Most states had an average of 6 to 11 passive modalities for every 10 active therapies. Passive modalities were used more often than active therapy in Arkansas and pre-reform California, where there were twice as many passive modalities as active therapies. Passive modalities were also used more frequently, relative to active therapy, in Louisiana, Maryland, and Massachusetts. Most evidence-based treatment guidelines recommend more active therapy for low back pain to help patients restore health and functioning, suggesting that passive modalities should be limited and performed at the acute stage of low back pain. Higher utilization of passive modalities in some states appears to be inconsistent with the evidence-based guidelines.

Disc Cases

Surgery

Workers with disc conditions in Arkansas and pre-reform Tennessee were twice or nearly three times as likely to get surgery as workers with such conditions in pre-reform California, pre-reform Florida, and pre-reform Texas. The percentage of disc cases with surgery was roughly in the range of 25–30 percent in 7 of the 16 states; lower in pre-reform California, pre-reform Florida, and pre-reform Texas (17–22 percent); and higher in Indiana (35 percent) and several southern states, including Arkansas, Georgia, Louisiana, North Carolina, and pre-reform Tennessee (33–45 percent). In Arkansas and pre-reform Tennessee, 40–45 percent of disc cases had spine surgery during the first year of treatment. No evidence-based treatment guidelines have provided clear recommendations either for or against surgery for cases with radiculopathy because of the lack of scientific evidence in the effectiveness of surgery. However, the large interstate difference in the rate of surgery needs to be further investigated.

Spinal fusions were infrequent in most states but were performed more often in Arkansas, Georgia, and Louisiana. In most states, fusions were performed in 1–5 percent of disc cases during the first year of treatment. In Georgia and Louisiana, 6–7 percent of disc cases had fusion performed during the first year of treatment.

Surgery was more likely to be performed early for disc cases in Arkansas, North Carolina, and Wisconsin but late in pre-reform California, pre-reform Florida, Louisiana, and pre-reform Texas. Among disc cases with surgery, less than 10 percent had surgery performed within six weeks postinjury in 7 of the 16 states. However, surgery was more

---

[7] In pre-reform California and pre-reform Texas, substantially more workers received physical medicine services by chiropractors, and the practice patterns of chiropractic care in those two states were substantially different from those in other states (Eccleston *et al.*, 2007).

likely to be performed early in Arkansas, North Carolina, and Wisconsin, where 18–19 percent of cases with surgery had the procedure within a six-week time frame. Surgery was also more likely to be early in Connecticut, Massachusetts, Michigan, Pennsylvania, and pre-reform Tennessee (14–15 percent of surgical cases). Among states where surgery was more likely to be performed early, the rate of surgery was higher in some states (Arkansas, North Carolina, and pre-reform Tennessee) but lower or typical in the other states listed. This suggests that in a state with a higher surgery rate, more cases that had surgery might have been marginal in terms of the need for surgery compared with a state with a lower or typical surgery rate, and some of these marginal cases not only had surgery but also had it early (within six weeks postinjury). Evidence-based treatment guidelines recommend considering surgical options only for patients with severe and persistent radicular symptoms after four to six weeks of conservative care. Based on our data, early surgery occurred more frequently in Arkansas, North Carolina, and pre-reform Tennessee, which appears to be inconsistent with the evidence-based treatment guidelines.

By contrast, 16–17 percent of disc cases with surgery had surgery performed after nine months postinjury in pre-reform California, pre-reform Florida, and pre-reform Texas. The figure was 21 percent in Louisiana, where the surgery rate was already higher than that of most states. More frequent late surgery raises questions about effectiveness of presurgical care, outcome of surgery, if done late, and resulting prolonged disability.

Diagnostic Radiology

MRIs were used early and often for disc cases in all states. Early MRIs, within four weeks postinjury, occurred substantially more frequently than what evidence-based treatment guidelines recommend. Among the 16 states, the percentage of disc cases that had MRIs ranged from 74 percent in Massachusetts to 90 percent in Arkansas. When provided, MRIs were more often performed early (within four weeks postinjury) in all states, especially in Arkansas, Illinois, Pennsylvania, and Wisconsin (51–56 percent of cases with MRIs). According to evidence-based treatment guidelines, MRIs may be useful in conjunction with other clinical findings for evaluation and diagnosis of disc disorders with suspected radiculopathy. However, evidence-based treatment guidelines do not recommend performing MRIs within the first four weeks of conservative care. Therefore, the more frequent early use of MRIs observed in many states studied was inconsistent with the evidence-based treatment guidelines.

X rays were also used early and often for disc cases in all states. The timing of X rays was often earlier than recommended in the evidence-based treatment guidelines. X rays were used in 69–85 percent of disc cases in all states except Massachusetts (57 percent). When provided, the services were performed early in all states: half of the cases with X rays had them within the first 6 to 15 days after the injury, and two-thirds to three-quarters had the first X ray within four weeks postinjury. Evidence-based treatment guidelines allow the use of X rays for cases with suspected radicular conditions but do not recommend X rays be performed during the first four weeks of conservative care. Our data show that early X rays occurred in 47–65 percent of disc cases in all states except Massachusetts (37 percent), which substantially deviates from evidence-based guideline recommendations. Multiple visits during which X rays were performed were also frequent in all states, with 25–45 percent of disc cases having two or more visits for X rays, except in Massachusetts (15 percent).

Nerve Testing

Nerve testing was used in fewer than a quarter of disc cases in most states but more frequently in pre-reform California, Michigan, Pennsylvania, and pre-reform Texas. The percentage of disc cases with nerve testing was between 20 percent and 26 percent in six study states, with the 16-state median of 21 percent. The figure was higher in Michigan (32 percent), pre-reform Texas (31 percent), Pennsylvania (28 percent), and pre-reform California (28 percent). Most cases with nerve testing had both electromyography (EMG) and nerve conduction velocity (NCV) tests. A small percentage of disc cases received NCV tests without EMGs, accounting for up to 2 percent of disc cases in all states in our study except pre-reform Texas (at 4 percent).[8]

Timing of nerve testing was earlier in Connecticut, Illinois, Michigan, and Wisconsin and later in pre-reform Florida, Georgia, Louisiana, Massachusetts, North Carolina, and pre-reform Tennessee. Nerve testing was more

[8] NCV testing without EMGs has not proven to be effective for evaluating cases with suspected radiculopathy. Evidence-based treatment guidelines do not recommend the use of such tests for evaluating and diagnosing disc disorders with radiculopathy. That was largely consistent with what we saw in the practice pattern of physicians.

likely to be performed early (within four weeks postinjury) in Connecticut, Illinois, Michigan, and Wisconsin (12–16 percent of cases with nerve testing) compared with the typical of 8 percent. Although evidence-based treatment guidelines do not recommend early nerve testing, we did not see clear evidence of inconsistency with the guidelines because early nerve testing occurred in only 4 percent or less of the disc cases in all states. In several states, nerve testing was more likely to be performed late, beyond six months postinjury. Those states include Massachusetts and the southern states of pre-reform Florida, Georgia, Louisiana, North Carolina, and pre-reform Tennessee.

Pain Management Injections

Workers with disc conditions in Georgia and Indiana were twice as likely to receive injections as workers in Connecticut and Massachusetts. The percentage of disc cases with injections was 40–50 percent in most states in our study. The figure was higher in Georgia and Indiana (59–62 percent), nearly double that in Connecticut and Massachusetts (31 percent). Some evidence-based treatment guidelines allow the use of injections for cases with radiculopathy but state that the effectiveness of injections is questionable or unknown. However, the large interstate difference in the rate of use of injections needs to be further investigated.

Workers who received injections were more likely to have them initiated early in Arkansas, Illinois, Indiana, and Wisconsin than in other states. Injections tended to be performed later in pre-reform California, pre-reform Florida, and Massachusetts. In most states, it was unusual for the first injection to occur within four weeks postinjury. Up to 10 percent of disc cases with injections had injections initiated that early in 11 of the 16 states. Injections were more likely to be initiated early in Wisconsin (23 percent of disc cases with injections), Illinois and Indiana (15–16 percent), and Arkansas (14 percent). Evidence-based treatment guidelines that allow the use of injections do not recommend performing the injections during the first four weeks of conservative care. By that standard, early injections might have been more frequent in some states than the evidence-based treatment guidelines recommend.

We also found that injections were performed later in pre-reform California, pre-reform Florida, and Massachusetts, where approximately one-third of disc cases with injections had the first injections after six months postinjury.

While most disc cases with injections had two or three visits for injections, some cases had four or more such visits, and four or more visits for injections occurred more frequently in Georgia, Illinois, Pennsylvania, and Wisconsin than in the other states studied. Although injections may be used repeatedly over time to reduce pain and facilitate therapeutic exercises for recovery, four or more visits for injections is considered to be indicative of possible overutilization of the service. Our data show that in most states we studied, more than 6 percent of disc cases had four or more visits for injections during the first year of treatment. The percentage was notably higher in Georgia, Illinois, Pennsylvania, and Wisconsin (8–9 percent). Connecticut and Massachusetts had only 2 percent of disc cases with four or more injections—a result of a lower rate of injections and less frequent multiple visits for injections.

Physical Medicine

Most workers with disc conditions used physical medicine services as part of conservative care. In most states, 79–86 percent of disc cases received physical medicine care provided by physical therapists or physicians. The percentage was somewhat lower in Arkansas, Massachusetts, Michigan, North Carolina, and pre-reform Tennessee (68–74 percent) and higher in pre-reform California (91 percent). In pre-reform Texas, the rate that physical medicine services were used among physical therapists and physicians, although among the highest (85 percent), was not dramatically different from that in most states in our study.[9]

Nonchiropractic physical medicine care was typically initiated within two to three weeks of injury but later in pre-reform Florida, Louisiana, Massachusetts, and North Carolina. The frequency of visits for nonchiropractic care was rather similar in most states but higher in pre-reform California. The median number of days from injury to first nonchiropractic physical medicine care was between 14 and 20 days in most states for disc cases but longer in pre-reform Florida, Louisiana, Massachusetts, and North Carolina (23 to 26 days).

---

[9] As mentioned earlier, substantially more workers in pre-reform California and pre-reform Texas received care from chiropractors, and the utilization patterns of chiropractic care in those two states were substantially different from those in other states (Eccleston *et al.*, 2007).

When receiving such care, workers typically made an average of 8 to 15 visits in all states except pre-reform California (19 visits).

Passive modalities were used more often than active therapy, especially in Arkansas and pre-reform California, which is inconsistent with the evidence-based treatment guidelines. In 6 of the 16 states, workers with disc conditions who had physical medicine received an average of 6 to 9 passive modalities for every 10 active therapies. Seven states had roughly the same number of services for each type. The utilization of passive modalities was notably higher relative to that of active therapy in Arkansas and pre-reform California, where a typical worker had 20 passive modalities for every 10 active therapies. Workers in Louisiana also received more passive modalities than active therapy compared with workers in the other study states. Most evidence-based treatment guidelines recommend limiting passive modalities and providing more active therapies for low back pain to help patients restore health and functioning. Higher utilization of passive modalities relative to physical therapy in Arkansas, pre-reform California, and Louisiana appears to be inconsistent with the evidence-based treatment guidelines.

IMPLICATIONS AND CONCLUSIONS

Medical care in workers' compensation represents a substantial opportunity for many state regulators to improve health care in a way that is consistent with a "win-win" approach from the perspective of employees, employers, payors, and providers. We say this because (1) this study found substantial interstate differences in the care delivered to workers with common low back condition, and (2) the study identified patterns of care received by injured workers that represent material departures from evidence-based treatment guideline principles. For several states where reforms have been undertaken in recent years, the results reported over the study period may serve as a baseline for monitoring relevant reforms.

Implications for Policymakers

In a number of states, some patterns of care delivered to injured workers (even where there is not substantial variability in clinical practices among the states) were not supported by evidence-based treatment guidelines. We made that observation especially in the rate of use and early use of diagnostic services (X rays and MRIs) for nonspecific low back pain cases and the early use of these same services for disc cases.

We also observed large interstate variations in medical practice in the areas of surgery and injections. For example, we found that for disc cases, the surgery rates were higher in Indiana and some southern states (Arkansas, Georgia, Louisiana, North Carolina, and pre-reform Tennessee) but lower in pre-reform California, pre-reform Florida, and pre-reform Texas. For workers with disc conditions who received surgical care, surgery was performed early in Arkansas, North Carolina, and pre-reform Tennessee and later in pre-reform California, pre-reform Florida, Louisiana, and pre-reform Texas.

Policymakers may better understand the strengths and weaknesses of their state's health care delivery system through comparisons with other states. We found low utilization patterns in Connecticut, Illinois, Indiana, Maryland, Massachusetts, and Wisconsin. In a few states, such as Louisiana, pre-reform Texas, and pre-reform California, we found strikingly high and unusual utilization patterns for some services.

Policymakers should examine how the economic incentives faced by providers in their states are shaping the substantial interstate variations in the medical care given to injured workers. Economic incentives can arise from state fee schedules and state laws about provider ownership and referral to provider-owned imaging and surgical facilities. The incentives may encourage the use of certain types of care or discourage the use of other types.

Implications for Clinicians

In general, this study shows that providers recognize the important clinical distinction between disc cases and cases with nonspecific low back pain. In all states, surgery is performed at a much lower rate for nonspecific low back pain. The study also shows empirically that substantially more MRIs, nerve testing, and injections were provided for disc cases than for cases with nonspecific low back pain. However, this study identified certain clinical utilization issues concerning the amount and timing of certain diagnostics and treatments.

The study shows practice norms for each state, and most importantly, for each of 16 larger states. Based on this study's descriptions of the care provided, clinicians may now compare their individual practice patterns with other providers in their state, as well as with other providers throughout the country. Although certain states in the study had similar utilization patterns, we observed some large practice differences among providers in certain states, and those differences may be educational for providers in those states.

For providers who administer pain medicine injections, it will become increasingly important to establish the clinical indications for utilization, including timing. The study found a substantial disparity among states in utilization and timing of injections for nonspecific low back conditions. For surgery, large differences occurred among states in terms of the amount and timing of surgery for disc conditions. In light of the diversity of practice patterns, it will become increasingly important to establish the clinical indications for surgery and the outcomes obtained by patients.

Implications for Payors

Because of the substantial variation in the pattern of medical services among states, insurers may have a substantial interest in developing relationships with individual providers and networks that are able to demonstrate cost-effective utilization patterns and good outcomes for injured workers. Better data on worker outcomes will be needed.

In an era of limited health care resources, identifying areas of overutilization can lead to potential opportunities for cost savings. For example, if the provider practices in a state with high utilization were to become comparable to those in states in the middle or low end of the range, that would represent a potential cost-saving opportunity in the high-utilization state. The high utilization patterns we found for certain states are striking and suggest opportunities for more-targeted utilization management activities. For instance, surgery rates were higher for disc conditions in Arkansas, Indiana, Michigan, North Carolina, and pre-reform Tennessee. Although few nonspecific low back pain cases had surgery, the surgery rates among those cases were higher in the same five states, with the highest rate of surgery in Louisiana (nearly 4 percent).

Louisiana had higher utilization of medical services for disc conditions and nonspecific low back pain, including X rays, MRIs, nerve testing, and injections. Conversely, several states had relatively low to medium utilization patterns, including Connecticut, Illinois, Indiana, Maryland, Massachusetts, and Wisconsin.

REFERENCES

AGREE Collaboration. Appraisal of guidelines for research and evaluation, AGREE instrument [document on the Internet]. 2001 [cited 2010 May 26]. Available from http://www.agreecollaboration.org/instrument/.

Airaksinen O, Brox J, Cedraschi, C, Hildebrandt, CJ, Klaber-Moffett, J, Kovacs, F, Mannion, AF, Reis, S, Staal, J, Ursin, BH, Zanoli, G 2006 'European guidelines for the management of chronic nonspecific low back pain', *European Spine Journal*, vol. 15 no. 2, pp. S192–S300.

British Medical Journal Publishing Group Summer 2007, *British Medical Journal clinical evidence*, London.

Cochrane Collaboration n.d., *Cochrane reviews* [document on the Internet], viewed 26 May 2010 http://www.cochrane.org/reviews/en/topics/51.html.

Dartmouth Atlas Project 2007, *The Dartmouth atlas of health care* [document on the Internet], viewed 26 May 2010 http://www.dartmouthatlas.org.

Eccleston S, Petrova P, Zhao X 2007, *The anatomy of workers' compensation medical costs and utilization,* 6th edn, 10 volume, Workers Compensation Research Institute, Cambridge, MA.

Glass LS, Harris JS (eds.) 2004, *Occupational medicine practice guidelines: Evaluation and management of common health problems and functional recovery of workers*, 2nd edn, American College of Occupational and Environmental Medicine, Elk Grove Village, IL.

Light, K 2005, *Right patient, right level, right operation*, San Francisco Spine Center, San Francisco, CA.

Van Tulder, M, Becker, A, Bekkering, T, Breen, A, Gil del Real, MT, Hutchinson, A, Koes, B, Laerum, E, Malmivaara, A 2006, 'European guidelines for the management of acute nonspecific low back pain in primary care', *European Spine Journal*, vol. 15, no. 2, pp. S169–S191.

Wang D, Mueller K, Hashimoto D, Belton, S, Zhao, X 2008 *Interstate variations in medical practice patterns for low back conditions*, Workers Compensation Research Institute, Cambridge, MA.

APTA
American Physical Therapy Association *

Appendix-A

Last Updated: 05/20/10
Contact: advocacy@apta.org

Workers' Compensation (WC) Resource Center State Information

AUTHRORITY/WC Home	CONTACT INFORMATION	NEWS/UPDATES	RESOURCES
Alabama **Department of Industrial Relations** **http://dir.alabama.gov/wc/**	**Alabama WC Directory** **http://dir.alabama.gov/wc/directory.aspx** **Phone numbers:** (334) 242-2868 or 1-800-528-5166 **Fax Numbers:** (334) 353-8262 -- Administrative/TPAs/Assessments/Self-Insurance/Education (334) 353-8228 -- Ombudsman/Drug Free/Medical (334) 353-0840 -- Claims (334) 353-8490 -- Compliance/Examiners		**Medical Section** **http://dir.alabama.gov/wc/Medical.aspx** **Utilization Management and Bill Screening** **http://dir.alabama.gov/wc/umbs.aspx** **Fee Schedules** **http://dir.alabama.gov/wc/FeeSchedules.aspx**
Alaska **Department of Labor and Workforce Development** ***Division of Workers' Compensation*** **http://labor.state.ak.us/wc/home.htm**	Phone: (907)-465-2790 Email Alaska DWC: workerscomp@alaska.gov	**Alaska WC News** **http://labor.state.ak.us/wc/home.htm** *Scroll down to "What's New"* **Alaska DWC Bulletins** **http://labor.state.ak.us/wc/bulletins.htm**	**Alaska Administrative Code: Title 8 Chapter 45 Section 82 – Medical Treatment** **http://www.legis.state.ak.us/basis/folioproxy.asp?url=http://wwwjnu01.legis.state.ak.us/cgi-bin/folioisa.dll/aac/query=%5bJUMP:'8+aac+45!2E082'%5d/doc/%7b@1%7d?firsthit** *See 8.45.082(i) for fee information* **Bulletin 09-06 Fees for Medical Treatment** **http://labor.state.ak.us/wc/bulletins/09-06.pdf** **Purchase Fee Schedule from Ingenix** **http://www.ingenix.com/**
Arizona **Industrial Commission** **http://www.ica.state.az.us/**	**Arizona WC Contacts** **http://www.ica.state.az.us/WorkersCompensation/WorkCmp_main.aspx** **Phone Numbers:** Phoenix: (602) 542-4661 Tucson: (520) 628-5181	**Arizona WC Home:** **http://www.ica.state.az.us/WorkersCompensation/WorkCmp_main.aspx**	**Physician's Fee Schedule** **http://www.ica.state.az.us/Director/DIR_FSSignUp.aspx**
Arkansas **Workers' Compensation Commission** **http://www.awcc.state.ar.us/**	**Arkansas WC Email Addresses** **http://www.awcc.state.ar.us/emailadd.html** *See: Medical Cost Containment Division*	**What's New at the Commission** **http://www.awcc.state.ar.us/news.html**	**Rule 099.30 Medical Cost Containment** **http://www.awcc.state.ar.us/ruleind.html** *Scroll down and select the rule*

	Telephone 1-501-682-3930 / 1-800-622-4472		*file* **Fee Schedule** **http://www.awcc.state.ar.us/ruleind.html** *Scroll down to Rule 099.30 and select (fee schedule)*
California **Division of Workers' Compensation** **http://www.dir.ca.gov/dwc/dwc_home_page.htm**	**California WC Contacts** **DWC Email Contacts** **http://www.dir.ca.gov/dwc/ContactDWC.htm** **Phone Numbers:** **http://www.dir.ca.gov/contactus.html** **Worker Hotline** (866) 924-9757 **Public information office** (415) 703-5070	**California WC Home** **http://www.dir.ca.gov/dwc/dwc_home_page.htm** *Scroll down to "What's New"*	**Medical Provider Page** **http://www.dir.ca.gov/dwc/MedicalProvider.htm** **Official Medical Fee Schedule** **http://www.dir.ca.gov/dwc/OMFS9904.htm**
Colorado **Division of Workers' Compensation** **http://www.colorado.gov/cs/Satellite/CDLE-WorkComp/CDLE/1240336932511**	**Colorado WC Contacts** **http://www.colorado.gov/cs/Satellite/CDLE-WorkComp/CDLE/1251567965675#wc** Phone (Main) (303) 318-8700 Fax (303) 318-8710 **Workers' Compensation** 633 17th Street, Suite 400 Denver, CO 80202 *In particular, Medical Cost Containment*	**What's new in the division of Workers' Compensation** **http://www.colorado.gov/cs/Satellite/CDLE-WorkComp/CDLE/1248095316832**	**Medical Providers Page** **http://www.colorado.gov/cs/Satellite/CDLE-WorkComp/CDLE/1248095316850** **Physical Medicine and Rehabilitation** **http://www.colorado.gov/cs/Satellite?c=Page&childpagename=CDLE-WorkComp%2FCDLELayout&cid=1251566954541&pagename=CDLEWrapper** **Rules of Procedure-General** **http://www.colorado.gov/cs/Satellite/CDLE-WorkComp/CDLE/1248095316862** **Medical Fee Schedule** **http://www.colorado.gov/cs/Satellite?c=Page&childpagename=CDLE-WorkComp%2FCDLELayout&cid=1251566953698&pagename=CDLEWrapper** **Medical Treatment Guidelines** **http://www.colorado.gov/cs/Satellite/CDLE-WorkComp/CDLE/1248095316866**
Connecticut **Workers' Compensation Commission** **http://wcc.state.ct.us/**	**Connecticut WC Email Contacts** **http://wcc.state.ct.us/email-contacts.htm** **Phone and Fax Contacts** **http://wcc.state.ct.us/wcc/wcc-offices.htm** **Fee Schedule Questions:** Marilou Lang 860-493-1559 Marilou.lang@ct.gov	**Subscribe to RSS news feed** **http://wcc.state.ct.us/rss/wcc-rss-news.htm** **News Page** **http://wcc.state.ct.us/news/news.htm**	**Fee Schedule Regulations** **http://wcc.state.ct.us/law/wc-regs/31-280-3.htm** Fee Schedule Contact Ingenix: 800-464-3649

Delaware **Division of Industrial Affairs** **Office of Workers' Compensation** **http://www.delawareworks.com/industrialaffairs/services/WorkersComp.shtml**	**John F. Kirk, Administrator – Office of Workers' Compensation** **http://phonedirectory.delaware.gov/egov/sw_phone_dir.nsf/495f98f6656810b08525740400577162/f192089cb4c7bdd58525741800695922!OpenDocument** Phone: 761-8200	**Subscribe to OWC Email Updates** **http://www.delawareworks.com/industrialaffairs/hcps/subscribe.shtml**	**Healthcare Management System Main Page** **http://dowc.ingenix.com/DWC.asp** *See introduction and fee schedule guidelines* *Fee Schedule Data and Guidelines*
District of Columbia **Department of Employment Services** **Office of Workers' Compensation** **http://www.does.dc.gov/does/cwp/view,a,1232,q,537428.asp**	Phone: (202)-671-1000	None	Resources not provided on website
Florida **Department of Financial Services** **Division of Workers' Compensation** **http://www.myfloridacfo.com/WC/index.htm**	Phone: (850)-413-1600 Or (800)-742-2214 Email Florida DWC Workers.compservice@MyFloridaCFO.com	**Sign up for Email notifications** **http://www.myfloridacfo.com/WCAPPS/Mail_List/Mail_List_Reg.asp**	**Office of Medical Services** **http://www.myfloridacfo.com/WC/provider/index.html** **Reimbursement Manuals** **http://www.myfloridacfo.com/WC/provider/reimbursement-manuals.html**
Georgia **State Board of Workers' Compensation** **http://sbwc.georgia.gov/portal/site/SBWC/**	**Georgia WC Contacts** **http://sbwc.georgia.gov/portal/site/SBWC/menuitem.2f54fa407984c51e93f35eead03036a0/?vgnextoid=8d2934a359b45210VgnVCM100000bf01020aRCRD** **CHIEF OPERATING OFFICER** Stan Carter 270 Peachtree Street, NW Atlanta, Georgia 30303-1299 404-656-2048 **CHIEF FINANCIAL OFFICER** Thomas M. Risko 270 Peachtree Street, NW Atlanta, GA 30303-1299 404-656-2314	**Georgia SBWC** *Scroll down to "news"* **http://sbwc.georgia.gov/portal/site/SBWC/**	**Procedure Manuals** **http://sbwc.georgia.gov/portal/site/SBWC/menuitem.2f54fa407984c51e93f35eead03036a0/?vgnextoid=2d5a34a359b45210VgnVCM100000bf01020aRCRD** **Fee Schedules** **http://sbwc.georgia.gov/portal/site/SBWC/menuitem.2f54fa407984c51e93f35eead03036a0/?vgnextoid=365a34a359b45210VgnVCM100000bf01020aRCRD** *(Note: Managed Care & Rehabilitation = catastrophic injuries)*
Hawaii **Department of Labor and Industrial** **Disability Compensation Division** **http://hawaii.gov/labor/dcd**	**Hawaii DCD Contacts** **http://hawaii.gov/labor/dcd/dcd-links/contact-information** Hawaii District Office Tel. (808) 974-6464 WC Facilitator Section Tel. (808) 586-9161 WC Insurance Section Tel. (808) 586-9166	None	**Administrative Rules and Fee Schedule** **http://hawaii.gov/labor/dcd/dcd-links/find-a-law** *See Chapter 15, Title 12 for rules* *Medicare Fee Schedule for fee information*
Idaho **Industrial Commission** **http://www.iic.idaho.gov/**	**Idaho IC Contacts** **http://www.iic.idaho.gov/bottom_navigation/contact.html** Phone: 208-334-6000 Fax: 1-208-334-2321	**Idaho IC Home** **http://www.iic.idaho.gov/**	**Medical Information** **http://www.iic.idaho.gov/medical/medical.html** **Rules of Administrative Procedure** **http://adm.idaho.gov/adminrules/rules/idapa17/17index.htm**

			See IDAPA 17.02.08 **Medical Fee Schedule** **http://www.iic.idaho.gov/medical/medical.html#feeschedule**
Illinois **Workers' Compensation Commission** **http://www.iwcc.il.gov/**	**Email Illinois WCC** **infoquestions.wcc@illinois.gov** Phone: Toll Free (within IL only) 866/352-3033 Chicago: 312/814-6611 Collinsville: 618/346-3450 Peoria: 309/671-3019 Rockford: 815/987-7292 Springfield: 217/785-7087 TDD: 312/814-2959	**Illinois WC News** **http://www.iwcc.il.gov/news.htm** **Subscribe to Email News** **Susan.piha@illinois.gov**	**Workers' Compensation Act** **http://www.iwcc.il.gov/workers.htm** **Fee Schedule** **http://iwcc.ingenixonline.com/IWCC.asp** **Frequently Asked Medical Questions** **http://www.iwcc.il.gov/faqmed.htm**
Indiana **Workers' Compensation Board** **http://www.in.gov/wcb/**	**Indiana WC Contacts** **http://www.in.gov/wcb/2340.htm** Phone: (outside Indianapolis only) (800) 824-COMP Local Switchboard (317) 232-3808	**Subscribe to WCB Email Updates** **http://www.in.gov/wcb/2413.htm**	Send email to Tony Webb to confirm no FS and where rules are located
Iowa **Iowa Workforce Development** **Division of Workers' Compensation** **http://www.iowaworkforce.org/wc/**	**Iowa WC Contacts** **http://www.iowaworkforce.org/wc/contact.htm** *In particular, Workers' Compensation Compliance Administrators* Phone: (515) 281-5387 or (800) JOB-IOWA	**News and Updates** **http://www.iowaworkforce.org/wc/newsandupdates.htm**	**Iowa Administrative Code Search** **http://search.legis.state.ia.us/nxt/gateway.dll/acts?f=templates&fn=default.htm** *See:* *IAC 876.10.3 regarding Health Service Dispute Resolution* No fee schedule – carriers pay "reasonable and necessary" or per contract
Kansas **Department of Labor** **Division of Workers' Compensation** **http://www.dol.ks.gov/WC/HTML/wc_ALL.html**	**Kansas WC Contacts** **http://www.dol.ks.gov/wc/html/wccontact_ALL.html** *In particular, Director's Office and Medical Services* Workers' Compensation Board Phone number: (785) 296-8484	None	**Medical Services & Fee Schedule Section** **http://www.dol.ks.gov/WC/html/wcmedfee_DBR.html**
Kentucky **Labor Cabinet** **Department of Workers' Claims** **http://www.labor.ky.gov/workersclaims/**	**Phone:** (502)-564-5550 X4578 **Email Kentucky DWC** **http://www.labor.ky.gov/footer/email.htm?ID=b0304224-c520-4170-99c1-dd673e2577cd**	**Kentucky DWC Home** **http://www.labor.ky.gov/workersclaims/** *See "What's New" in the Right Hand Column* **Communications Network** **http://www.labor.ky.gov/workersclaims/commnetwork.htm** *Sign up for emails to interested stakeholders by the Department of Workers' Claims*	**Medical Services and Cost Containment home** **http://www.labor.ky.gov/workersclaims/medicalservices/** **Statute** **http://www.lrc.state.ky.us/KRS/342-00/CHAPTER.HTM** *See:* *Section .035 re: Medical Fee Schedule* **Physicians Fee Schedule** **http://www.labor.ky.gov/workersclaims/medicalservices/physiciansfee.htm**
Louisiana	**Louisiana WC Contacts**	None	**See Fee Schedule (CPT Codes)**

Louisiana Workforce Commission **Workers' Compensation** **http://www.laworks.net/WorkersComp/OWC_MainMenu.asp**	**http://www.laworks.net/PublicRelations/PR_Contacts.asp** **Louisiana Workforce Commission** 1001 N. 23rd Street Baton Rouge, LA 70802 (225) 342-3111		**http://www.laworks.net/Downloads/Downloads_OWC.asp#Medical**
Maine **Workers' Compensation Board** **http://www.maine.gov/wcb/**	**Maine WCB Contacts** **http://www.maine.gov/wcb/contactus.htm** Office of Medical Rehabilitative Services Phone: (207)-941-4557	**Newsletters** **http://www.maine.gov/wcb/departments/execdirnewsletters/index.htm**	**Office of Medical Rehab Services** **http://www.maine.gov/wcb/departments/omrs/omrs/omrsindex.htm** **Utilization Review** **http://www.maine.gov/wcb/departments/omrs/omrs/ur.htm** **Medical Fee Schedule** **http://www.maine.gov/wcb/departments/omrs/omrs/mfs.htm**
Maryland **Workers' Compensation Commission** **http://www.wcc.state.md.us/**	**Maryland WCC Contacts** **http://www.wcc.state.md.us/Contacts_new.html** **Email WCC Support** **wccsupportserv@wcc.state.md.us** General Information/Intelligent Voice Response (IVR) Claim Info: (410) 864-5100 Outside Baltimore Metro Area Toll Free: 1 (800) 492- 0479	**WCC Notices and Announcements** **http://www.wcc.state.md.us/Adjud_Claims/Notices_and_Announcements/Current_Notices.html** **Subscribe to RSS feed** **http://www.wcc.state.md.us/rss_news.xml**	**Medical Fee Guide Information** **http://www.wcc.state.md.us/MFG/Medical_Fee_Schedule.html** *See:* *Medical and Surgical fees for rules* *Medical Services and Treatment – Reimbursement rates fee schedule*
Massachusetts **Labor and Workforce Development** **Department of Industrial Accidents** **http://www.mass.gov/?pageID=elwdagencylanding&L=4&L0=Home&L1=Government&L2=Departments+and+Divisions+(EOLWD)&L3=Department+of+Industrial+Accidents&sid=Elwd**	**Massachusetts WC Contacts** **http://www.mass.gov/?pageID=elwdmodulechunk&L=4&L0=Home&L1=Government&L2=Departments+and+Divisions+(EOLWD)&L3=Department+of+Industrial+Accidents&sid=Elwd&b=terminalcontent&f=dia_contact&csid=Elwd** Division of Healthcare, Finance and Policy (DHCFP) (617)-988-3206 (medical fees)	**News and Updates** **http://www.mass.gov/?pageID=elwdnewsandupdates&L=4&L0=Home&L1=Government&L2=Departments+and+Divisions+(EOLWD)&L3=Department+of+Industrial+Accidents&f=Department+of+Industrial+Accidents_more&sid=Elwd#top**	**Medical Providers Handling Insured Workers** **http://www.mass.gov/?pageID=elwdtopic&L=3&L0=Home&L1=Attorneys+and+Insurers&L2=Medical+Providers+Handling+Injured+Workers&sid=Elwd** **Medical Rates and Forms** **http://www.mass.gov/?pageID=elwdterminal&L=3&L0=Home&L1=Attorneys+and+Insurers&L2=Medical+Providers+Handling+Injured+Workers&sid=Elwd&b=terminalcontent&f=dia_medical_providers_rates_and_forms&csid=Elwd** *See:* *114.3 CMR 40.00* **114.3 C.M.R. 40.00 – Regulation (Including Fees)** **http://www.mass.gov/Eeohhs2/docs/dhcfp/g/regs/114_3_40.pdf**
Michigan **Department of Energy, Labor, and Economic Growth** **Workers' Compensation Agency** **http://www.michigan.gov/wca**	Phone: (888)-396-5041 **Toll Free Phone Guide** **http://www.michigan.gov/documents/wca_phone_map_05_126898_7.pdf**	**What's New Archive** **http://www.michigan.gov/wca/0,1607,7-191-26930---,00.html**	**Healthcare Services** **http://www.michigan.gov/wca/0,1607,7-191-26922---,00.html** **Rules, Manuals and Fees** **http://www.michigan.gov/wca/0,1607,7-191-26922-110009--,00.html**

	Email Michigan WC **wcinfo@michigan.gov**		
Minnesota **Department of Labor & Industry** **Workers' Compensation** **http://www.michigan.gov/wca/0,1607,7-191-26922-110009--,00.html**	**Minnesota WC Contacts** **http://www.dli.mn.gov/WC/Contact.asp** **Phone:** **St. Paul location:** (651) 284-5005; toll-free 1-800-342-5354; TDD (651) 297-4198 **Duluth location:** (218) 733-7810; toll-free 1-800-342-5354	**Compact Newsletter** **http://www.dli.mn.gov/WC/Compact.asp** **Sign Up for Emails** **http://www.dli.mn.gov/EmailLists.asp**	**Medical Benefits** **http://www.dli.mn.gov/WC/MedBen.asp** **Fees for Medical Services** **https://www.revisor.mn.gov/rules/?id=5221** *See:* *5221.4550 and 5221.4551 for Physical Medicine* **Treatment Parameters** **http://www.dli.mn.gov/WC/TpMain.asp**
Mississippi **Workers' Compensation Commission** **http://www.mwcc.state.ms.us/**	**Mississippi WC Key Contacts** **http://www.mwcc.state.ms.us/info/_keycontacts.asp** *See: Medical Cost Containment/ Fee Schedule Information* **Front Desk Switchboard:** Toll Free 866-473-6922 or 601-987-4200	None	**Claims Procedures Manual** **http://www.mwcc.state.ms.us/law-clms/Claims%20Procedures%20Manual.pdf** *See: Section II B – Paying and Reporting Medical Benefits* **Fee Schedule** **http://www.mwcc.state.ms.us/services/feeschedule.asp**
Missouri Department of Labor and Industrial Relations **Workers' Compensation Regulation Bureau** **http://www.labor.mo.gov/**	**Missouri Dept. and Division Contacts** **http://www.labor.mo.gov/contact_dolir.asp** Phone: (573)-751-4231 **Email Missouri DWC** **workerscomp@labor.mo.gov**	See Home Page **http://www.labor.mo.gov/**	**Workers' Compensation Law – Section 287.140** **http://www.moga.mo.gov/statutes/C200-299/2870000140.HTM** **Vocational Rehabilitation** **http://labor.mo.gov/DWC/Division_Units/Care_Unit/vocational_rehab.asp** **Physical Rehabilitation** **http://labor.mo.gov/DWC/Forms/WCR-7-AI.pdf** No Fee Schedule
Montana Department of Labor and Industry **Workers' Compensation Regulation Bureau** **http://erd.dli.mt.gov/wcregs/wcrhome.asp**	Phone: (406)-444-6541	None	**Administrative Rules** **http://www.mtrules.org/gateway/ChapterHome.asp?Chapter=24.29** *See:* *24.29.1585 and 1586* **Medical Regulations** **http://erd.dli.mt.gov/wcregs/medreg.asp** **Non-facility Fee Schedule** **http://mtwcfeeschedule.ingenix.com/overview.aspx** **Facility Fee Schedule** **http://erd.dli.mt.gov/wcstudyproject/mffsoverview.asp**

Nebraska **Workers' Compensation Court** **http://www.wcc.ne.gov/**	**Nebraska WCC Contacts** **http://www.wcc.ne.gov/contact_information.htm**	**What's New** **http://www.wcc.ne.gov/new_rss.xml** **Request Email Notifications** **https://www.nebraska.gov/WC/whatsnew.phtml**	**Fee Schedules** **https://www.wcc.ne.gov/apps/IPUBA0008Afrm.aspx**
Nevada Division of Industrial Relations **Workers' Compensation Section** **http://dirweb.state.nv.us/WCS/wcs.htm**	**Email Nevada WC** **mbrooks@business.nv.gov** Division Headquarters 400 West King Street, Suite 400 Carson City, Nevada 89703 Telephone: (775) 684-7260 Facsimile: (775) 687-6305	Select "Newsletters" from WC section home page **WC Section Email Enrollment Request** **http://dirweb.state.nv.us/WCS/handouts/electronicenroll.htm**	**Medical Information** **http://dirweb.state.nv.us/WCS/medical.htm** *Includes Medical Fee Schedule* **Healthcare Provider's Guide** **http://dirweb.state.nv.us/wcs/brochures/medical.pdf**
New Hampshire Department of Labor **Workers' Compensation** **http://www.labor.state.nh.us/workers_compensation.asp**	*See Workers' Compensation Home Page for further information* **Kathryn J. Barger - *Director, Wo* *Division*** Telephone (603) 271 1-800-27	**NHDOL News** **http://www.labor.state.nh.us/news_about_NHDOL.asp** **Sign Up for Email Alerts** **http://www.labor.state.nh.us/email_alerts.asp**	**Medical, Hospital, & Remedial Care: Title XXIII Section 281-A:23** **http://www.gencourt.state.nh.us/rsa/html/XXIII/281-A/281-A-23.htm** **Managed Care Rules** **http://www.gencourt.state.nh.us/rules/state_agencies/lab700.html** No Fee Schedule
New Jersey Department of Labor and Workforce Development **Workers' Compensation** **http://lwd.dol.state.nj.us/labor/wc/wc_index.html**	**Online Contact Form** **http://www.state.nj.us/labor/survey/contact.shtml** **New Jersey WC Contacts** **http://lwd.dol.state.nj.us/labor/wc/content/contact.html** Division of Workers' Compensation NJ Department of Labor and Workforce Development P.O. Box 381 Trenton, New Jersey 08625-0381 tel: (609) 292-2515, fax (609) 984-2515 General E-Mail: **dwc@dol.state.nj.us**	*See "What's New at the DWC" on the Workers' Compensation home page*	**Workers' Compensation Law** **http://lwd.dol.state.nj.us/labor/forms_pdfs/wc/pdf/wc_law.pdf** *See Article 2, 34: 15-15* No Fee Schedule
New Mexico **Workers' Compensation Administration** **http://www.workerscomp.state.nm.us/**	**New Mexico WCA Contacts** **http://www.workerscomp.state.nm.us/contact/index.php** Phone: 505-841-6000 :: In-state Toll Free: 1-800-255-7965	*See "News and Announcements" on the WCA home page*	**Healthcare Providers** **http://www.workerscomp.state.nm.us/partners/providers.php** **Rules Governing Payment for Healthcare Services (part 7)** **https://www.wcasubmit.org/fees/documents/rule7_integrated2009.pdf**
New York **Workers' Compensation Board** **http://www.wcb.state.ny.us/**	**New York WCB Contacts** **http://www.wcb.state.ny.us/content/main/Contact.jsp** NYS Workers' Compensation Board Customer Service Toll–Free Number (877) 632-4996	**Press Releases** **http://www.wcb.state.ny.us/content/main/PressRe/PressReleases.jsp** **Sign up for RSS feed** **http://www.wcb.state.ny.us/RSSFeeds/RSSfeeds.jsp**	**Healthcare Information** **http://www.wcb.state.ny.us/content/main/hcpp/hcpp.jsp** **Medical Care Fee Schedules** **http://www.wcb.state.ny.us/content/main/hcpp/FeeSchedules.jsp** **OT/PT – 4 Form** **http://www.wcb.state.ny.us/content/main/forms/otpt4.pdf**

North Carolina Industrial Commission **Workers' Compensation** **http://www.ic.nc.gov/**	**North Carolina WC Contacts** **http://www.ic.nc.gov/contact.html** Workers' Compensation HELP: (800) 688-8349 or (919) 807-2501	**News & Announcements** **http://www.ic.nc.gov/news.html#hot**	**Medical Fees Schedule** **http://www.ic.nc.gov/medfeeschdisclaimer.html** *See: "Physical Medicine Section 10" and "CPT Codes and Fees"*
North Dakota **Workforce Safety & Insurance** **http://www.workforcesafety.com/**	**North Dakota WSI Contacts** **http://www.workforcesafety.com/contact-us/** Customer Service: (701) 328–3800 Toll–Free: 1–800–777–5033 *(Note: Our customer service representatives are available from 7:30 a.m. – 5:00 p.m., Central Time, Monday through Friday, excluding holidays.)*	**Sign up for e-newsletter** **http://www.workforcesafety.com/enewsletter/** **Providers News/Updates** **http://www.workforcesafety.com/medical-providers/providernews/providernews.asp**	**Medical Providers** **http://www.workforcesafety.com/medical-providers/** **Utilization Review Guide** **http://www.workforcesafety.com/library/documents/brochures/managedcareguide.pdf** **Billings, Medical Payments and Fee Schedules** **http://www.workforcesafety.com/medical-providers/billingandmedicalpayments/billingandmedicalpayments.asp**
Ohio **Bureau of Works' Compensation** **http://www.ohiobwc.com/Default.aspx**	**Ohio WC Contacts** **http://www.ohiobwc.com/home/contactus/default.asp** The customer contact center is open from 7:30 a.m. to 5:30 p.m. EST. **Toll-free:** 1-800-OHIOBWC (1-800-644-6292) **TTY:** 1-800-BWC-4-TDD (1-800-292-4833) **Fax:** 1-877-520-OHIO (6446) **Mailing address:** BWC 30 W. Spring St. Columbus, OH 43215-2256 **Live Support Chat** **https://www.ohiobwc.com/bwccommon/contactus/WebChatForm.asp?txtRefererPage=http://www.ohiobwc.com/Default.aspx** *7:30 am – 5:30 pm M-F (EST) (excluding holidays)*	*See "What's New" on BWC Home Page*	**Medical Providers** **http://www.ohiobwc.com/provider/default.asp** **BWC Medical Guide** **http://www.ohiobwc.com/downloads/blankpdf/CD-106.pdf** **Fee Schedule Lookup** **http://www.ohiobwc.com/provider/services/agreement.asp** **Medical Prior Authorization Requirements** **http://www.ohiobwc.com/provider/services/authrequirements/default.asp**
Oklahoma **Workers' Compensation Court** **http://www.owcc.state.ok.us/**	**Oklahoma WC Contacts** **http://www.owcc.state.ok.us/Contact_Us.htm** Medical Phone: (405)-522-8794	**What's New** **http://www.owcc.state.ok.us/Whats_New.htm**	**Medical Services** **http://www.owcc.state.ok.us/Medical_services.htm** **Schedule of Medical and Hospital Fees** **http://www.owcc.state.ok.us/Agreement.htm** **Treatment Guidelines** **http://www.owcc.state.ok.us/guidelines.htm**
Oregon **Workers' Compensation Division** **http://wcd.oregon.gov/**	**Oregon WC Contacts** **http://wcd.oregon.gov/contactus.html** Phone: 503-947-7810 Toll-free: 800-452-0288 E-mail: workcomp.questions@state.or.us	**Sign up for Email updates** **https://service.govdelivery.com/service/multi_subscribe.html?code=ORDCBS** **What's New** **http://wcd.oregon.gov/wut_gnu.html**	**For Health Care Providers** **http://wcd.oregon.gov/rdrs/mru/mpindex.html** **Medical Services Rules** **http://wcd.oregon.gov/policy/rules/hist_010.html**

	Fax: 503-947-7581		**Max Payment Calculator** **http://www4.cbs.state.or.us/ex/wcd/maxpaycalc/index.cfm**
Pennsylvania Department of Labor and Industry **Bureau of Workers' Compensation** **http://www.portal.state.pa.us/portal/server.pt/community/workers'_compensation/10386**	BWC Phone: (717)-783-5421 **Email Pennsylvania BWC** **ra-li-bwc-helpline@state.pa.us**	**Publications** **http://www.portal.state.pa.us/portal/server.pt/community/publications/10443** *Scroll Down to "Newsletters"* *See BWC Home Page for Announcements*	**Medical Cost Containment Rules** **http://www.portal.state.pa.us/portal/server.pt?open=514&objID=553022&mode=2** *See Title 34, Part VII, Chapter 127* **Fee Schedule** **http://www.portal.state.pa.us/portal/server.pt/community/fee_schedule/10424**
Rhode Island Department of Labor and Training **Workers' Compensation** **http://www.dlt.ri.gov/wc/**	**Rhode Island WC Contacts** **http://www.dlt.ri.gov/wc/contactus.htm** *Send Workers' Compensation questions to our **Education Unit** at WCEdcUnit@dlt.ri.gov or call the Information Line at (401) 462-8100 and press option # 1.*	**View Information Letters** **http://www.dlt.ri.gov/wc/infoletters.htm** **Get Newsletters by Email** **WCWebmaster@dlt.ri.gov** *Include Name, Company and Phone number*	**Fee Schedule** **http://www.risingms.com/RIFee/Pages/default.aspx**
South Carolina **Workers' Compensation Commission** **http://www.wcc.sc.gov/**	**South Carolina WC Contacts** **http://www.wcc.sc.gov/contact/** Phone: 803-737-5700 **Insurance and Medical Services Contacts** **http://www.wcc.sc.gov/Insurance/**	See "What's New" on WCC Home Page	**Medical Services Division** **http://www.wcc.sc.gov/Medical/** *Order Medical Services Provider Manual Here* **Regulations** **http://www.scstatehouse.gov/coderegs/c067.htm** *See:* *Article 13*
South Dakota Department of Labor **Workers' Compensation Program** **http://dol.sd.gov/workerscomp/default.aspx**	**South Dakota WC Contact Form** **http://apps.sd.gov/applications/LD75UIBP/Secure/template/main.aspx?templateID=1&ID=12** Phone: 605.773.3681 Fax: 605.773.4211	**Subscribe to e-lerts** **http://apps.sd.gov/applications/LD75UIBP/Secure/template/main.aspx?templateID=1&ID=69**	**Rules and Fee Schedule** **http://dol.sd.gov/workerscomp/rulesfees.aspx**
Tennessee Department of Labor and Workforce Development **Workers' Compensation** **http://www.state.tn.us/labor-wfd/wcomp.html**	**Tennessee WC Contacts** **http://www.tn.gov/labor-wfd/wc_contacts.pdf** Phone 1-800-332-2667 (within Tennessee) or 615-532-4812 Fax (615) 532-1468 **Email WC Tennessee** wc.info@tn.gov	None	**Workers' Compensation Rules** **http://www.tennessee.gov/sos/rules/0800/0800-02/0800-02.htm** **Medical Fee Book** **http://www.tennessee.gov/labor-wfd/wc_medfeebook.pdf** **Utilization Review** **http://www.tn.gov/labor-wfd/wcfaq.html#WCutilizationreview**
Texas Department of Insurance **Division of Workers' Compensation** **http://www.tdi.state.tx.us/wc/indexwc.html**	**Email Texas WC Customer Service** **WorkersCompCustomerServices@tdi.state.tx.us** **Help For** **Toll-Free #**	**WC News Releases** **http://www.tdi.state.tx.us/news/index.html** **Sign up for email updates** **http://www.tdi.state.tx.us/alert/emailnews.html**	**Fee guidelines information** **http://www.tdi.state.tx.us/wc/fee/index.html** **Training module** **http://www.tdi.state.tx.us/wc/fee/documents/mfgmodule.pdf**

	Injured Employees **800-252-7031** DD Scheduling **512-804-4380** EDI Help Desk **888-4TXCOMP** MFDR **512-804-4812** Safety Hotline **800-452-9595**		
Utah Labor Commission – Division of Industrial Accidents **Workers' Compensation Program** **http://www.laborcommission.utah.gov/IndustrialAccidents/index.html**	**Email Utah WC** iaccd@utah.gov Phone: (801)-530-6800 In-State Toll Free (800)-530-5090	**Workers' compensation Bulletins** **http://www.laborcommission.utah.gov/IndustrialAccidents/Bulletins/index.html**	**Medical Fee Guidelines** **http://www.laborcommission.utah.gov/IndustrialAccidents/pdfs/Med_Fee_Guidelines__2008-9_3-26-08.6-08doc.pdf**
Vermont Department of Labor **Workers' Compensation System** **http://labor.vermont.gov/?TabId=114**	**Vermont WC Contacts** **http://labor.vermont.gov/Default.aspx?tabid=847**	**Sign up for Medical/Healthcare provider emails** **http://mail.state.vt.us/guest/RemoteListSummary/medcare**	**Medical/Healthcare Provider Information** **http://labor.vermont.gov/Default.aspx?tabid=151** **WC Rules 1-46** **http://labor.vermont.gov/Portals/0/WP%20Safety/Rules%201-46%204%2006.pdf** **WC Rule 40** **http://labor.vermont.gov/Portals/0/WP%20Safety/Rule%2040.pdf** **Medical Fee Schedule** **http://labor.vermont.gov/InfoCenter/Rules/WorkersCompensationRules/AMAAgreement51506/tabid/829/Default.aspx**
Virginia **Workers' Compensation Commission** **http://www.vwc.state.va.us/**	Phone: (877)-664-2566	**WCC Bulletin Board** **http://www.vwc.state.va.us/bulletin_board.htm**	**Rights and remedies for Healthcare providers** **http://www.vwc.state.va.us/medical_providers.htm** No Fee Schedule
Washington **Department of Labor and Industries** **http://www.lni.wa.gov/**	Provider Hotline: (800)-848-0811 Interactive Voice Response: (800)-831-5227	**Sign up for medical provider email news** **http://www.lni.wa.gov/Main/Listservs/Provider.asp** **Provider Bulletins** **http://www.lni.wa.gov/ClaimsIns/Providers/Billing/ProvBulletins/default.asp**	**Medical Providers** **http://www.lni.wa.gov/main/ForProviders.asp** **PT, OT and Massage** **http://www.lni.wa.gov/ClaimsIns/Providers/Manage/RTW/Therapy/default.asp** **Fee Schedules** **http://www.lni.wa.gov/ClaimsIns/Providers/Billing/FeeSched/** *See:* *Fee Schedules*

			Billing and Payment Policies *Updates and Corrections*
West Virginia Offices of the Insurance Commissioner **Workers' Compensation http://www.wvinsurance.gov/WorkersCompensation/tabid/73/Default.aspx**	**Email West Virginia WC MedicalRatesandPlans@wvinsurance.gov** Workers' Comp. Board of Review: 304-558-5230	None	**Rules http://apps.sos.wv.gov/csr/search.asp** *Search 85-15 (Vocational and Physical Rehabilitation) and 85-20 (Medical Management)* **Schedule of maximum allowed medical reimbursement http://www.wvinsurance.gov/Default.aspx?tabid=372**
Wisconsin Department of Workforce Development **Workers' Compensation http://www.dwd.state.wi.us/wc/default.htm**	**Wisconsin WC Contacts http://www.dwd.state.wi.us/wc/about_us/direct.htm** Phone: 608-266-1340 (Main Number) Fax: 608-267-0394 TTY 866-265-3142	See WC Home	**Medical Providers http://www.dwd.state.wi.us/wc/medical/** **Treatment Guidelines http://www.dwd.state.wi.us/wc/medical/DWD81.pdf** No Fee Schedule
Wyoming Department of Employment http://doe.wyo.gov/Pages/default.aspx	Phone: (307)-777-5476 **Email Wyoming DOE AskMeWC@state.wy.us**	**News and Events http://doe.wyo.gov/newsandevents/Pages/default.aspx**	**Service Providers Information http://doe.wyo.gov/serviceproviders/Pages/default.aspx** **Rehabilitation Therapy Guidelines http://doe.wyo.gov/ProductionDocuments/WSCD-CSS/Rehab%20Therapy%20Guidelines.pdf** **Fee Schedule http://soswy.state.wy.us/rules/RULES/7341.pdf** **Preauthorization Program http://doe.wyo.gov/serviceproviders/Pages/PreauthorizationProgram.aspx**

* **Note:** *This appendix was reprinted with permission of APTA. Marissa Webb, MA, updated it and added URLs on May 20, 2010.*

Appendix B

Interview Questions for

Current Perspectives in Clinical Treatment and Management in Workers Compensation Cases©

Chris Stout, PsyD; Matt Kruger, MS, CSCS; Jeff Rogers

Editors

Bentham Books

First and foremost, thank you for your participation in this project. We believe it will make an important contribution to the literature, and we are thrilled to have you play such a critical role. We have formulated this Questionnaire to be efficient as to not take too much of your time.

Please feel free to be completely honest, gloves-off, and even provocative if you so wish in your responses. You can choose to have your name associated with your comments, or you can have some or all or your comments be anonymous, or you can choose to have your name listed as a contributor, or not–it's all your preference as to what you feel comfortable with. Just let us know. We are looking to gather your opinions, stories, perspectives and wisdom.

Please do feel free to write as much as you wish, the space provided is NOT a limitation.

DEMOGRAPHIC INFORMATION:

1) Profession

☐ Surgeon/Physician, specialty ____________

☐ Case Manager

☐ Adjuster

☐ Vocational Counselor

☐ Employer

☐ Plaintiff Attorney

☐ Employer Attorney

☐ Judge

☐ Arbitrator

☐ Physical Therapist

☐ Athletic Trainer

☐ Psychologist

☐ Psychiatrist

☐ Other:

2) Please describe the nature of your work vis-à-vis workers compensation:

3) How many years have you worked in the area of workers compensation?

☐ 1 – 4

☐ 5 – 9

☐ 10 – 14

☐ 15 – 19

☐ 20 – 24

☐ > 25

4) Based on your profession, on average, annual basis, how many workers compensation cases do you manage, treat, represent, review, adjudicate, etc.? _____

5) What drew you to working with workers comp cases?

6) a) State(s) in which you work: ______________________________

b) If you work in more that one area, what state, region, and/or city do you find the most challenging to work with cases and why?

7) a) What is your annual salary that is generated as a result of your workers compensation work?

☐ > $500,000

☐ $350,000 - $499,999

☐ $200,000 – $349,999

☐ $100,000 - $199,999

☐ $75,000 - $99,999

☐ $50,000 - $74,999

☐ $25,000 - $49,999

☐ < $25,000

b) Of the amount noted in question 7a, what percentage is that of your total annual income?

☐ 100%

☐ between 75 – 99%

☐ about 75%

☐ between 50 – 74%

☐ about 50%

☐ 25 – 49%

☐ about 25%

☐ < 25%

8) What is your age? ________

9) What is your sex? ☐ Male ☐ Female

10) Level of Anonymity:

☐ None, please feel free to list my name with my comments, in the contributors list, and biography.

☐ Limited, please only list my name by my answers herein I so noted, and in the contributors list, and biography.

☐ Very limited, please DO NOT list my name by my answers herein, BUT YOU MAY list it in the contributors list, and biography.

☐ Total, DO NOT list my name by my answers herein, the contributors list, or biography

Brief 1 Paragraph Bio (if electing to have it included):

Current Perspectives in Clinical Treatment and Management in Workers Compensation Cases©

QUESTIONNAIRE

Again, please feel free to be completely honest, gloves-off, and even provocative if you so wish in your responses. You can choose to have your name associated with your comments, or you can have some or all or your comments be anonymous, or you can choose to have your name listed as a contributor, or not–it's all your preference as to what you feel comfortable with. Just let us know. We are looking to gather your opinions, stories, perspectives and wisdom.

Please do feel free to write as much as you wish, the space provided is NOT a limitation.

1) Do you feel spine/hand/shoulder/knee surgery is generally cost effective in treating injured workers? Why or why not? *(Feel free to distinguish your answer as to specific body part or collectively.)*

2) Do you feel surgery affects patient outcomes? Why or why not? *(Feel free to distinguish your answer as to specific body part or collectively.)*

3) What should spine/hand/shoulder/knee surgery procedures cost? *(Feel free to distinguish your answer as to specific body part or collectively.)*

4) What is your response to the data that suggest that spine surgeries have not improved patient outcomes but have nevertheless increased in frequency?

5) When I think of work related injuries, I think….*(Feel free to distinguish your answer as to specific body part or collectively.)*

6) Describe the "ideal" workers comp patient from your perspective:

7) How do you view the role of the MD in workers comp cases?

8) How do you view the role of the surgeon in workers comp cases?

9) How do you view the role of the pain medicine physician in workers comp cases?

10) How do you view the role of the Case Manager in workers comp cases?

11) How do you view the role of the Adjuster in workers comp cases?

12) How do you view the role of the Vocational Counselor in workers comp cases?

13) How do you view the role of the Patient in workers comp cases?

14) How do you view the role of the Employer in workers comp cases?

15) How do you view the role of the Plaintiff Attorney in workers comp cases?

16) How do you view the role of the Employer Attorney in workers comp cases?

17) How do you view the role of the Judge in workers comp cases?

18) How do you view the role of the Arbitrator in workers comp cases?

19) How do you view the role of the Physical Therapist in workers comp cases?

20) How do you view the role of the Athletic Trainer in workers comp cases?

21) How do you view the role of the Psychologist/Psychiatrist in workers comp cases?

22) How do you view the role of the Chiropractor in workers comp cases?

23) What do you estimate the rate/level of fraud is in workers compensation, and from what source(s)?

24) Do you believe attorneys help workers comp patients? How or why not?

25) What other factors (e.g., pharmacological) may impact workers compensation care and how?

26) Out of an average 100 cases, what number would you estimate are factitious/fraudulent or malingering?

27) Out of an average 100 cases, what number would you estimate are malingering?

28) What is the hardest part of your job in working with workers comp cases?

29) What is the most satisfying part of your job in working with workers comp cases?

30) Please describe how you would improve the current workers compensation system and/or describe what you would consider to be an ideal model from your perspective.

31) Please, while maintaining patient confidentiality, describe an interesting or challenging case or two that you feel is representative of your work with workers compensation cases or the system.

Please feel free to add any additional commentary that you feel would be important to note or clarify that has not yet been addressed herein:

Is there anyone you would recommend we contact to also participate as a contributor to the book? If so, please list their name, phone, and email:

(Please email this questionnaire once completed to Chris.Stout@ATIPT.com and fax just your signature page below to his attention at 630.759.6702. Thanks!)

Signature: __________________________ **Name Printed:** ____

Date: ___________________

Rev: 11/16/09

Appendix C: Fee Schedules for Workers' Compensation

OWCP (Federal) Medical Fee Schedule

http://www.mtclibraries.com/lib/table.php?id=rm28782%22)
Online fee schedule (applies to FECA, EEOIC and LHWCA; a modified version is used for the FBLBA)

AL - Alabama WC Provider Fee Schedules

http://dir.alabama.gov/wc/services.aspx
Ordering information

AK - Alaska WC Provider Fee Schedule

http://www.shopingenix.com/modules/default/
Ordering information

AR - Arkansas WC Medical Fees Schedule

http://www.awcc.state.ar.us/medfeetoc.html
Online Rule 30 Medical Fee Schedule

AZ - Arizona WC Fee Schedule

http://www.ica.state.az.us/
Ordering information

CA - California WC Medical Fee Schedules

http://www.dir.ca.gov/dwc/OMFS9904.htm
Ordering information for Official Medical Fee Schedule
Other fee schedules available online

CO - Colorado WC Medical Fee Schedule, Rule 18

http://www.coworkforce.com/dwc/Rules/Rules%20pdf/RulesLinksTable.asp
Online fee schedule

CT - Connecticut WC Practitioner Fee Schedule

http://wcc.state.ct.us/memos/2006/2006-01.htm
Ordering information

DE – Delaware

http://www.delawareworks.com/industrialaffairs/services/documents/DE_Final_Draft_092507_FUDASST_Print_110707_Request.pdf

FL - Florida WC Reimbursement Manuals

http://www.fldfs.com/WC/publications.html
Online fee schedules

Chris E. Stout, Matt Kruger and Jeffrey Rogers, (Eds)

GA - Georgia WC Medical Fee Schedule

http://sbwc.georgia.gov/00/channel_modifieddate/0,2096,11394008_34361078,00.html
Ordering information

HI - Hawaii WC Medical Fee Schedule

http://hawaii.gov/labor/dcd/dcd-links/find-a-law
Online fee schedules (click on "Subtitle 3 Disability Compensation Division")

ID - Idaho WC Customary Medical Charge Value Table

http://www.iic.idaho.gov/medinfo/medinfo.htm
Online fee schedule

IL - Illinois WC Fee Schedule

http://iwcc.ingenixonline.com/iwcc.asp
Online fee schedule

KS - Kansas WC Medical Fee Schedule

http://www.dol.ks.gov/wc/html/wcmedfeesched_DBR.html
Online fee schedule

KY - Kentucky WC Medical Fee Schedule

http://www.labor.ky.gov/workersclaims
Ordering information

– Memo regarding corrections to the 2005 fee schedule

http://www.labor.ky.gov/workersclaims/homepage_repository/Important_Information.htm

LA - Louisiana WC Medical Fee Schedule

http://www.laworks.net/Downloads/Downloads_OWC.asp
Online fee schedule

MA - Massachusetts WC Fee Schedules

http://www.mass.gov/?pageID=eohhs2terminal&&L=4&L0=Home&L1=Consumer&L2=Insurance+(including+MassHealth)&L3=Workers'+Compensation&sid=Eeohhs2&b=terminalcontent&f=dhcfp_consumer_wc_faqs&csid=Eeohhs2
Online fee schedules

MD - Maryland WC Medical Fee Schedule

http://www.wcc.state.md.us/MFG/Medical_Fee_Schedule.html
Online reimbursement guidance

ME - Maine WC Medical Fee Schedule

http://www.maine.gov/wcb/departments/omrs/omrs/mfs.htm
Online fee schedule

MI - Michigan WC Medical Fee Schedule

http://www.michigan.gov/wca/0,1607,7-191-26922-86583--,00.html
Online fee schedule

MN - Minnesota WC Medical Fee Schedule

http://www.doli.state.mn.us/workcomp.html
Online fee schedule

MS - Mississippi WC Medical Fee Schedule

http://www.shopingenix.com/modules/default/
Ordering information

– Frequently Asked Questions

http://www.mwcc.state.ms.us/services/feeschedule.asp

– Fee schedule addenda

http://www.mwcc.state.ms.us/services/feeschedule.asp

MT - Montana WC Fee Schedules

http://erd.dli.mt.gov/wcregs/medreg.asp
Online fee schedules

NC - North Carolina WC Medical Fee Schedule

http://www.comp.state.nc.us/ncic/pages/feesched.asp
Online fee schedule

– Notes for processing medical bills

http://www.comp.state.nc.us/ncic/pages/medbill6.htm

ND - North Dakota WC Medical Services Fee Schedules

http://www.workforcesafety.com/medical-providers/feeschedule/feescheduleagreement.asp
Online fee schedules

NE - Nebraska WC Fee Schedules

http://www.wcc.ne.gov/fee_schedules.htm
Online fee schedules

NM - New Mexico WC Fee Schedule

https://www.wcasubmit.org/fees/
Ordering instructions

– Rule 7 – Payment of Medical Services

http://workerscomp.state.nm.us/rules/index.php

NV - Nevada WC Medical Fee Schedules

http://dirweb.state.nv.us/WCS/wcs.htm
Online fee schedules (select "Medical" from menu on left)

NY - New York WC Inpatient & Outpatient Fee Schedules

http://www.wcb.state.ny.us/content/main/hcpp/FeeSchedules.jsp
Online inpatient/outpatient facility fee schedules, ordering instructions for medical fee schedule

OH - Ohio WC Billing and Reimbursement Manual

http://www.ohiobwc.com/provider/services/brmdefault.asp

OK - Oklahoma WC Schedule of Medical and Hospital Fees

http://www.owcc.state.ok.us/Fee%20Schedule.htm
Online fee schedule

OR - Oregon Medical Fee & Relative Value Schedule Rules

http://www.cbs.state.or.us/wcd/policy/rules/hist_009.html
Online fee schedule

PA - Pennyslvania WC Fee Schedule

http://www.dli.state.pa.us/landi/cwp/view.asp?a=138&Q=58551&landiNavDLTEST=|852|1065|1306|
Online fee schedules

– Pennsylvania Charge Classes by Zip Code

http://www.dli.state.pa.us/landi/cwp/view.asp?a=138&q=190242&landiNavDLTEST=|852|1065|1306|

RI-Rhode Island WC Fee Schedule

http://www.dlt.ri.gov/wc/infomedfeesched.htm
Ordering information

SC - South Carolina WC Fee Schedules

http://www.wcc.state.sc.us/Medical/
Online fee schedules and ordering information

TN - Tennessee WC Fee Schedule

http://www.state.tn.us/sos/rules/0800/0800-02/0800-02.htm
Online fee schedules

TX - Texas WC Medical Fee Guideline

http://www.tdi.state.tx.us/wc/indexwc.html
Online fee schedules

UT - Utah Medical Fee Guidelines

http://laborcommission.utah.gov/Provider%20Page.html

Online fee schedules

VA - Virginia WC Rule Regarding Reimbursements

http://www.vwc.state.va.us/medical_providers.htm
Explanation of employer's liability for medical charges

VT - Vermont WC Fee Schedule, Rule 40

http://labor.vermont.gov/Workers'%20Compensation%20Rules/tabid/311/Default.aspx
Online fee schedules

WA - Washington Fee Schedules

http://www.lni.wa.gov/ClaimsIns/Providers/Billing/FeeSched/default.asp
Online fee schedules

WI - Wisconsin WC Fee Schedules

http://www.dwd.state.wi.us/wc/insurance/radiology/radiology_database.htm
Online Hospital Radiology fee schedules

– Ordering information for medical fee schedules

http://www.dwd.state.wi.us/wc/insurance/radiology/databaselist.pdf

WV - West Virginia WC Fee Schedules

http://www.wvinsurance.gov/wc/medical/index.htm
Online fee schedules

WY - Wyoming WC Fee Schedules

http://wydoe.state.wy.us/doe.asp?ID=741
Online fee schedule

As of this writing (July 2010), the following four states to not have a fee schedule:

IN – Indiana

MO – Missouri

NH - New Hampshire

NJ - New Jersey

Appendix D: Workers' Compensation Publication List

- Matthew J. Kruger MS, CSCS, CPT (March, 2009) Physical demand levels in individuals completing a sports performance-based work conditioning/hardening program after lumbar fusion. **Invited Presentation at NASS-PA**

- James Allivato, ATC; Wade Meyer, PT, DPT, Chris E. Stout, PsyD (2009) The Role of Athletic Trainers in Selecting Outcome Measures For Rotator Cuff Repair Patients Participating in a Supervised Work Conditioning/Work Hardening Program **NATA Annual Meeting**

- Wade A. Meyer PT, DPT, CSCS Matthew J. Kruger MS, CSCS, CPT (2008) Resistance Training Volume -- Comparison Of Rotator Cuff Repair Patients In Physical Therapy Vs. Initial Training Volume Of Work Conditioning/Work Hardening Program **National Strength and Conditioning Association International Conference on Strength Training**

- Wade A. Meyer PT, DPT, CSCS Matthew J. Kruger MS, CSCS, CPT (2008) Resistance Training Volume -- Comparison Of Rotator Cuff Repair Patients In Physical Therapy Vs. Initial Training Volume Of Work Conditioning/Work Hardening Program **Illinois Physical Therapy Association Annual Meeting**

- Keith Cole, PT, DPT, MBiomedE, Matt Kruger, MS, CSCS, Dylan Bates, PT,MSPT,CSCS, Greg Steil , EP, Mike Zbreski, MS, CSCS Physical demand levels in individuals completing a sports performance-based work conditioning/hardening program after lumbar fusion. **The Spine Journal 2008 outstanding paper**

- Jamie Stark, PhD, CSCS, HFI, Mike Zbreski, MS, Matthew Kruger, MS, CSCS Advanced Rehabilitation Following Lumbar Fusion: An Evidence Based Approach. (2007) **Biomechanics Journal**

- Jamie Stark, PhD, CSCS, HFI, Mike Zbreski, MS, Matthew Kruger, MS, CSCS (2007) A Two-Component Model Of Resistance Training Volume And Intensity To Optimize Outcomes In Workers' Compensation Lumbar Fusion Patients. **NSCA Annual Meeting** (Accepted; Abstract ID# N/A)

- Jamie Stark, PhD, CSCS, HFI, Mike Zbreski, MS, Matthew Kruger, MS, CSCS (2007) Workers' Compensation Indemnity Settlement Costs Vary By Functional Outcome Following Sports Performance Based Rehabilitation In Spinal Fusion Patients. **ACOEM AOHC 2007** (Accepted; Abstract ID# N/A)

- Jamie Stark, PhD, CSCS, HFI, Mike Zbreski, MS, Matthew Kruger, MS, CSCS (2007) Workers' Compensation Indemnity Settlement Costs Vary By Functional Outcome Following Sports Performance Based Rehabilitation In Rotator Cuff Repair Patients. **ACOEM AOHC 2007** (Accepted; Abstract ID# N/A)

- Jamie Stark, PhD, CSCS, HFI, Mike Zbreski, MS, Matthew Kruger, MS, CSCS (2007) Case Closure: Does Having a Functional Capacity Evaluation Matter? **ACOEM AOHC 2007** (Accepted; Abstract ID# N/A)

- Jamie Stark, PhD, CSCS, Mike Zbreski, MS, Matt Kruger, MS, CSCS. (2007) Floor-to-Waist Weight and Resistance Training Volume Are Better Predictors of Functional Outcome than Core Training Volume in Workers' Compensation Lumbar Fusion Patients. **World Spine IV (NASS Affiliate)** (Accepted; Abstract ID# 172239)

- Jamie Stark, Mike Zbreski, Matthew Kruger. (2007) Resistance Training Volume During

Rehabilitation Predicts Functional Outcomes In Workers' Compensation Rotator Cuff Repair. **FASEB 2007 Annual Meeting (American Physiological Society)** (Accepted; Abstract ID# 7184)

- Jamie Stark, Mike Zbreski, Matthew Kruger. (2007) Overhead Press Lift Weight During Rehabilitation Predicts Functional Outcomes In Workers' Compensation Rotator Cuff Repair Patients. **FASEB 2007 Annual Meeting (American Physiological Society)** (Accepted; Abstract ID# 7187)

- Jamie Stark, Mike Zbreski, Matthew Kruger. (2007) Floor-to-Waist Lift Weight During Rehabilitation Predicts Functional Outcomes In Workers' Compensation Rotator Cuff Repair Patients. **FASEB 2007 Annual Meeting (American Physiological Society)** (Accepted; Abstract ID# 7192)

- Jamie Stark, Mike Zbreski, Matthew Kruger. (2007) Development of Relative Loading Metrics for Analysis of Core Resistance Training Volume. **FASEB 2007 Annual Meeting (American Physiological Society)** (Accepted; Abstract ID# 7194)

- Jamie Stark, Mike Zbreski, Matthew Kruger. (2007) Isotonic Core Resistance Training Volume does not Predict Functional Outcomes in Workers' Compensation Lumbar Fusion Patients. **FASEB 2007 Annual Meeting (American Physiological Society)** (Accepted; Abstract ID# 7195)

- Jamie Stark, Mike Zbreski, Matthew Kruger. (2007) Isometric Core Resistance Training Volume does not Predict Functional Outcomes in Workers' Compensation Lumbar Fusion Patients. **FASEB 2007 Annual Meeting (American Physiological Society)** (Accepted; Abstract ID# 7197)

- Jamie Stark, PhD, Brent Henry, MS, Mike Zbreski, MS, Tyler Hanley, BS, and Matt Kruger, MS. (2007) Combined Physical Therapy and Work Conditioning Increases Patient Satisfaction. **APTA National Conference** (Accepted; ID# 292866)

- Jamie Stark, Mike Zbreski, Matthew Kruger (2007) Resistance Training Volume During Rehabilitation Predicts Functional Outcomes In Workers' Compensation Rotator Cuff Repair Patients. **ACSM National Conference** (Accepted; ID# 07-SA-3335-ACSM)

- Jamie Stark, PhD, CSCS, HFI, Mike Zbreski, MS, Matthew Kruger, MS, CSCS Adequate Resistance Training Volume and Floor-to-Waist Lift Weight Required for Optimal Outcomes in Workers' Compensation Lumbar Fusion Patients (Unpublished manuscript)

- Jamie Stark, PhD, CSCS, HFI, Mike Zbreski, MS, Matthew Kruger, MS, CSCS Relative Contributions of Resistance Training Volume and Floor-to-Waist Lift Weight Required to Optimize Outcomes Benchmarks in Workers' Compensation Lumbar Fusion Patients (Unpublished manuscript)

- Jamie T Stark, PhD; Matthew J Kruger, MS; Mike G Zbreski, MS; Anthony A Romeo, MD. (2006) Overhead Press Weights Used During Rehabilitation Predict Functional Outcomes In Workers' Compensation Rotator Cuff Repair Patients. **ASES Closed Meeting** (accepted; WEB515)

- Jamie T Stark, PhD; Matthew J Kruger, MS; Mike G Zbreski, MS; Anthony A Romeo, MD. (2006) Resistance Training Volume During Rehabilitation Predicts Functional Outcomes In Workers' Compensation Rotator Cuff Repair Patients. **ASES Open/Closed Meeting** (accepted; WEB509)

- Jamie Stark, PhD, CSCS; Mike Zbreski, MS; Matthew Kruger, MS, CSCS. (2006) Identifying Maximum Medical Improvement For Back Injury Rehabilitation Utilizing Sports Performance Based Work Conditioning/Hardening Following Physical Therapy. **NSCA Annual Meeting** (Abstract)

- Jamie Stark, PhD, CSCS, HFI, Matthew Kruger, MS, CSCS, Mike Zbreski, MS, Dylan Bates, MSPT, CSCS, Greg Steil, BS. (2006) Workers' compensation indemnity settlement costs vary by functional outcome following sports performance based rehabilitation in spinal fusion patients. **NASS 21st**

Annual Meeting (Accepted; ID # 154731)

- Jamie Stark, PhD, CSCS, HFI, Matthew Kruger, MS, CSCS, Mike Zbreski, MS, Dylan Bates, MSPT, CSCS, Greg Steil, BS. (2006) Identifying maximum medical improvement for back injury rehabilitation utilizing sports performance based work conditioning/hardening following physical therapy. **NASS 21st Annual Meeting** (Accepted; ID# 155635)

- Jamie Stark, PhD, CSCS, HFI, Matthew Kruger, MS, CSCS, Mike Zbreski, MS, Dylan Bates, MSPT, CSCS, Greg Steil, BS. (2006) Equivalent functional outcomes for single and multiple level lumbar fusion workers' compensation patients following rehabilitation. **Spine Across the Sea Annual Meeting** (accepted [combined abstract/presentation]; ID# 150996 -and- ID # 150983)

- Jamie Stark, Matthew Kruger, Mike Zbreski, Dylan Bates, Greg Steil. (2006) Resistance Training Volume During Rehabilitation Predicts Functional Outcomes In Workers' Compensation Lumbar Fusion Patients. **ACSM National Conference** (accepted; ID# 06-SA-3604-ACSM)

- Jamie T Stark, Matt Kruger, Mike Zbreski, Dylan Bates, Greg Steil. (2006) Floor-to-waist lift weight and volume during rehabilitation predicts functional outcomes in workers' compensation lumbar fusion patients **FASEB (American Physiological Society)** (Abstract)

- Jamie T Stark, Matt Kruger, Mike Zbreski, Dylan Bates, Greg Steil. (2006) Pre-program function predicts outcomes in workers' compensation post-lumbar fusion patients **FASEB (American Physiological Society)** (Abstract)

- Jamie T Stark, Matt Kruger, Mike Zbreski, Dylan Bates, Greg Steil. (2006) Resistance training volume during rehabilitation predicts functional outcomes in workers' compensation lumbar fusion patients FASEB (American Physiological Society) (Abstract)

- Stark, JT, Kruger, M, Bates, D, Lorenz, M, Steil, G (2005) Sports performance based strength training improves spinal fusion outcomes. **Eurospine Conference** (Abstract).

- Stark, JT, Kruger, M, Bates, D, Lorenz, M, Steil, G (2005) Sports performance based strength training improves spinal fusion outcomes. **NSCA National Conference** (Abstract).

- Kruger, M, Bates, D, Lorenz, M, Steil, G (2004) An outcome study: 2 year RTW rates post Sports Performance based Work Conditioning/Hardening Program for post-lumbar fusion patients. **Spine Across the Sea**

- Kruger, M, Bates, D, Lorenz, M, Steil, G (2004) Strength Training based rehabilitation improves RTW rates for post-lumbar fusion patients. **ISSLS**

- Kruger, M, Bates, D, Lorenz, M, Steil, G (2004) Strength and Conditioning based rehabilitation improves both outcomes and economic factors in injured workers. **NSCA National Conference**

- Matt Kruger, M.S.,CSCS, Greg Steil EP,B.A., Dylan Bates MSPT, CSCS, Shawn Rankin MSPT, CSCS, Phillip Lorenz, BS, Mark A. Lorenz, MD (2004). Does functional capability in a Sports Performance based Work Conditioning/Hardening Program correlate with RTW capabilities at 1-yr follow-up with worker's compensation subjects s/p lumbar fusion? **NASS 19th Annual Meeting** (Abstract)

- Kruger, M, Bates, D, Lorenz, M, Steil, G (2003) Outcomes of a strength training based rehabilitation system for injured workers post-lumbar fusion. **World Spine II**

- Kruger, M, Bates, D, Lorenz, M, Steil, G (2003) Strength Training in a different setting – Outcomes with injured workers status post-lumbar fusion surgery. **NSCA National Conference**

- Kruger, M, Bates, D, Lorenz, M, Steil, G (2003) Strength Training based rehabilitation improves functional outcomes for post-lumbar fusion patients – **ISSLS**

- Matt Kruger, M.S.,CSCS, Greg Steil EP,B.A., Dylan Bates MSPT, CSCS, Shawn Rankin MSPT, CSCS, Mark A. Lorenz, MD (2002). Sports performance-based work conditioning/hardening with subjects' status after lumbar fusion: an outcome based study. **NASS 17th Annual Meeting**

Author Index

A

B

C

D

F

G

Chris E. Stout, Matt Kruger and Jeffrey Rogers, (Eds)

H

J

K

L

M

N

O

P

R

S

T

W

Subject Index

A

B

C

D

E

Chris E. Stout, Matt Kruger and Jeffrey Rogers, (Eds)

T

U

W

Made in the USA
Las Vegas, NV
13 April 2026

45266697R00164